D1452724

Florence Nightingale's

NOTES ON NURSING: WHAT IT IS AND WHAT IT IS NOT

&

NOTES ON NURSING FOR THE LABOURING CLASSES

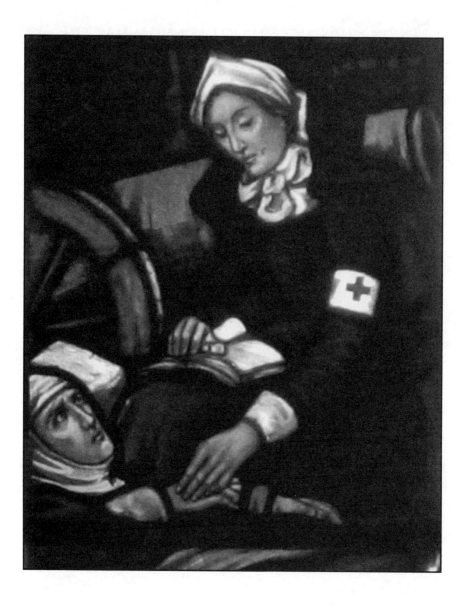

Florence Nightingale's

NOTES ON NURSING: WHAT IT IS AND WHAT IT IS NOT

&

NOTES ON NURSING FOR THE LABOURING CLASSES

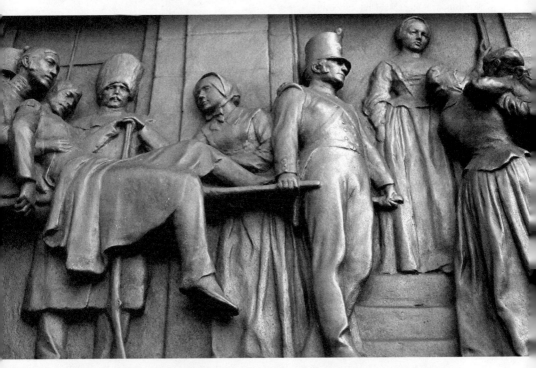

Commemorative Edition with Historical Commentary

EDITED BY

VICTOR SKRETKOWICZ

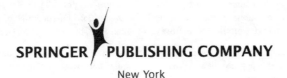

SPRINGER PUBLISHING COMPANY

New York

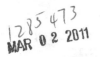
Springer Publishing Company, LLC
11 West 42nd Street
New York, NY 10036
www.springerpub.com

Acquisitions Editor: Margaret Zuccarini
Project Manager: Becca Mosher
Cover Design: David Levy
Composition: Publication Services, Inc.

ISBN: 978-0-8261-1842-4
E-book ISBN: 978-0-8261-1843-1

10 11 12 13 / 5 4 3 2 1

Library of Congress Cataloging-in-Publication Data

Nightingale, Florence, 1820-1910.
 [Notes on nursing]
 Florence Nightingale's Notes on nursing : what it is and what it is not & Notes on nursing for the labouring classes : commemorative edition with historical commentary / edited by Victor Skretkowicz.
   p. ; cm.
 Other title: Notes on nursing : what it is and what it is not & Notes on nursing for the labouring classes : commemorative edition with historical commentary
 Includes bibliographical references and index.
 ISBN 978-0-8261-1842-4 (alk. paper)
 1. Nursing. I. Skretkowicz, Victor. II. Nightingale, Florence, 1820-1910. Notes on nursing for the labouring classes. III. Title. IV. Title: Notes on nursing : what it is and what it is not & Notes on nursing for the labouring classes : commemorative edition with historical commentary.
 [DNLM: 1. Nursing. 2. Nursing Care. WY 100 N688n 2010]
 RT40.N5 2010
 610.73—dc22
                                                                                                2010010111

Contents

Foreword – by Barbara Dossey
   International Co-Director, Nightingale Initiative for Global Health
   Ottawa, Ontario, Canada, and Arlington, Virginia *vii*
Acknowledgments *xiii*
Preface – About This Edition *xv*

Part One **Introduction to This Edition** **1**

A Brief History 4
 The First Version (January 1860) 5
 The Second Version (The Library Standard Edition: July 1860) 6
 The Third Version (April 1861) 7
Planning and Publishing 10
 1. The First Version (January 1860) 10
 2. The Second Version (The Library Standard Edition: July 1860) 14
 3. The Third Version 21
  i. The 1861 Edition 21
  ii. The 1868 Edition 29
  iii. The Unpublished 1875 Edition 32
Conclusion 38
Editor's Notes 40

Part Two **Notes on Nursing: What It Is and What It Is Not**
   (1860 Library Standard Edition) **45**

Preface 49
Digest [Nightingale's Summary of the Contents] 51
Notes on Nursing: What It Is and What It Is Not
 (Based on the Second Version, the Library Standard Edition,
 published July 1860) 61
Editor's Notes 285

Contents

Part Three **Notes on Nursing for the Labouring Classes (1868 Edition)** **297**

Notes on Nursing for the Labouring Classes (1868 Edition)   299
Editor's Notes   413

Part Four **1875 Additions**   **415**

Baby's Food   417
Disease from Air and Sewers   420
Steady Degeneration   427

Appendix: First Edition—Guide to Identification   **431**
Index   **443**

Foreword

This foreword is dedicated to the memory of
Dr. Victor Skretkowicz (August 26, 1942–July 22, 2009)

As I began to write this foreword on July 28, 2009, I received a phone call that Dr. Victor Skretkowicz passed away on July 22 after a long illness. As a Nightingale scholar, it was a privilege to be introduced to Victor's primary research in *Florence Nightingale's Notes on Nursing (Revised with Additions)* in 1996 and then to have been invited to write the foreword for his 2010 publication. Reading Victor's book took my breath away, and I was in awe of his findings on Florence Nightingale's masterwork of nineteenth-century literature on social reform. Victor's commitment to researching *Notes on Nursing* and his findings, details, and differences in the first version, second version, and third version are astonishing, as you will soon read.

Victor was an accomplished researcher of biographical and cultural history for over 30 years. He was an author and editor, publishing widely in early romance and Renaissance literature, and he was the 2004 research director of the electronic *Dictionary of the Scots Language*. On his retirement in 2007 as a senior lecturer in the English department at the University of Dundee, international experts in Renaissance literature from the United States, Germany, and around the United Kingdom gathered at the University of Dundee at a Romance Conference in his honor. Victor lived his life with extraordinary purpose, passion, enthusiasm, and determination. All who knew Victor were touched and knew that they had encountered a very special and rare person.

With the 2010 publication of Dr. Victor Skretkowicz's *Florence Nightingale's Notes on Nursing* and *Notes on Nursing for the Labouring Classes* in Florence Nightingale's (1920–2010) centenary year, nurses and others will recognize this extraordinary woman whose dedication and determination helped to shape the course of modern global healthcare and holistic and integral relationship-centered care.[1,2,3] Nightingale's vision in *Notes on Nursing* contained the basic elements for all that nursing could be; it is a vision to which contemporary global nursing still aspires.

Nightingale's ideas and years of studying the prevention of disease, as well as her Crimean War (1854–1856) experiences, helped her to shape *Notes on Nursing,* which was written to assist women to care for their families as well as themselves in the home. *Notes on Nursing* is a book more on prevention or wellness rather than sickness; it includes much of Nightingale's theosophical and philosophical ideas in very practical terms. She also wrote as a person who had suffered with a debilitating bout of Crimean Fever in 1855, with further fever episodes on her return to England in 1856 that led to her chronic illness with major symptoms until 1887. Today her illness is recognized as chronic brucellosis.*

Shortly after Nightingale published her first version, the 79-page *Notes on Nursing,* she expanded this work in a second version of 229 pages, and it became a touchstone for the emerging profession of nursing. Her major challenge was to outline this new field of nursing that had no theories from which to draw. She feared that the student nurses, called probationers, would become too medical, and she predicted the problem of educating tradesmen's and farmers' daughters, as well as not having educated women to teach or mentor them. She also contended that the educated women could be health missioners who were needed to teach the population at large, "to care for its own health."

Nightingale saw healing as a lawful process; like all physical phenomena, it is regulated by nature and is the manifestation of God. Nursing must discover the laws of healing—such as proper nourishment, ventilation, cleanliness, and quiet—and thus be able to cooperate consciously in the restorative process. "Nature alone cures, and what nursing has to do . . . is to put the patient in the best condition for nature to act upon him."

Nightingale's *Notes on Nursing* is a classic and timeless text for today, both locally and globally. It has a modern message; many of the concepts that she suggested are just now being integrated with traditional medicine. Today these are referred to as caring-healing modalities, alternative/complementary therapies, and integrative practice—for example, healing environments, color, light, music, pets, relaxation, nutrition, and exercise.[3] Although much has changed in healthcare delivery since 1860, in many parts of the world nurses are still faced with poor working conditions just as in Nightingale's time, where many disparities exist. With our global nursing shortage, many countries lack adequate nurses and healthcare workers to deliver professional services; medications, equipment, and protocols are also in short supply.[4]

---

* Today, Crimean fever, also called Malta or Mediterranean fever, is included under the generic name *brucellosis*. Brucellosis exists worldwide and remains endemic in many parts of the underdeveloped world.

Nightingale's *Notes on Nursing* message and vision for health and wellness are referred to today in global public health terms as social, environmental, and health determinants.[5] *Social determinants of health* are the economic and social conditions under which people live that determine one's health. Disease and illness are often a result of detrimental social, economic, and political forces. *Environmental determinants of heath* are any external agents (biological, chemical, physical, social, or cultural) that can be linked to a change in health status that is involuntary, such as breathing secondhand smoke, whereas active tobacco smoking is a *behavioral determinant*. *Health determinants* are those factors that determine the level of health and a sense of wellbeing; they include physical environment (food, water, air pollution, home/workplace environment), social environment (family composition, friends, religion, race/gender, socioeconomic status and conditions, education, occupation/profession), and personal behaviors (healthy eating, exercise, stress management).

Another concept throughout *Notes on Nursing* that nurses use today is called the *precautionary principle*. The precautionary principle implies that when an activity raises threats of harm to human health or the environment, precautionary measures shall be taken, even if some cause-and-effect relationships are not fully established scientifically.[6] The emphasis is on "suspects"; if there is a suspicion about anything that is harmful, the person or thing is removed from the environment. The emphasis is on accepting zero, not minimal or moderate, contamination and pollution of our environment. In the *Notes on Nursing* section, Nightingale gives us an example of the precautionary principle:

> The senses of nurses and mothers become so dulled to foul air that they are perfectly unconscious of what an atmosphere they have let their children, patients, or charges, sleep in. But if the tell-tale air-test [Dr. Angus Smith's air test] were to exhibit in the morning, both to nurses and patients and to the superior officer going round, what the atmosphere has been during the night, I question if any greater security could be afforded against a recurrence of the misdemeanour . . . And oh; the crowded national school! where so many children's epidemics have their origin, what a tale its air-test would tell! We should have parents saying, and saying rightly, "I will not send my child to that school, the air-test stands at 'Horrid.'" And the dormitories of our great boarding schools! Scarlet fever would be no more ascribed to contagion, but to its right cause, the air-test standing at "Foul."[7]
>
> Another example is . . . If you think a patient is being poisoned by a copper kettle, cut off all possible connection to avoid further injury . . .[8]

Florence Nightingale's *Notes on Nursing* is nursing's legacy to assist nurses in developing a consciousness related to healing—physical, mental, emotional, social, and spiritual. The World Health Organization defines this healing consciousness as *decent care*. Decent care is a set of values that place individuals, in their social and cultural contexts, at the center of the caring process.[9] The International Council of Nurses has recently released a modern version of Nightingale's book, *Notes on Nursing: A Guide for Today's Caregivers*,[10] that gives many modern examples to assist in the delivery of decent care.

Nightingale saw the first priority of nursing as devotion to human health—of individuals, of communities, and of the world. Nurses are presented with new common health concerns for humankind and global health imperatives; they are not isolated problems in far-off countries. With global warming and the globalization of the world, there are no natural or political boundaries that can stop the spread of disease.

Starting in the 1880s, Nightingale began to write that it would take 100 or 150 years to have nurses educated to transform hospitals and healthcare. Nurses today are 21st-century Nightingales that she knew would arrive in the future. In 2010, Nightingale's centenary year, many initiatives (see Resources) will occur around the world to unite 15 million nurses and many midwives that together will be 35 million strong and will be working with other healthcare workers, communities, and nongovernmental organizations (NGOs). Together we can achieve a healthy world by 2020.

Dr. Victor Skretkowicz's important research distinguishes the three versions of *Notes on Nursing* for the 21st century. His research increases nurses' understanding of the Nightingale legacy, the legacy that has deepened personal commitment to improving health throughout the world. Our role in today's events will be part of tomorrow's future. We must challenge ourselves to learn to communicate to a wider audience. This means to share our nursing stories and learn to write clearly and powerfully—not only for our colleagues, but also for patients, consumers, and other health care professionals—about how we as nurses integrate caring and healing.

Each of us must look forward, not backward. Exciting work lies ahead. How are we going to write our chapter of nursing history at the beginning of the 21st century? What is our role at the local, national, and international levels? What germinating seeds are we going to leave for others? What is our next innovative and creative education, practice, or research endeavor? What is our leadership role in the health care system? And finally, I ask, "Can you hear Nightingale's voice?"

Barbara Dossey, PhD, RN, AHN-BC, FAAN
International Co-Director, Nightingale Initiative for Global Health
Ottawa, Ontario, Canada, and Arlington, Virginia

Notes

1. B. M. Dossey (2010). *Florence Nightingale: Mystic, Visionary, Healer. Commemorative Edition.* Philadelphia: F. A. Davis.
2. B. M. Dossey, L. C. Selanders, D. M. Beck, and A. Attewell (2005). *Florence Nightingale Today: Healing. Leadership, Global Action.* Silver Spring, MD: Nursesbooks.org, 2005.
3. B. M. Dossey (2008). Integral and holistic nursing. In Dossey and Keegan, L. *Holistic Nursing: A Handbook for Practice* (5th ed.). Sudbury, MA: Jones and Bartlett, pp. 7–16.
4. International Council of Nurses (ICN) (2004). The Global Shortage of Registered Nurses: An Overview of Issues and Action. Accessed July 28, 2009 at http://www.icn.ch/global/shortage.pdf.
5. *Nightingale Initiative for Global Health.* Available at http://www.nightingaledeclaration.net. Accessed July 28, 2009.
6. C. Raffensperger and J. Ticker (1999). *Protecting Public Health and the Environment: Implementing the precautionary principle.* Washington, D.C.: Island Press.
7. F. Nightingale (1860). *Notes on Nursing: What It Is, and What It Is Not.* London: Harrison and Sons, p. 10.
8. Ibid., p. 70.
9. T. Karpf, N. Tashima, and C. Crain (2008). *Restoring Hope: Decent Care in the Midst of AIDS.* London: Palgrave MacMillan.
10. International Council of Nurses (2009). *Notes on Nursing: A Guide for Today's Caregivers.* Edinburgh: Baillie Tindal.

Website Resources

www.nightingaledeclaration.net
www.2010IYNurse.net
www.watsoncaringscience.org
www.facebook.com/wcsi.care
www.www.flickr.com/photos/wcsicares
www.Heartmath.org
www.glcoherence.org

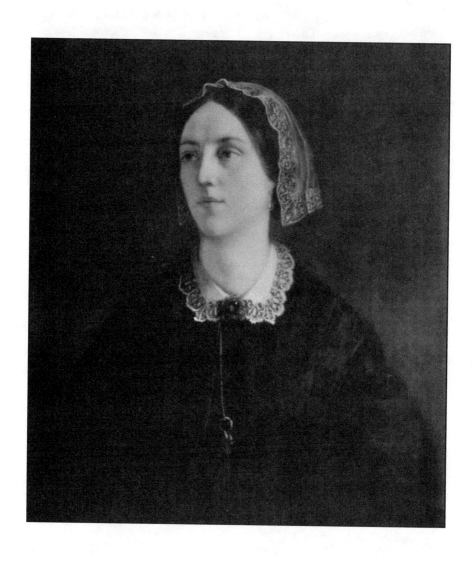

Acknowledgments

This volume owes its existence to Margaret Zuccarini, executive acquisitions editor of the Springer Publishing Company. It could not have been done without her understanding and generous support.

I wish to reiterate my thanks to the trustees of the Henry Bonham Carter Will Trust and the British Library for permission to publish materials from the Nightingale manuscript collection. The Wellcome Trust both funded the bibliographical research and granted permission to quote from the archives of the Wellcome Institute for the History of Medicine. It is also a pleasure, once again, to thank the Florence Nightingale Museum Trust and the museum staff for their help.

Other organisations to contribute assistance of a more sustaining nature include the Scottish government, NHS Tayside, the Scottish Motor Neurone Disease Association, the Marie Curie Cancer Care, and Macmillan Cancer Support. My son, and especially my wife, have given countless hours and their unstinting devotion. It is to them that I wish to dedicate this book.

V. S.

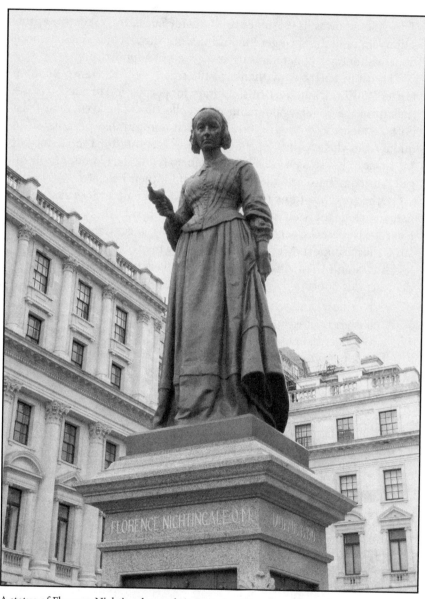

A statue of Florence Nightingale stands in Waterloo Place, London. Arthur George Walker, sculptor. PHOTO COURTESY OF CRAIG BELCHER.

Preface

About This Edition

The rationale behind publishing a commemorative reprint of an influential book by an iconic figure may seem transparent. It provides a basis to reflect on the long dead author's achievements and shortcomings, and to reassess the qualities of the written work. In the mid-1980s my wife, a nurse and academic, first introduced me to Florence Nightingale's *Notes on Nursing* and to the relevance of her ideas in the contemporary world. I was immediately intrigued about the extent of this continuing influence and, particularly from my own perspective, about the bibliographical history of this work.

My own career has focused on the historical, political, cultural, and rhetorical contexts of English language and literature. Most of my research is on writing from the sixteenth, seventeenth, and nineteenth centuries. It deals with the processes involved in transforming authors' drafts and manuscript copies of multiple versions of texts into books that were printed using loose, hand-set type. *Notes on Nursing* fitted all of my research criteria, and when I began studying the historical background and publishing history of the text, it soon became evident what an important and influential piece of literature it is.

The numerous editions and reprintings of *Notes on Nursing* reflect a welcome and burgeoning renaissance of interest in Florence Nightingale and "the most popular and enduring of her books."[1] It is not one book, but three, each with a different text. The first two versions, although markedly different, were published in 1860 under the same title, *Notes on Nursing: What It Is, and What It Is Not.* In 1861 she published a third version, *Notes on Nursing for the Labouring Classes.* A revised edition of this came out in 1868. In 1875 Nightingale prepared fresh material to add to a further edition, but this never appeared in a printed version.

During the 1980s precious few, if any, understood in detail the relationships of the texts. The most significant conclusion of my research into this was that no single text represented the author's ideas. This not uncommon editorial problem can be approached from either of two directions. The one I used in my 1992 edition was to construct

---

Internal cross-references (to pages in this volume) use the actual page numbers—where the pages fall in this volume—given at the feet of pages.

a composite "complete" edition. I therefore based the text on the second version, described on the title-page as a "New Edition, Revised and Enlarged." Although different in tone and diction, the most significant additions to *Notes on Nursing for the Labouring Classes* in 1861 and 1868, plus the passages written in 1875, were spliced into the text.[2] This was the first time the 1875 additions were incorporated in any edition. Unobtrusively printed within square brackets, these were preceded by the date of their source to maintain editorial and historical transparency.

In this edition, however, I use the alternative and by far preferable method of editing a multiversion text. This is to describe the variant versions and their bibliographical and social history, and to print the full texts of the second and third versions in their final form. The rationale for using these two versions is that they represent, between them, the complete published work of Nightingale's *Notes on Nursing*. A second edition of *Notes on Nursing for the Labouring Classes,* which included some minor revisions to the original text, was published in 1868, and as this represents the most complete text, it will be used for this edition. Because this commemorative edition represents the second and third versions in unadulterated form, the 1875 additions are printed separately.

The research-based introductory material, however, documents the genesis and evolution of all versions of the text and contains the historical, cultural, bibliographical, and other contextual material needed to understand the rationale behind this edition. One of the purposes of this new edition is to draw attention to the history of *Notes on Nursing* since it was first published over one hundred and fifty years ago. As the text continues to be cited with increasing frequency in nursing scholarship, lack of discernment in this matter can lead to unwarranted conflict of opinion. Because the first and third versions have been reproduced in enormous numbers, most authors have ready access to a copy of one or the other. They are cited out of convenience and clearly without any awareness of the practical considerations involved in the choice of a reliable text.

A problem arises because these versions of the text, so regularly used by students and researchers, are not the ones that Nightingale designed for nurses of an equivalent caliber and standard. There is an immediately perceivable disparity between today's formally educated nurses and the readership to whom Nightingale directed the first and third versions of *Notes on Nursing.* The first was written mainly for domestic servants who cared for the sick and injured in private homes; the third was written especially for those who lived in country cottages or who cared for the sick—and for the babies—who lived in them. Table A, which Nightingale printed in her text (see p. 284), is based on the census of 1851. It showed that thousands of those who nursed in domestic service were in their teens; some were as young as five. These domestic servants certainly did not possess the formal credentials of a trained nurse and were not drawn from that small and select band who attended at that time, or even later, a Nightingale-inspired training institution.

Only the second version of *Notes on Nursing*, published as the Library Standard edition in July 1860, was intended for use as a reference work by professionals. This contains by far the fullest and most scientifically oriented text, and it begins with the comprehensive "Digest" of its contents, listing with a great degree of accuracy the headings that fill the margins of the book. In its day, it was expensive to produce and purchase. Designed to occupy a place on the library shelves of the influential and the wealthy, the deluxe format of this second edition gave the book respectability and permanence—but its literary and meditative qualities jarred against Nightingale's growing preoccupation with social reform. As her thoughts shifted away from the privileged toward achieving the widest possible dissemination of her ideas among the masses, she excerpted from this second version the most generally applicable sections for *Notes on Nursing for the Labouring Classes*. The Library Standard edition was never reprinted.

The unavailability of the text of the Library Standard edition has clearly led to some unfortunate conclusions about the development of the work. Without an understanding of the rationale behind the different versions, and entirely oblivious to the procedure of simplification and reduction undertaken to produce *Notes on Nursing for the Labouring Classes*, editors and scholars have perpetuated the unsupportable belief that Nightingale's latest version is the most complete. This theory, and all it implies, is wrong. The fullest and most sophisticated text is that of the undiluted second version, the Library Standard edition, which is reproduced in its original form in this edition.

Nightingale's later additions, which originated in this second version, are considerable and important. She prepared "Minding Baby," which, along with other additions, was incorporated into her 1861 edition of *Notes on Nursing for the Labouring Classes*. "Minding Baby" was never published separately (see page xxxi in the 1992 edition). In 1868 concrete evidence in support of some of her precepts, along with a small amount of supplementary material, was also included in a new edition of this text. In future years it was this edition that formed the basis for the many reprints of *Notes on Nursing*.

After 1868, when *Notes on Nursing for the Labouring Classes* was reprinted, Nightingale continued to develop material that she intended to add to later editions. In 1875 she composed nearly 3,000 words on nutrition and sewers that for many decades did not appear in print. Within these handwritten, manuscript drafts, reference to the appropriate page number of the 1868 edition (or 1874 reprint of it), indicates where in the printed text she wanted the new material to be inserted. This provides evidence of Nightingale's intention to include these unpublished additions in a later edition. For various reasons she never saw this through the press. As Nightingale's desire to publish these passages is beyond doubt, they are included in this book.

This commemorative edition of *Notes on Nursing: What It Is and What It Is Not* will be the first time that it has appeared in its original form since it was published in July 1860. Together with *Notes on Nursing for the Labouring Classes* and the additional material presented, it provides today's educated readership with the nearest possible "authoritative, complete and unexpurgated" version of one of the bestselling, globally circulated texts of the nineteenth century.

V. S.

Notes

1. Mark Bostridge, *Florence Nightingale the Woman and Her Legend* (London: Viking, 2008).
2. Victor Skretkowicz, *Florence Nightingale's Notes on Nursing (Revised, with Additions)* (London: [Royal College of Nursing] Scutari press, 1992: repr. London: Bailliere Tindall, 1996).

Part One

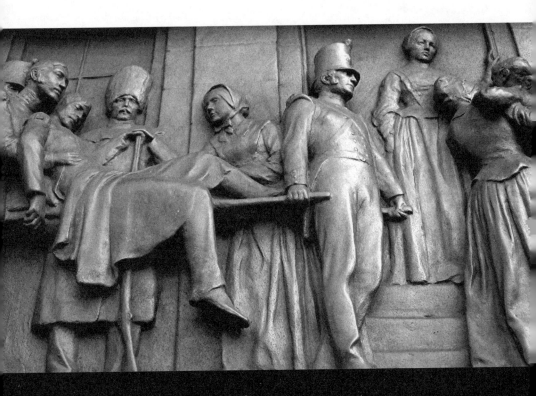

Introduction to This Edition

Florence Nightingale was born on May 12, 1820. She died 100 years ago on August 13, 1910. Among the mountains of her surviving manuscript and printed output, *Notes on Nursing* is the one item of truly exceptional merit—a masterpiece in the literature of nineteenth century reform. It is unlike any other work of this type because the author combines unprecedented first-hand experience in health care with an instinct for organization, wit, and creative expression.

What gives *Notes on Nursing* its enduring quality is not that exposure of the evils of overcrowding and need for sanitary reform that so strongly characterize the writings of Charles Kingsley, Charles Dickens, and Elizabeth Gaskell. Rather, Nightingale confronts these issues in a positive manner, complaining less, and doing much more. If, for example, the disposal of human waste is a problem among the healthy populace, it becomes an even more acute one for the sick. By tackling this and other social difficulties in the miniature and isolated society of the bedroom by suggesting to others how they might contribute to the restoration of health in their one bedridden patient, she sets in motion wheels that she understands to be the primary impulse toward "making the Earth healthy," knowing full well it would take "many thousands of years" (below, p. 64).

Notes on Nursing does not belong to that class of literature that seeks immediate legal reform of social ills, though such were the objectives that Nightingale strived for and achieved as an activist within the political forum. It could even be argued that her long-sighted perspective toward achieving world health removes from this work any semblance of social relevance. It is difficult to imagine a more limited interpretation of Nightingale's aims. In fact, her self-control in avoiding narrow controversy over specific issues is awe inspiring: she is not disengaged from them, she has a broader purpose. In her preface (below, p. 49) she argues that "every woman must, at some time or other of her life, become a nurse," and wonders aloud, "how immense and how valuable would be the produce of her united experience if every woman would think how to nurse." The careful phrasing of "think how to nurse" is a perfect example of Nightingale's determination to shun knee-jerk reaction and the quick fix. She inspires contemplation—and with the understanding and humility of being the one woman who has, more than anyone before her, thought how to nurse, she concludes, "I do not pretend to teach her how, I ask her to teach herself, and for this purpose I venture to give her some hints."

Notes on Nursing does not offer rapid solutions to the causes of abominable living conditions on the grand scale, but Nightingale knows that intellectual advancement necessarily precedes social reform. That is the aim of her book, which she keeps short, direct, and filled with insight. She strikes out to advance the dignity of woman through encouraging her to "think how to nurse" and by virtue of the universal applicability of the hints she ventures to give, dignifies mankind.

A Brief History

In *Notes on Nursing* Florence Nightingale sets out her principles of care for the sick and the injured. Simultaneously witty, scathing, ironic, wry, dictatorial, anecdotal, and factual, her book is a model of clarity that few other writers on the subject have been able to emulate successfully.

While she was working on *Notes on Nursing*, Nightingale corresponded with Harriet Martineau, an uncompromising professional writer eight years her senior. In a letter to Martineau of July 29, 1860, she included a rare appraisal of her own work: "The only possible merit of my little book is that there is not a word in it, written for the sake of writing, but only forced out of me by much experience in human suffering."[1] Notwithstanding the numerous official reports, research on hospital design and organization, and the personal writings she previously committed to print for private circulation, this is the first book that Nightingale wrote for general consumption by a broad reading public. Corrections and rewriting in the snippets of drafts that survive support her modest confession that composition did not flow easily or without deliberation. It is an enormous tribute to its author's tenacity that, despite this difficulty, *Notes on Nursing* reads so easily that it has become a classic among English essays.

At the same time that new developments in nursing are eroding and supplanting many of the practices advocated by Nightingale, the breadth and sensitivity of her general principles are still being lauded for their permanence. The mixture of admiration and nostalgia that has long perpetuated a regular outpouring of editions of *Notes on Nursing* is now also accompanied by a growing and justifiable historical interest. Nursing education, which properly begins in 1860 with Nightingale's success in establishing a training school at St. Thomas's Hospital, has developed a new and sophisticated appreciation of its origins. Inevitably it is to Nightingale's own so-called "little book" that many students and historians of nursing are obliged to turn for illumination. This introduction attempts to provide a degree of understanding about what the book *Notes on Nursing* consists of, and to indicate a measure of its immense popularity.

The First Version

From the time it was first published, early in January 1860, *Notes on Nursing: What It Is, and What It Is Not* exercised an enormous impact on society. In two months at least 15,000 copies, bound in cardboard covered in charcoal colored medium-fine bead-cloth,[2] had been published to sell at the price of two shillings. Adhesive booksellers' labels, inked stamps, or embossed seals that survive in early copies indicate that it was marketed throughout the four corners of Britain, as far apart as Dublin, Aberdeen, Brighton, and Plymouth.

The last of the book's 80 pages was initially blank but later on was used for the printer's name and address (the colophon). Library catalogues therefore describe the book as having 79 pages, or 79 plus one (pp. 79,[1]). In all copies, the London publisher's name and address, initially in the form "HARRISON, 59, PALL MALL,/ BOOKSELLERS TO THE QUEEN," appears at the foot of the title-page, but the date that one might expect to follow this is missing. In consequence, many of the reprints produced during this century err in stating that the first edition was published in 1859 rather than 1860. Publisher's advertisements printed on the end-papers and fly-leaves of many copies do contain dates in them: 1860, 1864 (January), 1873, 1883, 1891, and 1897. In a still later copy, Harrisons style themselves "BOOKSELLERS TO HIS MAJESTY THE KING." There could be no clearer indication that *Notes on Nursing* remained in print until after Queen Victoria's death on January 22, 1901, and into the reign of Edward VII. Indeed, my own recent study of roughly 100 copies demonstrates that they even continued to be printed from the original setting of type.

The earliest of the modern reprints and photographic reproductions (facsimiles) of this first edition appeared in 1946.[3]

Interest in *Notes on Nursing* is practically global. Right from the beginning, copies were taken into continental Europe. In 1860, an Italian translation with a preface dated "Marzo"—March—was published simultaneously in Turin, Milan, Florence, and Nice (it was later in 1860 that Nice passed from Sardinian to French control). A translation into Danish was published at Copenhagen in 1861, and in the same year a Swedish translation came out in Gotenborg.[4]

In America, where English laws on copyright did not apply, two publishers invested in their own distinct editions in 1860: D. Appleton and Company in New York, and W. Carter in Boston.[5] The New York edition was astonishingly successful. On June 9, 1860, the sanitary reformer Sir Edwin Chadwick (1800–1890) wrote to Nightingale that he had seen indications in the American papers that *Notes on Nursing* had been published in a cheap form that achieved wide circulation.[6] Its popularity demanded that it be frequently reprinted: there are records of copies from 1861, 1876, 1878, 1879, 1883, 1888, 1890, 1891, 1896, 1898, 1901, 1902, 1906, 1908, 1909, 1910, 1912, 1916, 1920, 1922, 1926, 1929, 1932, 1936, 1938, and 1940, and there may well have been others. A photographic reproduction or facsimile, still in print, was first published in 1946.

The Boston edition, reprinted in 1990, begins with two biographical sketches of Nightingale. The first is unsigned, but the second by Ingleby Scott is extracted without acknowledgement from an article entitled "Representative Women. The Free Nurse. Catherine Mompesson: Mary Pickard: Florence Nightingale," published in the periodical *Once A Week* on March 17, 1860 (pp. 258–262). This edition, unlike the New York edition, was published only once. It was a luxury edition for a limited clientele and was in stark contrast to the New York edition. Carter, the Boston Publisher, had the hardback binding, extravagant in itself, covered in red cloth, with a frontispiece illustrating Miss Nightingale seated and reading, with an image described as "the jewel presented to Miss Nightingale, by Queen Victoria" embossed on the front. In 1990 the Nightingale Society published a facsimile of this edition that makes comparison of the two American editions possible. The Boston edition was translated into German and published in New York by N. Müller in 1860.[7]

J. M. Scudder included *Notes on Nursing* in his popular compendium *Domestic Medicine* (Cincinnati, 1863), later entitled *A Familiar Treatise on Medicine*, and revised as *The Eclectic Practice of Medicine for Families*. This was subsequently called *The Eclectic Family Physician*, which was in its fifth revision and had 22 editions in 1924.

The Second Version

It is no longer generally known that within 16 months Nightingale wrote three quite different versions of her so-called "little book." The second version of *Notes on Nursing: What It Is, and What It Is Not* was described on the title page as "REVISED AND ENLARGED": it contains a substantially longer text to which an extensive "Supplementary Chapter" is added. Because a completely new setting of type was necessary, this book may be distinguished from the first edition by Nightingale's own designation of it as the Library Standard edition. Now a hardback in larger print, the text is swelled to include 16 preliminary pages and 224 pages of text. The preliminaries include nine pages of "DIGEST", a detailed catalogue of the contents keyed into the topic headings that appear in the margins of the text. Of this edition, 2,000 copies, in two entirely different bindings, came out in July 1860. Some were bound in elegant, very hard maroon or blue boards with a tight wavy pattern, the corners embossed with crosses of St. Michael and joined by decorative straps. This deluxe format was advertised in 1861 inside the back cover of the third version (see below). It was described as "extra cloth," that is, in an extra quality cloth binding, "price 6s." The others, in black or blue-black semi-hard covers, with scroll-work at the corners, were probably priced at five shillings.

This text forms the basis of the translations into German (Leipzig, 1861), French (Paris, 1862; second edition, 1869), Dutch (Amsterdam, 1862—new edition, Rotterdam, 2005; Haarlem, 1863), Czech (Prague, 1874), and after a gap, into Finnish (Helsinki, 1938).[8] It is the fullest version, and for that reason provided the textual foundation of my composite edition,[9] which has been translated into Norse (Oslo, 1997) and Japanese (Tokyo, 1998). Similarly, because the Library Standard edition is the most complete version of *Notes on Nursing: What It Is and What It Is Not*, it will form the basis of the first part of this edition.

The Third Version

Determined to make her work more accessible and attractive to members of working households, Nightingale cut down and rewrote the Library Standard edition for the diminutive cheap third version. The first edition of this third version, with its new title of *Notes on Nursing for the Labouring Classes*, was published in April 1861 in a cramped little 96-page volume, bound either in thin blue paper and selling at six pence, or pink flexible cloth at seven pence. The old title of *Notes on Nursing: What It Is, and What It Is Not*, used for the two earlier versions, was removed from the title-page and relegated to the first page of the text. All the marginal notes disappear. The text concludes with chapters called "Convalescence" and "What Is A Nurse?," adapted from sections of the "Supplementary Chapter" of the Library Standard edition. A third chapter, "Minding Baby," is new, although its origins lie in the "Conclusion" of the first two versions: part is a paraphrase of the section headed "Children: their greater susceptibility to the same things" (below, p. 246 and p. 401). Death-bed scenes in "Observations which might be made by the sick bed" (Library Standard Edition, see p. 266) now appear at the end of "Chattering Hopes and Advices" (*Notes on Nuring for the Labouring Classes*, see p. 382). The "Note Upon Employment of Women," which originates in the Library Standard edition and stresses the significance of the profession, here also incorporates most of the previously separate "Note as to the Number of Women Employed as Nurses in Great Britain."[10]

When this third version, *Notes on Nursing for the Labouring Classes*, went into a second edition in 1868, a number of short additions to the text required the type to be reset into 114 pages. With increased margins and more spacing between the overcrowded lines, it looked much clearer and became far easier to read. At the end a recruitment advertisement, the "Appendix on Method of Training Nurses under the Nightingale Fund at Saint Thomas's Hospital, London" replaced the "Note Upon Employment of Women" (see below, p. 410).

An unfortunately misleading note appears on the reverse of the title page: "This Edition has been made for the use of the Labouring Classes, with some abridgement, with considerable additions, and with a supplementary Chapter on Children." The note is dated September 1867, and signed "F.N." Although this could be interpreted as indicating that a major rather than minor revision was carried out in 1867, with only slight exceptions all of these changes had already been made and been published in 1861. The statement on the revisions functions as a promotional device, perpetuating the illusion of freshness among a readership that hung upon this author's latest word.

The success of the 1868 version of *Notes on Nursing for the Labouring Classes* can be measured by the number of copies produced from this same setting of type during the next 41 years. Reprints survive from 1876, 1883, 1885 (when copies are numbered as being among the "SIXTY-THIRD THOUSAND" printed), 1888 ("SIXTY-SIXTH THOUSAND"), 1890 ("SIXTY-EIGHTH THOUSAND"), 1892 ("SEVENTIETH THOUSAND"), 1894 ("SEVENTY-SECOND THOUSAND"), and 1898 ("SEVENTY-FOURTH THOUSAND"). A translation into German was published in Leipzig in 1878, in which it is specified that it was based on the 1876 reprint; and in 1887 a condensed Italian rendering appeared in Lucca.[11]

In 1909 the same body of type that was first used in 1868 was called into service for the last time. The words "for the Labouring Classes" are left out of the title, which is shortened to *Notes on Nursing*. It is probable that the original version, the first 1860 edition with the title *Notes on Nursing: What It Is, and What It Is Not*, had finally gone out of print and there was now no danger of confusing the two. The symbol of the Red Cross (on a white disk), which adorns the front of the red hardback binding, separates the title from the name of the author. Extra wide margins give this volume the appearance of being considerably larger than preceding copies of this version. Although the book actually ends at

p. 111, omitting from the end of the volume the three-page "Appendix on Method of Training Nurses under the Nightingale Fund," the table of contents retains the reference to the appendix at p.112. A copy in the Nightingale Museum still has the price inside the front cover—one shilling and sixpence.

The next edition produced by the original publisher, Harrison & Sons, is that of 1914, some four years after Nightingale's death on August 13, 1910. The Editors' Note begins soberly, "Until this autumn Britain had not been engaged in a European war since the Crimean War." British involvement from August 4, 1914 in the armed conflict of World War I assured a new readership.

The editors make the extraordinary claim that their 1914 edition is an exact reprint of the first edition of *Notes on Nursing for the Labouring Classes* (1861): "The edition now reprinted, that of 1861, gives the book with Miss Nightingale's latest corrections," which include "three new chapters: 'Convalescence,' 'What is a Nurse?' and 'Minding Baby'" (p. 5). This is terribly misleading, for the text reprinted is clearly not that of 1861. The extra material found in the 1868–1909 edition of *Notes on Nursing for the Labouring Classes* is present, but the "Appendix on Method of Training Nurses" is not. This combination only exists in the 1909 text, of which this is a new edition in a far more attractive format, a substantial hardback bound in pale grey-brown buckram, and with large, modern-looking type. It was reprinted in 1924.

Concealing the fact that the 1914 edition reproduces the recent 1909 text, and stating instead that it represents the first edition of *Notes on Nursing for the Labouring Classes* is one of the earliest indications of a rising antiquarian interest in the book. It is a kind of sales gimmick with power to appeal to those whose tastes are stimulated by the hint of authenticity. As with so many sales pitches, it stretches the truth.

An example of how such misinformation can be perpetuated from one edition to another occurs in the 1952 reprint. In the foreword by Lucy J. Ottley, President of the Royal College of Nursing, the information in the 1914 Editors' Note is repeated in good faith (though without reference to the source): "the 1861 edition of the book is used, containing three new chapters and some rearrangement of the original matter of the 1859 [i.e., January, 1860] edition, all carried out by Florence Nightingale herself" (p. 5). Not knowing the history of *Notes on Nursing*, and clearly desirous of presenting the genuine article, Ottley paraphrases the 1914 statement. In doing so, she reflects an unreserved belief in its authenticity, completeness, and integrity, which gains in authority from being endorsed by Harrison and Sons, Nightingale's own publisher. Alas, as records for printing and publishing were never preserved,[12] by 1914 not even the Harrisons knew that the book was first published in 1860, or what constituted the different published versions.*

Unfortunately, Ottley's intention to reproduce the 1861 edition is belied when she twice repeats a telltale misprint that was first introduced when the type was reset for the 1914 text. Up to that point in the book's 54-year history, in all three versions, the second paragraph of the "Conclusion" had read, "A patient may be left to bleed to death in a sanitary palace." In 1914 the printer left the first "a" out of "palace," changing it to the more pedestrian "place" (p. 143). The impact of Nightingale's ironic expression vanishes in 1914 as if it had never even existed. And the presence of "sanitary place" in Ottley's "Foreword" (p. 7) and text (p. 140) confirm the use of the 1914 edition, or one derived from it, as printer's copy in 1952. Further, in Ottley's 1952 edition, the subtitle, "What It Is, and What It Is Not," also disappears from the first page of the text.

Planning and Publishing

1. The First Version

The Nightingale manuscripts in the British Library are mounted in huge green leather scrap books, catalogued under the designation Additional Manuscripts (MSS. Add.). Among the multitude of letters and papers in this collection a few key documents survive that cast light upon the early stages of planning and preparing the text. Much of the material they contain has never before appeared in print.

---

*Publisher's Note: Follows a memorandum, inserted by the Editor into the running text. The Editor's exact intention is unknown. It is an extract from C. R. Harrison and H. G. Harrison, M.A., *The House of Harrison[:] Being an Account of the Family and Firm of Harrison and Sons* (London: Harrison and Sons, 1914), p. 42:

After the Crimean War the sum of £1,000 was paid to Florence Nightingale for her Notes on Nursing. We may well suppose that at the time of its first publication, when Miss Nightingale's self-sacrificing devotion was fresh in everybody's mind, the book would be eagerly taken up and find a ready sale, but the modest little publication has done much more than that: giving advice on the technical details of the art of nursing in the simplest language, it was alive with womanly sympathy and inspired by the soul of Christian charity; it was quickly appreciated for its intrinsic merit and originality, and has become a classic for all time; it has been reprinted again and again, keeping its original form, and it still finds a sale to this very day.

The earliest indication that Nightingale intended to publish a book on nursing is in a note to her from her close adviser, Dr. John Sutherland, on February 10, 1859. She evidently asked him to examine and criticize a short piece containing the outline of what would become *Notes on Nursing*. He replied:

> The paper on Nursing. I have looked it over but would like to do so two or three times before returning it. At first sight I should say that it would be improved by making it more preceptive, and less doctrinal. A number of years ago there were some very good little books on the subject which fairly represented the then state of knowledge, but the public did not appear to relish their contents and they have ceased to be heard of.[13]

Two days later, on February 12, Sutherland sent Nightingale his extensive and encouraging comments. They place us right at the beginning of the project when the approach, the readership, and the style are not yet fixed:

> The enclosed proof is of course merely a collection of ideas & experience for use. I would soften down the doctrines in the first page, because they would be disputed by some men of name & the general tenor of the criticism would I fear set the M.D.s against you and stave off improvement. It is very important not to offend the doctors.
>
> If I were you I should go on with it. Get out all your ideas on the subject of nursing & all your experience. Never mind the arrangement. The great thing is to get the ideas into tangible shape. There are many in these papers very valuable & which indicate others. I should feel disposed also to go more into detail, & to distinguish between the different classes of nursing, for instance Hospital Nursing, Domestic nursing by hired nurses, & Domestic nursing by Mothers, sisters &c. And I put in a petition for a few words on that kind of nursing that most nearly touches my feelings— namely nursing the poor in their own houses & how Charitable women could go about it quietly, unostentatiously & without letting their left hand know what is done by their right hand. You might draw such a picture of the work as would draw all hearts to it.
>
> Well then having got in Harrison's type all you wish to say. How to use it?
>
> The present form contains as it appears to me the basis of a paper similar to your Liverpool paper. It stirs up the question and draws attention to it. It would set a number of people thinking, & it would give them elements of thought. It might be well to consider whether it would not help on this good work to read such a paper next time at Bradford. But more will be required. If you come to teach nursing to the class of people from whom

nurses are taken you will have to be simpler and write in precepts, illustrating your precepts where required by a few easy sentences requiring little thought but appealing to the one element that every good nurse must have namely common sense. This strikes me as the general plan of such a manual, most conducive to forward the work. Why should you not make it a legacy to the Fund?

At all events go on, put together all your thoughts in any order they come & you can easily cut out & arrange afterwards. It will be the least fatiguing process in your present state of health.

As you *intend* to get "Common things" introduced into the schools, don't forget that also.

God bless you & give you strength in such a work. I am yours ever

JS[14]

Although in his initial response Sutherland called what he was sent a "paper on Nursing," he now makes it clear that what he is examining is not a manuscript in Nightingale's handwriting, but a proof. A proof consists either of printed strips of paper ("galley proof") or pages ("page proof") returned to an author to check prior to final printing and publication. It is at this stage, when they could more easily read their work, that many nineteenth-century authors made very substantial additions and emendations.

When Sutherland refers to "your Liverpool paper," he has in mind one or both of the two papers entitled "Sanitary Construction of Hospitals" and "Hospital Construction" that Nightingale wrote for delivery to The National Association for the Promotion of Social Science at Liverpool in October of 1858.[15] Together these two essays occupy only 20 pages in the 1858 *Transactions* of the National Association, and when reprinted they became the first 22 pages of *Notes on Hospitals* (1859). It might be conjectured that this "proof" is only at most half the size of one paper, roughly five pages. In so far as this very brief "basis of a paper" seems literally to have consisted of the "notes" out of which the book was to grow, it may have served Nightingale as a working draft, and never actually have been published in that form.

Sutherland's reference to "Harrison's type" indicates that the company of Harrison and Sons, the publisher of the finished volume, was already involved at this preliminary stage of the projected work. Harrison did not serve Nightingale well, and she lived to regret that she had not taken Edwin Chadwick's advice when he suggested a different publisher. In a letter of June 9, 1860, Chadwick laments Harrison's inexcusably high cost of two shillings, implying that this prevented the book from reaching the poorly paid. By contrast, the Americans, by whom he means Appleton and Company, New York, had published a cheap edition, "and have obtained the circulation there which in the hands of some intelligent publishers, such as the Routleges whom I once mentioned,—they might have obtained here."[16] This was to be a long running saga.

Sutherland's insistence that Nightingale write simply and in precepts for "the class of people from whom nurses are taken" should not be interpreted as a pejorative comment upon the intellectual power or education of professional nurses, slender though their training may have been. His reference is not to this group of nurses, but rather to those little-educated domestic servants whose duties included nursing and "minding baby" within the home.

On June 8, 1859, four months after receiving Sutherland's critique, Nightingale wrote to Dr. William Aitken on the subject of the terrible effect of unexpected noise on patients. In this letter, in the library of the Wellcome Institute for the History of Medicine, she emphasizes that it is

> . . . distressing to the Patient to have any noise behind him which he can-not *see*—A Patient dying or coughing or who required much fidgetting attendance would make the bed back to back with him, almost uninhabit-able—Noise which a Patient cannot *see*(!) always partakes with him of the character of *Suddenness* & injures him—This is, believe me, the fruit of long experience with the sick . . . I enclose for your own private eyes a little Pam-phlet I wrote on Nursing, (which is really "Confidential,")—perhaps the article *Noise* will illustrate what I have said about Patients—[17]

Nothing more is known of the "little Pamphlet I wrote on Nursing" that she mentions in this letter. It may well be the "proof" to which Sutherland alludes, for Nightingale's remarks are directly related to the substantial section entitled "Noise" in *Notes on Nursing*. The wording in part of the section "People Overhead" (below, p. 143) is almost exactly the same.

Progress on *Notes on Nursing* continued into the latter part of the year. Dr. Charles West's lecture, "On Sudden Death in Infancy and Child-hood," to which Nightingale so enthusiastically refers as "just published," did not appear in *The Medical Times and Gazette* until November 26 (see below, p. 247, and note). When the book was completed, it went to the printer, and proofs were corrected and returned. Anticipating publica-tion, Harrison advertised *Notes on Nursing* in the *Publishers' Circular* from December 14 to 31, 1859. On Wednesday December 28, 1859, Nightingale was able to promise Edwin Chadwick a copy of the finished product "in a few days." She writes:

> I hope in a few days, if the printers are faithful, you will see (by a copy of a little thing of mine you will receive) that I have taken your suggestions as to setting down a few plain hints to teach people to nurse themselves—[18]

In this letter she expresses herself in words that parallel those of the preface: "I do not pretend to teach her how, I ask her to teach herself."

Harrison and Sons, the present printing company descended from Nightingale's publishers, assure me that no company records exist from this period. Nonetheless, the approximate date of publication can be ascertained from the combination of this letter to Chadwick and the earliest known presentation copy of *Notes on Nursing*. On Sunday January 1, 1860, Nightingale's cousin, Beatrice Shore Smith, Lady Lushington, became the proud recipient of the autographed copy that is now in the Florence Nightingale Museum, St. Thomas's Hospital. At the top of the title page Nightingale has written, "For my dear Beatrice from her loving FN / New Year's Day 1860." Given that delivery from the printers was anticipated "a few days" from December 28, this Sunday inscription attests to a publication date during the first week of January.

The word "notes" in the title is one of Nightingale's favorite ways of describing the concise chapters of her works. She had previously used it in *Notes on Matters Affecting the Health, Efficiency, and Hospital Administration of the British Army* (1858), in *Subsidiary Notes as to the Introduction of Female Nursing into Military Hospitals in Peace and in War* (1858), and in *Notes on Hospitals* (1859). In these books the title appropriately describes a disjointed structure consisting of observations on loosely connected topics. By contrast, *Notes on Nursing* is smaller and much better organized.

The first version concludes with an appendix containing another "note," the "Note as to the Number of Women employed as Nurses in Great Britain." Two tables based upon the census of 1851 (the next was not till 1861) give the distribution of these nurses by age and location. Apart from the typography, these tables are identical to those that accompany the shorter form of this note in *Subsidiary Notes*, privately printed by Harrison in 1858. This same appendix reappears at the end of the second published version of *Notes on Nursing*, in which Nightingale further demonstrates her skill in adapting earlier material to new circumstances.

2. The Second Version

Some time before March 4, 1860, Nightingale discussed the second and third versions with her publisher Harrison, who quibbled about the nature and cost of any alterations. In a letter to Sutherland she complains about these unhappy negotiations. The letter itself is undated, but the postscript added "Mar 4 /60" indicates that she probably wrote it the day before. She indignantly reports that Harrison has given her no indication of the outstanding success of the first edition, of which he has published over 15,000 copies at the price of two shillings. He offers to purchase the copyright from her: that the first edition continued to be reprinted without change for a further 42 years strongly suggests that she sold it to him. This would reinforce his reticence to publish another edition to compete with the one he now owned:

Harrison has now made me "an Offer" as he says—

He refuses to print a cheaper Edition for a twelvemonth, (before which ~~time~~ he says it would spoil the sale of the present one).

He consents to print a 5/ [*i.e., five shilling*] Edition of 2000 copies—which he says he shall not be able to sell off in less than 2 years—[In Harrison's veracity let who will trust]

He consents to do so only on the ~~ground~~ condition that I shall *add* to it but not *alter* & that I receive nothing for it—while he says he shall lose.

He tacitly submits to my having granted the right of translation, which indeed he was told I should do, whether *he* gave leave or not.

Finally, he offers me 500 guineas for the Copyright.

Upon all this I feel that it is founded upon a roguery—viz. the having gone on selling an Edition of at least 15,000 copies, by his own shewing—without giving any sign of life to me—& then saying that he can't publish a cheaper Edition *on the Score* of his not wishing to spoil the sale of this roguery.

I am quite willing to "add & not alter" in the 5/ proposed Edition—For indeed I have nothing I want to alter.

FN

But Nightingale's postscript reflects her continued irritation:

It seems to me that the whole question turns upon this: would *the trade* consider it a fair thing to call fifteen thousand copies, (at least,) of a 2/ pamphlet an Edition?

And is there not danger of such a sale of a pamphlet being a "nine days' wonder," without producing any permanent good effect, while to publish in addition a cheap Manual for the uneducated and a Library Standard Book for the educated *would* produce a real permanent effect?[19]

This extraordinary letter helps put into perspective many of the misunderstandings about the editions that originate in Sir Edward Cook's *Life of Florence Nightingale* (London, 1913), and which prevail today. Because the information provided by this official biographer could be expected to be reliable, he has exercised continuous influence over bibliographical accounts of Nightingale to the present day.

In Cook's Appendix A, a chronologically arranged description of Nightingale's printed writings, he gets the date, the number of pages, and the price of the first version wrong. Under publications for 1859, his entry reads: "*Notes on Nursing: What it is and what it is not. By Florence Nightingale.* London: Harrison (1869). Octavo, pp. 70. Issued at the end of December 1859, at the price of 5s."[20] Not only is 1869 a misprint for 1859, but in addition we know that the book was not published until after New Year's Day, 1860. Another misprint is "pp. 70," where the correct number of pages is 79, or if the final blank is counted, 80. In the body of his text, Cook again gives the price as five shillings, but goes on to state that "15,000 copies were sold in a month, and a cheaper edition at 2s. quickly followed."[21]

The only possible source for Cook's figure of 15,000 copies, together with a price of five shillings, is Nightingale's letter to Sutherland, printed above. This letter was written not one, but two months after publication. Nowhere does it refer to numbers actually sold as opposed to published.

No "cheaper edition at 2s. quickly followed": the original sold at that price. What did follow was the second version, Library Standard edition, of which we know that copies in "extra Cloth" cost 6 shillings, and can therefore surmise that those in the cheaper binding represent the 5 shilling copies proposed in discussions. On p. 223, this volume advertised that "A cheaper Edition is also published, price Two Shillings, in limp cloth." Cook's variation on this in Appendix A, under the 1860 entry for the Library Standard edition, is that "Simultaneously, a 'Popular Edition' was issued, in limp cloth, price 2s."[22] Here at least he echoes the note on p. 223, although he adds the idea of simultaneity—no new two shilling "Popular Edition" was ever published in addition to the already much reprinted first version. Detailed analysis of the three versions and the typography in them demonstrates this without a doubt. Cook has compounded into a confused amalgam the publisher's advertisements from December 1859, the information in Nightingale's letter, and the publisher's blurb at the end of the Library Standard edition.

Because the handwritten text sent to the printer in 1859 appears no longer to exist, we cannot examine the thought processes that went into the original composition of *Notes on Nursing*. However, some drafts of short passages composed for the Library Standard edition, as well as for the later printed versions, do survive.[23] There are also several pages of material written in 1875 but not published at that time that are printed in this edition (the passages begin on p. 417).

The nature and significance of Nightingale's revisions in the second version are fascinating, and reward close examination by giving a clearer insight into her intentions. They seem to be of two types: those that represent the development of ideas and those that reflect the care and attention she pays to her style of writing and her concern about how best to express herself.

The style of the writing in the first version had been effusively praised in *The Quarterly Review* for its clarity and economy:

> There is not a sentence of fine [*i.e.,* pretentious] writing, and hardly a super-fluous word. The amount of meaning conveyed in the shortest and sharpest way gives the impression of wit [*i.e.,* great intelligence]; and the complex influence of this stimulating style, and the pathos of the topic treated, is the genuine operation of genius.[24]

The author of this unsigned review was Harriet Martineau, whom Nightingale in a letter of June 18, 1860, thanked for her advice given "in your 'Quarterly'," and to whom she sent copies of all three versions of her "little book" as they came out.[25]

It would be surprising if Martineau's friendship with Nightingale did not bias her judgment in favor of the work, but perhaps her disregard of what might now be noticed as glaringly "fine writing" stems from her familiarity with a style now lost to common use. It is true that much of *Notes on Nursing* consists of punching, dogmatic, and eminently clear statements. On the other hand, running together sentence after sentence in order to create a cumulative impact, as in the passage on "Well-instructed lifeless victims" in "Children in London" (below, p. 273), is now seldom practiced outside of novels. The work is filled with emphatic phrases that are detached from any main sentence, nowadays rarely found outside the realms of snappy journalism. And it is punctuated throughout with dashes, using dashes in lieu of full-stops, and with redundant dashes after commas, after semicolons, and after colons. Nightingale tinkered with this punctuation in the 1861 and 1868 editions, adding and subtracting commas or semicolons, and only sporadically removing commas before dashes. Her token grammatical propriety serves only to slow the tempo of the sentences and remove the original vigorous rhythms. For this reason, I have decided to preserve the punctuation of the second version where it cannot be misconstrued, as its looseness combines with the content and a number of old-fashioned spellings to give *Notes on Nursing* its preeminently Victorian flavor. Alterations have been kept to a minimum; for example, at the beginning of Chapter V a comma is added after e.g., thus standardizing the form.

Although Nightingale strived to express herself with precision, at times she forced herself to settle for second best. Sometimes it was simply not appropriate to express in writing what she really wanted to say. She wanted, for example, to stress something that remains dear to the heart of today's nursing community, that nursing is a profession. Where Nightingale in her manuscript wrote, "Nursing is a profession, a specialty," the printed version has only the simpler "Nursing is a specialty" (see below, p. 124). This falls in a paragraph that Nightingale rephrased several times, but because there is no indication that she intended these particular words to be cut out, she must have decided to delete them at some later stage, perhaps at the last minute when she was correcting proofs.

One fairly obvious reason for this change would be to avoid the duplication of diction that is present in the draft. "Nursing is a profession, a specialty" almost immediately precedes "doctors are now set free for their professional duties," a clash not only of words but of ideals. Given the proximity of the expressions, Nightingale was forced to choose between one assertion or the other. We may come near to discerning the truth behind her opting in favor of the doctors rather than the nurses in the final version if we recall the practical Sutherland's letter of February 12, 1859. He warns Nightingale to "soften down the doctrines . . . because they would be disputed by some men of name & the general tenor of the criticism would I fear set the M.D.s against you and stave off improvement. It is very important not to offend the doctors." Precious few doctors would at that time have granted nursing the status of a profession. As this expanded edition was particularly intended to catch their attention and gain their support, the potentially offensive and contentious phrase, "Nursing is a profession," was not printed.

Another incomplete manuscript fragment contains an addition to what at that early stage Nightingale called the "Appendix," but which became the "Supplementary Chapter" in the Library Standard edition. Evidently a preliminary version of "What Is A Nurse?" already existed before she composed this short passage. It begins with the words "When you reflect," and ends with "to observe the," which in the printed text covers one short paragraph and the beginning of the next (see below, p. 264).

Comparison with the Library Standard edition reveals that, before settling upon the final wording, alterations to the draft were made at two different times. The printed version of the clause reads, "the prevailing impression is that almost any woman will do for a nurse, provided she is thus 'sober' and 'kind.'" The first change was made while Nightingale was still in the process of composing. She substituted the word "kind" for the original wording, "honest & chaste," which she then crossed out. In doing this, she avoided repeating the identical words from the previous paragraph, a criticism of naïve "ladies," who "generally give the definition of a good nurse as 'sober, honest, and chaste.'" The word "kind" is a genuine substitute for "honest and chaste," for in that era it meant "well-bred." Where "kind" might today describe a nurse's caring attitude and her kindness towards others, in Nightingale's language it refers to a certain social background, and the ethics and morality commonly associated with it.

The second change took place between the time the draft was completed and publication, again possibly when the pages were in proof. In a parenthesis that follows the words "sober" and "kind," Nightingale originally wrote her observation that "Mrs. Gamps are not considered desirable now." This material was omitted from the printed text. Mrs. Sarah Gamp is that poorly-educated, heavy-drinking private midwife and nurse who attends to the sick, the dying, and the dead in Charles Dickens's *Martin Chuzzlewit*, published in 1843–1844, and popularized throughout Britain and in America by Dickens's dramatic readings. The model for Mrs. Gamp was hired by Dickens's friend Miss Burdett-Coutts to take care of her comfortably well-off invalid friend Miss Meredith. Dickens's parody suggests that she must have been wholly insensitive and absolutely repulsive. Nightingale's principal aim in writing *Notes on Nursing* was to get these domiciliary nurses, whether hired or amateur, to improve their demeanor toward their patients, alerting them to their patients' needs as well as to their own shortcomings. And though many advocates of formal schools of nursing in hospitals came more and more to disparage untrained Mrs. Gamps, Nightingale in her curious way realized the importance of domestic nurses, and never abandoned them. She had, after all, begun that way herself.[26]

In redirecting the Library Standard edition toward professional hospital nurses, Nightingale clearly distinguished between the two separate classes of nurses, as had Dickens. For his 1850 edition Dickens added a preface to *Martin Chuzzlewit*, in which he declared:

> in all my writings, I hope I have taken every possible opportunity of showing the want of sanitary improvements in the neglected dwellings of the poor. Mrs. Sarah Gamp is a representation of the hired attendant on the poor in sickness. The Hospitals of London are, in many respects, noble Institutions; in others, very defective. I think it not the least among the

instances of their mismanagement, that Mrs. Betsy Prig [Sarah Gamp's asso-
ciate from St. Bartholomew's] is a fair specimen of a Hospital Nurse; and
that the Hospitals, with their means and funds, should have left it to private
humanity and enterprise, in the year Eighteen Hundred and Forty-nine, to
enter on an attempt to improve that class of persons.

A far more aggressively hostile condemnation of hospital nurses was
published as a letter to *The Times*, April 13, 1857, by "One Who Has
Walked A Good Many Hospitals." This provoked a rigorous defense by
John Flint South, Senior Surgeon of St. Thomas's, of the high standard of
nurses produced through the apprenticeship training given in London
hospitals. In *Facts Related To Hospital Nurses* (1857), Flint denounced
the movement to develop schools of nursing, attacking a still earlier critic
of drunken and debauched nurses, "whoever he or she may be," the
author of *The Institution of Kaiserwerth on the Rhine, for the Practical
Training of Deaconesses* (1851) (p. 21). There is a strong possibility he
knew full well that this author was Nightingale herself.

Dickens's serious interest in this subject involved him as a member
of the Association for the Improvement of the Infirmaries of
Workhouses, founded in March of 1866. By 1867 he felt able to add to his
preface that hospital nurses had "since greatly improved through the
agency of good women."[27] Clearly the establishment of the Nightingale
School in 1860 had begun to have its desired effect.

The omission of "(Mrs. Gamps are not considered desirable now)"
from the Library Standard edition of *Notes on Nursing* may once again
reflect Nightingale's desire to avoid repetition—Mrs. Gamp is alluded to
in the preceding section, the description of "A nurse without the nurse's
calling." After reciting a list of blunders calculated to drive any patient to
distraction, Nightingale points an accusing finger towards her readers:
"Yet these things are not done by drinking Mrs. Gamps, but by
respectable women, receiving their guinea a-week in private families."
Not until the third version did Mrs. Gamp disappear from *Notes on
Nursing* altogether.

In 1867 Dickens' reformist cynicism was greatly in sympathy with
the efforts of those "good women" who had measurably improved
hospital nursing. Nevertheless, it is clear from her "Note Upon Some
Errors in Novels" (see below, p. 277) that Nightingale had long before
turned against the exaggerations, vagueness, and errors of fact that
abound in the fiction of less realistic writers.

In the first edition of *Notes on Nursing* (p. 75), Nightingale had
restricted her criticism of novelists to those who depict "ladies
disappointed in love or fresh out of the drawing-room turning into

the war-hospitals to find their wounded lovers." The Florence Nightingale Museum, St. Thomas's Hospital, possesses the copy that Nightingale inscribed to her lifelong friend, "Selena Bracebridge[,] from the Authoress." In the margin beside this passage, Nightingale identifies one such offensive novel, *Sword and Gown*, which was both serialized in *Fraser's Magazine*, of which Nightingale was a reader (volumes 59 and 60, April to November 1859), and also published in book form. This melodrama of the Crimean War, by the popular fiction writer George Alfred Lawrence, portrays a deathbed love scene between a wounded hero, Royston Keene, and his nurse, an old flame and now a Sister of Charity, Cecil Tresilyan. The novelist lauds Cecil's characteristic "defiance of conventionality" when she utterly abandons her duties to spend the night in her lover's bed: "no one came in to molest them: there was work enough and to spare, that night, for all in Scutari. The thought of interruption never crossed Cecil's mind for an instant" (further quotation is given below, p. 292).

Lawrence's novel is far from subtle, yet one has to appreciate the distinction tacitly drawn in portraying Cecil not as one of Nightingale's nondenominational, paid army nurses, but very specifically as a volunteer "in the gay robe of a Sister of Charity," the Order founded in 1633 by St. Vincent de Paul. Nightingale would nonetheless have been appalled by such powerful advocacy of dereliction of duty, and such seductively described immoral and irresponsible behavior. She had no sooner overcome Mrs. Gamp's gin-filled teapot than she encountered the problem of Cecil Tresilyan's hormones boiling over! It is precisely this overt clash between self-interest, well-intentioned or not, and the selfless if not self-sacrificing altruism demanded by nursing that determined whether its practitioners could be classed as professionals.

3. The Third Version

i—The 1861 Edition

Nightingale's purpose in preparing her third version, *Notes on Nursing for the Labouring Classes* (1861), was to make her work widely available in the cheapest possible form. This meant cutting down the text and ensuring that it was relevant to her new readership. One way to do this was to remove a large proportion of the literary and other allusions. Thus, both the original criticism of novelists and the "Note Upon Some Errors in Novels" are omitted. The reference to Mrs. Gamp is neutralized and shortened to "Yet these things are not done by drinking old females, but by respectable women" (p. 86; in 1868–1909, p. 101). The other passage, which in the manuscript drafts of the Library Standard edition had mentioned Mrs. Gamp, disappears as well. Although there is nothing wrong with the idea that a good nurse should be described as " 'sober, honest, and chaste' and 'sober' and 'kind,' " Nightingale in her marginal note had designated these two short paragraphs as "A lady's definition of a nurse." This category being both too restrictive and too overtly against the class bias toward which this revision is directed, both paragraphs became superfluous to the requirements of the laboring classes edition.

In order to get what she wanted into a much-contracted space, Nightingale tried to moderate her self-consciously literary pretensions. She simplified some of her arguments, reduced some of the less than objective passages, and eliminated some of the difficult ones. In "What Is A Nurse?" as it appears in the second version, one of the marginal headings refers to "A man's definition of a nurse": "no man, not even a doctor, ever gives any other definition of what a nurse should be than this—'devoted and obedient'" (below, p. 262). The fun of reveling in such sexist sarcasm becomes a luxury in the stripped-down laboring classes text, from which all the marginal headings disappear. Even so, an air of resigned irritation can still be detected in the bland and simplified version that remains, "Yet we are often told that a nurse needs only to be 'devoted and obedient.'"

A certain rationale exhibits itself here in Nightingale's choice of what to cut and what to keep. She drops her intention to embarrass the male doctors, presenting the modified definition of a nurse as a globally accepted error rather than a specifically "male" one. In spite of this, the general principle loses none of its impact, for she only sacrifices a weaker remark in order to retain a stronger. Both versions of "What Is A Nurse?" still follow on with the trenchant comment, "This definition would do just as well for a porter. It might even do for a horse. It would not do for a policeman."

Such outrageous outbursts of Nightingale's wry wit and mischievous sense of humor form one of the delights of reading *Notes on Nursing*. Although her words retain their simplicity, her instinct for sarcasm makes her clutter her argument with unrelated and irrelevant images. The comic conjunction of ideas in "nurse," "porter," "horse," and "policeman," stressed by being placed at the end of each statement, obscures rather than clarifies her meaning. She introduces but never addresses the anomaly of why "It would not do for a policeman," and assumes that the meaning of what she writes is transparent, which it is not. From the perspective of a strict logician, she is utterly wrong to indulge in this distracting habit; but it is in her nature to do so, and that in itself speaks volumes about her irrepressible sense of humor, a little remarked upon side of her personality.

A second type of change made in preparing the text of *Notes on Nursing for the Labouring Classes* was to substitute illustrations of the unhealthy practices of ordinary people, where previously she had criticized the pretentious habits of the rich. It was alleged, for example, in the Library Standard edition, that fashionable "young ladies" made themselves willing victims of consumption through overzealously caring about the appearance of their figures and their "complexion." Such unladylike "young ladies" refused to eat in public, though many in private gorged themselves on exceptionally rich pound cake. They also tried to control their weight by taking aperients, that is, laxatives. When they fainted through lack of nourishment, as seemed inevitable, if not fashionable, they sniffed a socially acceptable stimulant rather than submit to hunger and eat:

> Insufficient and unwholesome food is an auxiliary in some people to the work of consumption. For the "fashion" of not eating is still in vogue among "young ladies," and they make up for it, not unfrequently, in their own rooms, by tea and pound cake.
> The object of spoiling her digestion is still further forwarded by many a young lady by the practice of taking continual and powerful aperients—still "to improve her complexion;" or, if the process of exhaustion is far advanced, by taking eau-de-Cologne, sal-volatile, or ether (p. 40).

In *Notes on Nursing for the Labouring Classes* this passage is greatly contracted and its meaning quite changed. Here Nightingale gives her words more universal application by referring, not to the vanity of socialites, but rather to all groups of women. The dreaded consumption is still advanced through poor eating, but by seeking common forms of relief in taking aperients and strong, habit-forming drinks, they exacerbate their already debilitated state:

> Insufficient and unwholesome food is an auxiliary in some people to the work of consumption.
> The object of spoiling her digestion is still further forwarded by many a woman by the practice of taking continual and powerful aperients; or, if the process of exhaustion is far advanced, by taking opium, gin, or some other cordial (p. 31).

A third kind of adjustment was to simplify diction, as in the opening sentence of Chapter I, where she altered the word "canon" to the more easily understood "rule." As this exercise in critical purging naturally extended to the simplification of difficult ideas, the two familiar, if not famous, paragraphs with which the first and second versions of the book open became its victims. When they were first published, they had served to set the tone of the work as one in which any nineteenth-century reader of intellectual orientation, and with an interest in the classics, would reap considerable delight. But whereas the subtle ingenuity of the argument once made a grand opening for an educated audience receptive to its rhetorical exhibitionism, now it had outlived its purpose. It was an impossible introduction to a work designed for a nonliterary and poorly educated readership.

Nightingale's father had taught her classical languages, rhetoric, and philosophical debate, all of which are fundamental to the art of beautiful writing, or poetry. Such training in expression and in the arts of persuasion teaches an understanding of varying psychological dispositions, imparting to speaker and writer the knowledge of how to control the emotions of various types of audiences. This accounts in part for the powerful, mesmerizing effect of Nightingale's fascinating prose style.

Given that her mind had been trained in the rhetorical and argumentative style of the classics and the Bible, perhaps it is understandable that Nightingale became inherently incapable of writing with the sustained clarity and simplicity of scientific language. Recall Sutherland's advice given on February 12, 1859, after he had looked at the first stages of her work: "be simpler and write in precepts, illustrating your precepts where required by a few easy sentences requiring little thought." He never changed his mind on the importance of simplifying the content, of not allowing the style of expression to obtrude upon the meaning, and of backing up every point with obvious examples. In fact, on June 15, 1874, when he was being badgered to make suggestions for a major revision of *Notes on Nursing for the Labouring Classes*, his frank and devastating reply was that "The real objection to the book is that it contains too much of a very profound discussion."[28] Nightingale was never able to satisfy him on this point. To have done so would have meant suppressing the instinctive vitality in her writing that preserves this book from reading with the drabness of a government report. We must recognize, therefore, that it was despite, rather than because of her nature that Nightingale set about simplifying her prose style for a less educated and less privileged readership than she was accustomed to addressing.

Having power to dominate and guide the direction of her reader's response, Nightingale had opened the first two versions of her book in a calculated and positive manner. Rather than begin with an opinion that might invite disagreement, she cleverly put her thesis in the form of a question: "Shall we begin by taking it as a general principle . . . ?" By asking "Shall we" at the outset, she immediately involved the reader in tacit agreement with her hypothesis that disease is a "reparative process," not a debilitating one.

A trained rhetorician who opens an argument with a weak and unsupported generalization anticipates objections: "If we accept this as a general principle we shall be immediately met with anecdotes and instances to prove the contrary." This is not an acknowledgement that her opening remarks are invalid; rather, it sweeps aside objections by stating the obvious: there will always be someone who will disagree. To protect her hypothesis about disease, she creates a diversion, advancing an equally provocative proposition against which the inevitable objections will also be raised: "all the climates of the earth are meant to be made habitable for man, by the efforts of man." With the contentious first statement safely in the background where it remains undisputed, the reader is led to believe that, if this second principle can be defended, then the truth of the first is automatically demonstrated.

Nightingale's envisaged attack on this second statement, "the objection would be immediately raised,—Will the top of Mont Blanc ever be made habitable?," is one to which she has a prepared refutation: "Our answer would be, it will be many thousands of years before we have reached the bottom of Mont Blanc in making the earth healthy." She glosses over all distinctions in this ingenious conflation of ideas, amalgamating part of the first statement, "a reparative process," with part of the second, "earth . . . made habitable for man," and creating out of them a third, "making the earth healthy."

Through this verbal wizardry or sophism, man's involvement in the reparative process of disease is equated with making the top of Mont Blanc not habitable, as in the challenger's question, but healthy, which is far more plausible. Then, in a crushing grand finale, Nightingale blends the language of her own question with that of her own answer to create a single dismissive metaphor: "Wait till we have reached the bottom before we discuss the top." The questions have been asked, and the answers given. She stamps her authority over her reader, and secures for herself the working definition that she reasserts in the fourth paragraph: "The reparative process which Nature has instituted, and which we call disease. . . ."

Nightingale recognized this complex, playful argument to be an inappropriate and unattractive opening to the "Labouring Classes" version of her text. She accepted that it clashed with the more basic forms of expression familiar to her anticipated readership, and did the only thing she could with it—cut it out.

Similar motivation led her to drop the first two sentences of "What Is A Nurse?" from *Notes on Nursing for the Labouring Classes*. This stunning opening passage, only published in the Library Standard edition, possesses real genius, and has a touch of artistic magic about it:

> This book takes away all the poetry of nursing, it will be said, and makes it the most prosaic of human things. My dear sister, there is nothing in the world, except perhaps education, so much the reverse of prosaic—or which requires so much power of throwing yourself into others' feelings which you have never felt,—and if you have none of this power, you had better let nursing alone.

Despite their superficially simple appearance, in these two sentences Nightingale uses her art to its utmost potential. The delicacy of expression and elegantly balanced rhythms seen here typify much of her style of writing. But such calculatedly ornate presentation disguises her uncompromising, ruthless, and at times psychologically brutal treatment of her reader.

In beginning "This book takes away all the poetry of nursing," Nightingale convincingly pretends to give a coolly objective assessment of her work. Coming abruptly upon "it will be said," the reader realizes that this was only another hypothetical charge, that in agreeing he has been wrong-footed, and that he must reverse his opinion. In this way Nightingale disables the reader's initial instinct to interpret what he reads. Now he is forced to disapprove both of those who might dislike the book, and also of anyone so intellectually blinkered as to conceive that Nightingale could be capable of debasing nursing into "the most prosaic of human things." In manipulating her reader in this fashion, she is a brilliantly successful, though exhausting writer.

Her opening literary metaphor distinguishes between an enlightened, mystical quality in poetry, and an inferior, demystified, rational quality associated with prose; between this articulate exposition of the mysteries of the art of nursing, and a sterile catalogue of "dos" and "don'ts." As if to further contradict whatever preconceptions her reader might hold by using poetic techniques within her own prose, Nightingale demonstrates the fallacy of this distinction. In the second sentence, the rhetorical iron fist with which she shames her reader is immediately followed by the softness of her warmly intimate address, "My dear sister." She gently massages the reluctant reader toward an idealistic view of nursing: "there is nothing in the world . . . so much the reverse of prosaic." Education is put forward only as a noble but short-lived exception.

In his famous "O what a rogue and peasant slave am I!" speech (II.ii.576), Shakespeare's Hamlet stands in awe of an actor who projects himself into a character's feelings, even though he has not personally experienced them. Nightingale uses a similar idea to demonstrate that nursing, in requiring the same rare ability, is far superior to education. Unlike education, she argues, only nursing addresses that immensely difficult problem, hitherto by universal consent faced only by poets, playwrights, and actors, whose art "requires so much power of throwing yourself into others' feelings which you have never felt." Through inspired use of logic, rhetoric, and literary theory, she proves conclusively what no one had ever before even begun to imagine: that nursing is the equal of the sublime art of poetry. Lastly, from her authoritative position as creator and high priestess of this newest of the arts, she utters a dire warning from the depth of her enormous and painful experience: "if you have none of this power, you had better let nursing alone."

Nightingale knew that such a compact, demanding, and at times even threatening style of writing was not now the way to proceed. Her idealized "dear sister" of the Library Standard edition, just possibly able to understand this prose-poetry, is certainly not within the group to whom she now addresses her attention.

It is self-evident that, despite her efforts to simplify the language and concepts in *Notes on Nursing for the Labouring Classes*, parts of the original were written in such an idiosyncratic style that its author could never entirely eradicate from them her peculiar combination of wit and intellect. Although the individual words could not be simpler, the simultaneous clarity and obscurity of Nightingale's literary language must have baffled many nineteenth-century readers of whatever class. Sutherland was right to comment that, in the end, "it contains too much of a very profound discussion."

As if to support his opinion, "What Is a Nurse?" still begins with an abstract metaphor: "The very alphabet of a nurse is to be able to read every change which comes over a patient's countenance, without causing him the exertion of saying what he feels." Whereas the word "alphabet" means "A,B,C" or "basic knowledge," when placed as it is here in conjunction with "read" it takes on the meaning of "letters through which to communicate in words" (the Library Standard text had "alphabet" and "interpret"). A contrast is developed between the nurse, literate in reading her patient's feelings as expressed in the silent language of facial expression, and the barely vocal patient's "exertion of saying what he feels." This subtle combination of words and ideas is followed by one so ridiculous as deliberately to embarrass the reader: "What would many a nurse do otherwise than she does, if her patient were a valuable piece of furniture or a sick cow?" Every one knows the answer to this gamesome riddle because it is painfully obvious: "pay closer attention." But no help is forthcoming from this arrogant, even insulting, author. With a reply befitting the sphinx, she enigmatically answers another of her own controversial questions: "I do not know," she writes, "Yet a nurse must be something more than a lift or a broom." She leaves us with another little poem to think about.

When Nightingale sent two copies of *Notes on Nursing for the Labouring Classes* to her mother, she wrote a separate note dated April 21, 1861, in which she explained the origins of the new chapter "Minding Baby." It was, she says, something

> which I was ordered to write by a Schoolmaster at Peckham, Mr. Shields, who had made my book a text book for his children and said that the girls went home and removed dung-heaps from before their parents' doors & opened their parents' windows at night (to the great discomfiture of the latter) but that the "strongest motive" was to tell the girls to do this for the sake of "Baby"—and so I must write a chap. about "Minding Baby."

In a postscript, she adds, "A great part of the 2nd Chapter 'Health of Houses' and part of the first Chap. are also new. And I was thinking of the Lea Hurst cottages all the time I wrote them."[29]

It is certainly true that the additions in the first two chapters are less poetic and more objective in style than much of the writing in the earlier versions. Even so, they are largely expressed in generalities, which is the direction toward which some of the emendations turned. For example, the very specific "three cases of Hospital pyaemia, one of phlebitis, two of consumptive cough," become only "six cases of serious illness" (see below, p. 99). Other changes altered the tone from up-market to down-market. Thankfully, she could find no justification for retaining the puzzling grammatical metaphor, "For diseases, as all experience shows, are adjectives, not noun substantives" (see below, p. 109).

In "Minding Baby" Nightingale reaches new heights of poetic creativity and rhetorical purpose, once more altering the tone and style of her address to fit an entirely new audience. When she begins, "And now, girls, I have a word for you," she is not simply being disarmingly colloquial. She is trying every trick she knows to create a sympathetic bond with her young audience, winning them over by expressing a great deal of respect: "Do you know that one-half of all the nurses in service are girls of from five to twenty years old? You see you are very important little people" (see below, p. 403). No documentation seems to record whether the new approach succeeded with these young nurses, but the generally favorable reception accorded to the contents of the volume seems to have outweighed any latent criticism of this calculated change of language.

There is nothing to suggest that "Minding Baby" was not an outright success, even though its appearance in very small print would have made it difficult for the young to read. It was slightly more legible in the clearer 1868 edition. Shortly after the publication of this volume, Nightingale revealed in a letter to Henry Bonham Carter, quoted below, that "Minding Baby" had actually been written for separate printing as a booklet, and she expressed her anger that it was never issued as such.

ii—The 1868 Edition

On November 28, 1868, several months after the publication of the 1868 edition, Henry Bonham Carter, the Secretary to the Nightingale Fund, expressed his concerns about its price and the format in which it was issued: "Can you tell me what Agreement you have with Harrison respecting 'Notes on Nursing'? I should like to see a cheaper edition in better print than the last."[30] Nightingale's candid reply of November 30 puts the entire history of the publishing of *Notes on Nursing*, and her long standing quarrel with her publisher, into context:

> I am sorry to say I have no agreement whatever with Harrison's ("Notes on Nursing")[.] The M.S. [manuscript] was parted with to him when I was very ill & when dear A. H. Clough was so also—without any Agreement.[31]
>
> The alterations & slight improvement in type in the New Edition were made at my own request, & only consented to by him because the old d/6 [sixpence] Edition was out of print.
>
> I do not believe that Harrison's will do anything cheaper or anything he is asked.
>
> E.g. He has been asked over & over again by different persons to publish the Chapter on "Minding Baby"—(which I wrote for him separately—) separately—He gets over every such request by simply taking no notice.
>
> An "eminent Publisher" (as newspapers say) stated that Harrison's might have sold the 2/ [two shilling] edition at /9^d [nine pence]—& generally that I had been ill used. & that Harrison must have made a great deal of money.
>
> But as the "Unprotected Female" is fond of calling herself "ill-used," I have held my tongue.
>
> Obviously having no redress.[32]

Because Nightingale had no contract with Harrison, he had total control over publication. From his commercial viewpoint, it was obviously more profitable to continue reprinting the two shilling first version in great quantity, while allowing this cheap third version to go out of print. This ran counter to the author's impatient desire to achieve wider dissemination of her work, but she had no rights whatsoever. Her hands were completely tied.

The alterations to the text of the 1868 edition must have been ready by September 1867, the date of Nightingale's prefatory note on the back of the title page. Corrected proof sheets of parts of the volume with the date October 28 stamped on them survive in the British Library. They are marked "1st," indicating that another set was still to follow after the alterations made at this juncture were set in type. On the title page the year 1867 has been altered to 1868.[33]

Nightingale's manuscript drafts of three entirely new passages survive. One, on purifying village wells, was for "Health of Houses" (below, p. 320); the second, on crinoline fire deaths, for "Noise" (below, p. 340); and the third, for "Chattering Hopes and Advices," on telling patients the truth about their illnesses (below, p. 375).[34]

On the back of the "village wells" fragment Nightingale wrote the following irritated notes to Sutherland. Taken out of context they have little meaning except to indicate the pressure she was capable of exerting through the liberal application of verbal vitriol: "Which means nothing but this—that you're too lazy to look at it"; "You've looked at it for just 5 minutes"; "on Wednesday."

The draft on crinoline fire deaths is in Sutherland's hand, and differs somewhat from the printed version. On May 20, 1867, Nightingale had written to William Farr requesting information for this revised text. She asked him, "What would be a safe statement as to Deaths from clothes catching fire in women at the 'fashionable' *ages* to put into my text?" Farr replied, "We are at work on the violent deaths. And I enclose you an extract from our Tables—as far as they go. You will be able to trace the sexes— through the 'Ages'—& to show how the unhappy butterflies are burnt."[35]

On May 23, Farr wrote again:

You know how imperfectly our coroners do their duty—& how negligent they are in stating the cause of Death precisely—as they are instructed by the Registrar General.

Hence we do not get the returns of all the deaths by Clothes-taking-fire—distinguished. Upon looking into the matter—I am inclined to believe that nearly all the women burnt to death—in "manner not stated"—are burnt in their clothes—& through their clothes taking fire.

You will see that at 60 & upwards—the poor old women are burnt in great numbers—through falling asleep &c &c

I enclose you a Table complete for the year 1866. Note the boys drinking scalding water—out of tea-pots & kettles—in greater numbers than girls.[36]

Using Farr's information, Sutherland composed the draft, which Nightingale then modified to her own livelier style. She reduced his tedious phrasing, "From a return prepared by the registrar General for the years 1863–64 it appears that in these two years," to only a few crisp words: "In two years, 1863–4." But the factual center part of the paragraph (below, p. 340) repeats Sutherland's draft almost verbatim.

Another addition to the 1868 *Notes on Nursing for the Labouring Classes* is the "Appendix on Method of Training Nurses Under the Nightingale Fund at Saint Thomas's Hospital London" (below, p. 410). This was prepared by Henry Bonham Carter, and submitted to Nightingale. When she wrote on June 4, 1867, thanking him "for your Appendix to 'Notes on Nursing,' which I adopt," she altered the phrasing of the probationer's four-year commitment after training from "binding her to enter into hospital service" to "binding her as a nurse for the sick poor." She deferentially asked Bonham Carter if this would do. Then, on November 6, 1867, she forwarded the proofs of his appendix (his "fag end") for criticism and correction.

The heavily emended British Library proofs of the appendix contain an early draft. Later, when second proofs had been extensively revised, a shortened version was published. Material contained only in the first proofs draws directly upon the summary of training nurses at Saint Thomas's, published in Nightingale's pamphlet *Suggestions on a System of Nursing for Hospitals in India* (1865). Borrowing from this, Bonham Carter included a paragraph describing the reluctance of the Committee of the Nightingale Fund to give out certificates on completion of training—but Nightingale marked it for deletion:

We do not give the woman a printed certificate, but simply enter the names of all certified nurses in the register as such. This was done to prevent them, in the event of misconduct, from using their certificates improperly. When a nurse has satisfactorily earned the gratuity attached to her certificate the Committee, through the Secretary, communicate with her and forward the money.

The implications for social history in a second altered passage are little short of extraordinary: they bear witness to the gradual unfolding of a significant event, the closing of the midwifery ward at King's College Hospital after an outbreak of puerperal fever in the late autumn of 1867.

In addition to the advertisement for nursing at St. Thomas's, the proofs that Nightingale sent Bonham Carter on November 6 have a second section devoted to midwifery training at King's College Hospital. Quite clearly it was Bonham Carter's intention to foster this program, which received sponsorship from the Nightingale Fund. That only the third paragraph is scored through by Nightingale signifies that at this moment in time the impending disaster had not yet begun to exert its malign influence:

2. As to King's College Hospital, where women are trained in the practice of Midwifery.

From the nature of midwifery training it is not practicable to exact the same system at King's College Hospital Midwifery ward as in the regulated wards of St. Thomas's Hospital.

The class of duties required of midwifery nurses is also different, but the principles and methods of selection and of training are much the same, as also the conditions of admission and of service. A form of application for admission will be supplied by the Lady Superior of St. John's House, King's College Hospital, London, W.C.

[*This paragraph is deleted in the proof.* For these trained midwifery nurses, who are exclusively for the *poor,* we find there is now a demand by ladies' committees and other institutions (chiefly benevolent), which pay them a salary.]

At King's College Hospital instruction is given in midwifery and matters connected with the diseases of women and children, during the time of the special training in midwifery.

By the time the 1868 edition of *Notes on Nursing for the Labouring Classes* was published, all trace of this section of the advertisement had disappeared. So also had the midwifery ward at King's College Hospital. Nightingale's correspondence reveals that she was aware of trouble by mid-November, that by December 2 she was considering the politics of closing the midwifery ward, and that by mid-January she had entirely severed her ties with the hospital.[37] The evolution of the appendix reflects this sad sequence of events. With the section on midwifery cut out, the published appendix continues, as in the proofs, with the proposal to train girls from the large union schools.

iii—The Unpublished 1875 Edition

The scarcity of material appertaining to the planning and writing of any of the three versions of *Notes on Nursing* is compensated for by the surviving documents related to the proposed but unpublished edition of

1875. Preserved along with the other manuscript drafts already cited are the revised texts of three new and substantial sections.

In the first, an addition to "Health of Houses," Nightingale describes the relationship between disease and air from sewers, and suggests remedies in more careful construction (see below, p. 420). She intended the second and third for the conclusion of her chapter, "What Food." The second warns particularly of the sale of substandard and diluted milk, and prepared baby foods (see below, p. 417). The third concerns the "stomach habits which make our race degenerate" (below, p. 427): "Is there any wonder," she asks, "that, between smoking & drinking, boys & girls (who are going to be fathers & mothers) destroy first their own constitutions," then pass them on to their children? There is no question in her mind who must shoulder most of the blame: "It is the fault of drinking: it is the fault of tobacco: it is the fault of mothers . . . it is the fault of mothers . . . it is the fault of mothers."

This passage concludes with a scenario that relates industrial strife and business failure to a decline in the health of factory workers, whose already "weak brains are farther stupefied by tobacco or drink." Nightingale did not remain oblivious to the dramatic rise in organized labor and its disputes—the Trades Union Congress was founded in 1868. In fact, she comments in the first *Labouring Classes* edition (1861) that proper ventilation of "badly constructed work-places" "*would* be worth a 'Trades' Union,' almost worth a 'strike' " (below, p. 312). The clear implication of this is that she does not consider many of the reasons given for strikes to be particularly worthy, particularly if motivated by what she interprets to be greed: inflationary pay for less work. In this discussion, Nightingale focuses on what she sees as one of the social causes of industrial unrest. Because the mills are healthier to work in than ever before, she blames the workers' own poor choice of diet for rendering them susceptible to agitators. With their brains addled by strong tobaccos and alcoholic drink, she inquires, do they not "become a prey to 'Agitators,' & think that, by driving trade & manufactures [manufacturing businesses] away from England, where it will not so soon return, they can raise wages? get a higher wage for shorter hours of work?"

Although it is regrettable that this interesting passage is not further developed, the original correspondence related to the first two new sections does survive, and adds considerably to our understanding of them.[38] On May 22, 1874, Nightingale sent Sutherland a copy of "*My Small*" 1868 edition so that he could begin making "additions and corrections." Though this copy had blank leaves bound between the pages, she requested that *"you* should kindly make your additions & criticisms *on separate sheets:* & leave *me* to enter them on the interleaved copy."[39] Given this instruction, Sutherland accordingly drafted four suggestions on the back of the black bordered writing paper she had used since the death of her father on January 10, and promptly returned it.[40] He qualified the 1861 insertion on "washing the walls and ceilings with quick-lime wash" (below, p. 325), adding, "with the precaution of first scraping off the old whitewash." On the problem of sewage from country cottages (below, p. 321), he brought to her attention that "you might put in dry earth closets." His draft of this section reads

> Of late years what is called the "dry earth system" has been beneficially for country cottages where drainage & water supply are not common suitable. This consists in using common garden earth instead of water for closets. It is safest to place dry earth closets outside cottages altogether. They have if properly used none of the dangers of cesspits, and the earth is always useful as a manure.[41]

The most substantial passage in this note is about the relationship between typhoid fever and sewer air, and on this, as well as on the subject of babies' milk, he wrote the following anecdotal accounts which eventually became the basis of the unpublished additions:

> I dont know if I told you years ago about the typhoid in the Royal Hibernian School. I got at the cause (sewer air) at once, & one of the experiments was having a handkerchief blown up out of a drain by a blast of sewer air.
> A remedy was applied & the fever immediately ceased, and I was told the other day that the "local authority" says that ever since "the old gentleman" (meaning me the rascals) waved his handkerchief over the sewer the fever had been charmed away. They never will allow that their own remedied neglects had any influence in the result. This is the latest dodge.
> I will send you whole instructive case when it is finished. We are still trying to complete the school improvements. What I have told you is in confidence.
> In the section *Minding Baby*
> You might dwell on the necessity of providing babies with first class milk. I have been working out the causes of the enormous death rates among children in India, as you will see in the next blue book. Now there is reason (not yet conclusive) for attributing a large share of this to starvation. Milk is used, & it is produced by animals often fed on excrementatious matters & bad as it is, it is diluted by the sellers to such an extent as to render it scarcely of any use.

Nightingale was livid that Sutherland, who had already expended an enormous amount of energy upon her projects, dealt with this request so quickly, and with such brevity. On June 15 she him sent this stern reprimand:

Dear Dr. Sutherland,
    After keeping me & Harrisons *a year and a half* waiting, you keep the copy sent *one hour* & return me about *half an hour's* work in suggestions. (on my own little sheet)
    I have rather more to do each day than can be done in the 24 hours. And this is my busiest time.
    Unless you can do something more for me—I think I shall give up the idea of furnishing Harrisons—which I only promised upon *your* sugges-tion & *promise* repeatedly renewed to help—with a new Edition. He has sent for it again & again.
    I now send you back these poor little 'scrimpie duds.' I think ms. *p. 2*, that a most effective & useful addition might be made *to Chapter "Health of Houses"* about *Sewer Air, Schools, Houses, Fever, Pr. of Wales*, if you would give me the data, I would put them into form. If not, not. [*Indeed I thought* that *this* was to have been the *main part* of the *addition*.]
    You can take out your own story of the "handkerchief," if you like it. Je n'y tiens pas.

To term his efforts "scrimpie duds" (which seems to mean "tiny, raggy scraps"), and return them for additional information, epitomizes the snarling but effective working relationship that she shared with Sutherland. She invites him to "take out," that is, "extract from this draft for further development," his important anecdote of the handkerchief, pejoratively referring to it as a mere "story," and closes with the French throw away line, "Je n'y tiens pas"—"It's all the same to me!" Such pretended indifference is mischievously provocative, calculated to make Sutherland feel guilty.

Sutherland retaliated by once more replying on the back of her sheet of note paper. He knew this irritated her, and his defiant Italian *"Ecco"*—"so there!," suggests that he hoped at least for the moment to persuade her to contain her wrath:

There is nothing like writing on the back of your scold. Ecco.
    Your impression appears to be that since the very careful consideration which was given to the book there has been great progress in sanitary work. But there has been none—We have known every principle we are ever likely to know for the last 30 years—or more. All that you ever can do with

your book is to use a bit of fresh thread to take up a loop, or else you must unravel the whole stocking & begin again to knit for the mere amusement. The real objection to the book is that it contains too much of a very profound discussion. When I suggested your having the fresh proofs, it was merely that you might see whether you would alter any thing of the Nursing part & you said no. That was all.

The context provided by this argument, coupled with Sutherland's advice to Nightingale, suggests that another, undated note of his filed among the drafts belongs to this point in the sequence. On one side, it contains the beginning of what would become the new section on milk (below, p. 417), and on the other, further advice about her request for information on current developments in sanitary work:

> I don't think you want much alteration for a new edition so far as Sanitary work is concerned.
> It does not do to overload the pages of a book with this object.
> Curiously enough however there is scarcely any of it in ordinary books of hygiene.
> I have put down a few points, and would merely suggest for consideration whether a very simple way of making it useful for a school would not be to print separately the chapters on Health of houses & Minding baby.
>
> JS.[42]

Nightingale has drawn a vertical line through both sides of the letter, with the exception of the final four lines, which she highlights with lines in the margin.

Sutherland's efforts won him no mercy. She switched on her most hurtfully humorous charm, and on June 18 asked in a pretentiously polite way for more facts. At some later time, both in this letter and in Sutherland's extensive reply of the same day, Nightingale deleted a large number of words, phrases, and lines, adding her own emendations. These reflect her economical practice of editing her correspondence for use as early drafts of the revised text. The text given here is in its original form, the only change being Nightingale's alteration in the first line of the rather bland "coming to" to the more sarcastic "trying":

> Dear Dr. Sutherland
> Excuse me for ~~coming to~~ trying you once more:
> If you would give me the *bare data* about *Sewer Air* coming into the *houses*
> – *how it comes*} briefly & generally

- *how it can be prevented* }
- as exemplified too often alas! in *London*
- in my own house or in *a grand country house by the sea* where the *heir to the throne* was all but murdered
- in what was attempted to introduce as *Legislation* via Mr Stansfield
- in *Caius College Cambridge or some similar instance*
- in some instances of *Schools* like the *R. Hibernian*
- in some of the numberless instances of *Typhoid* & *Typhus,* like *Lord Elcho's children,* from this cause:
- saying briefly *how the Sewer Air comes in*
- & generally *how it is to be prevented:*

you w^d much oblige Yours to command FN

The principal alterations that Nightingale made in adjusting this for inclusion in her drafts are diplomatic in their nature: "in *Caius College Cambridge*" becomes "Colleges at Universities," and the reference to "*Lord Elcho's children*" is neutralized in "even among noblemen's children." Exclusion of specific and potentially embarrassing references such as these is an example of the precautions taken to preserve the anonymity of victims of unfortunate circumstances. She may well have learned of Lord Elcho's personal tragedy at first hand, for as early as 1862 she had prepared a speech in memory of Thomas Alexander, Director-General of the Army Medical Department, which Lord Elcho read on her behalf at a public ceremony in September.[43]

Faced by this list of demands, Sutherland knows he has been outfoxed, and relents without further resistance, even to the extent of using fresh paper. Selecting sheets of War Office letterhead for this exercise, he writes an extended and detailed commentary on the problems his old enemy has faced him with. But he takes advantage of his opening paragraph to make her aware of his displeasure, beginning abruptly with a pained question:

What on earth am I to do? Your last "favour" was a fierce attack on a very humble person because your questions were not answered on separate papers. Here is a whole lot of questions on one paper & I am "fixed."

However. You cannot get any reply that will cover all your cases. Just as you could not get a diagnosis & treatment that would cover every case of illness. The only general part is that sewer air comes from sewers & that if it gets into houses it will do mischief, & further that it can be kept out by certain engineering details amongst others by relaying the whole sewerage & draining of districts. Sewer air comes essentially from bad sewers & the "cases" of bad sewers would fill volumes. In your own street one of the main causes is half a mile away.

All you can do is to advise that the cause of the sewer air should be sought in the defective construction of sewers & drains; & that so far as concerns the house itself that all ~~sewer~~ house drain pipes should be cut off from the street sewer by efficient trapping & that all house drain pipes should be ventilated by pipes carried above the roof, & all cistern overflow pipes cut off from the W.C. pipes.

The cause of the P. of W.s [*that is, the Prince of Wales's*] attack has never been decided by any competent enquirer. It was sewer air I believe, but how it got there is not settled till this day.

The Cambridge case is a muddle of the same kind & for the same reason. The Hibernian School is the only case that has been examined in our sense. But you had better not name it otherwise than as a large public School. Our work gave rise to great ill blood & Mr. Lowe behaved very badly. We had to fight for dear life about it, but we would not yield a step. The facts are that for 10 years gastric fever existed in the School, the disease was traced to sewer air from foul sewers. The sewers were ventilated & the water pipes cut off from them & since then there has been no gastric fever. They would not allow the sewer to be relaid because it condemned the work of a Govt Board & hence I should be loathe to certify that the place is safe especially as they had 4 deaths from Scarlet fever last year out of 30 cases?

Lord Elcho's house ought to have been carefully examined. I dare say it is neither better nor worse than others in St James Square[.]

You might say that the only way to prevent such calamities is to enable local boards to examine & certify the plans of all house drainage & water supply in order to be sure that no drains are carried down inner walls, that they are all trapped & ventilated & that the water cisterns have no direct connection with the soil pipes.

Now please arrange this on as many bits of paper as necessary for its passes [*passed?*] me.

Sutherland concludes his letter with a cut-away sketch of the sewer and ventilation system required in a house with a toilet on each of four stories. Rather than rearrange this letter on separate pages, as Sutherland facetiously recommends, Nightingale makes her preliminary adjustments to the text on the letter itself. She next writes it out in full, along with the other drafts of materials compiled for the new revision, and puts it into the form printed in this edition (below, p. 420).

Conclusion

This brief history of the writing and publishing of *Notes on Nursing* attempts to set the work within the context of Nightingale's life and times.

The main thrust is to show how seriously Nightingale looked upon her "little book," and how she persevered in trying to make it more accessible to the widest audience possible.

That the influence of her work spread farther than even she could have anticipated is owing in part to the efforts of those who held her opinions in high esteem. On May 8, 1861, Harriet Martineau expressed such very great satisfaction when she received her copy of *Notes on Nursing for the Labouring Classes* that she ordered copies to distribute as broadly as she could:

> I could not help reading it all through again—all the old part,—as well as the new: & I think I like it better than ever. I have ordered a batch of copies; & the parson & the Arnolds & I shall soon see that every body here has it who can at all profit by it. It is a great boon.[44]

This letter was written from Ambleside, Martineau's retreat on Lake Windermere, where she numbered among her neighbors two generations of the Arnolds, of whom the younger was Matthew, the poet and social critic.[45]

In one form or another the "little book" was quoted and paraphrased wherever authoritative advice was to be given on the subjects she covered. The variety of contexts in which it appears is not without its amusement. The hugely successful *Book of Household Management* (1862) by Mrs. Isabella Beeton, and her husband's *Beeton's Dictionary of Practical Recipes* (1870) both include passages on food, noise, and children drawn from various editions. Mrs. Beeton's 1861 preface reassures her readers that the chapters on medical subjects were contributed "by an experienced surgeon," a gentleman. Experienced or not, he most certainly does not remain a detached reporter. Even given Nightingale's reputation, it is still surprising that the Beetons have represented her in a dramatic portrayal, speaking words that only approximate those she actually wrote (compare below, p. 84):

> "It is another fallacy," says Florence Nightingale, "to suppose that night air is injurious; a great authority told me that, in London, the air is never so good as after ten o'clock, when smoke has diminished; but then it must be air from without, not within, and not air vitiated by gaseous airs."

And when this "experienced surgeon" comes across Lord Melbourne's misogynistic complaint against women and their rustling crinolines, he springs to their defense:

Miss Nightingale denounces crinoline, and quotes Lord Melbourne on the subject of women in the sick-room, who said, "I would rather have men about me, when ill, than women; it requires very strong health to put up with women." Ungrateful man! but absolute quiet is necessary in the sick-room.[46]

This unexciting paraphrase is mellower than the original phrasing of the Library Standard edition (see below, p. 129). It is designed to elicit the reader's sympathy through the gratuitous addition of the exclamation "Ungrateful man!", and entirely suppresses Nightingale's brutal frankness in joining Lord Melbourne in condemning noisy nurses: "I am quite of his opinion." The Beeton circle wants no part in such controversy, choosing to ignore the distinction drawn between good and poor nurses.

Nightingale has suffered more than enough through distortion, and through her book being offered by Harrison in different versions to the reading public. This edition seeks to enlighten the reader in relation to the mysteries that surround these various versions of the text. In addressing the historical problems posed by *Notes on Nursing*, and considering them from the perspective offered by applying a literal interpretation of the subtitle, *What It Is and What It Is Not*, the deficiencies of earlier texts are explained. This commemorative edition of *Notes on Nursing: What It Is and What It Is Not*, together with the 1868 edition of *Notes on Nuring for the Labouring Classes*, and the 1875 additions, represents the most complete and unadulterated version of Nightingale's much loved and precious "little book."

EDITOR'S NOTES

1. British Library MS. Add. 45788, fol. 91b. Fols. 29–57 contain Nightingale's correspondence with Martineau (1802–1876) during the preparation in 1859 of her *England And Her Soldiers*. This book popularized the facts contained in Nightingale's *Mortality of the British Army* (1859), and Nightingale underwrote the costs of its publication.
2. This description of the cloth follows the guidelines in G. T. Tanselle, "The Bibliographical Description of Patterns," in *Studies in Bibliography*, xxiii (1970), 71–102.
3. This and the following bibliographical details are based on those in *The British Library Catalogue*; the Library of Congress, *The National Union Catalog: Pre-1956 Imprints*; W. J. Bishop and S. Goldie, *A Bio-bibliography of Florence Nightingale* (London, 1962); and Sir E. Cook, *The Life of Florence Nightingale* (London, 1914), especially ii. 439–442. Instructions on how to distinguish copies of the first edition from one another are given at the end of this book in the Guide to Identification. For a full description, see V. Skretkowicz, "Florence Nightingale's *Notes on Nursing*: The First Version and Edition," *The Library*, 6th Ser. xv (1993), 24–46.

4. The publication details given here follow those on the respective title pages. The Italian translation by Sabillo Novello was published "Torino Fratelli Bocca, Librai di S.S.R.M.; Milano, Gaetano Brigola; Firenze, E. Goodban; and Nizza, Societa Tipografica"—the license to publish on the verso of the title page is dated "Nizza 1860" (pp. 96). The Danish version was published in "Kjöbenhavn, / Forlagt Af Den Gyldendalske Boghandling (F. Hegel) / Thieles Bogtrykkeri / 1861" (pp. iv + 157); and the Swedish, translated by E[mily] N[onne]n, with a forward by Charles Dickson dated June 1, 1861, was published at "Göteborg / Handelstidningens Bolags Tryckeri, 1861" (pp. viii + 120).

5. The relationships between the texts are described in V. Skretkowicz, "The New York, Boston, and London Editions of Nightingale's *Notes on Nursing*," *Notes on Nursing Science* iv (1991), pp. 2–8.

6. British Library MS. Add. 45770, fol. 122–122b.

7. Library of Congress *Catalog*, NN 0266002. The facsimile of the New York edition is published by Dover Books; that of the Boston, edition by the Nightingale Society, Carmel, California.

8. The German translation by H. Bunsen, with a Forward by "Sch. Sanitäts-Rath Dr. S. Wolff in Bonn," was published in "Leipzig: / F. A. Brockhaus. / 1861" (pp. xvi + 224). The French, with an introduction by M. Daremberg, and preceded by a letter to Daremberg by M. Guizot, was published in Paris "A La Libraire Academique / Didier Et Ce., 1862", and again in 1869 (pp. xlviii + 308). The Dutch translation by [Anna dor.] Busken Huet[-Van Der Tholl], with an address to the reader by Professor G. E. V. Schneevoogt (dated Amsterdam, November 21, 1862), was first published in Amsterdam (no copy seen), and again in 1863 in Haarlem by J. J. Weeveringh (pp. 239). This omits the entire "Supplementary Chapter." Paulina Králova's Czech translation was published in Prague, "Nakladatel J. Otto Knihkupec./ 1874" (pp. 188). This was published as volume cxiv in Sofie Podlipská, editor, Ženská Bibliotéka. The 1938 Finnish translation is by Aune Brotherus, published by Porvoo, Helsinki.

9. *Florence Nightingale's Notes on Nursing (Revised, with Additions)* (London: [Royal College of Nursing] Scutari Press, 1992; repr. London: Baillière Tindall, 1996).

10. Cook, *Life of Florence Nightingale*, ii. 441, notes a reprint in 1865, which I have not come across.

11. This German translation is by Dr. Paul Niemeyer (Leipzig / F. A. Brockhaus / 1878), the preface dated November 1877 (p. x + 210). The note at the foot of p. 1 refers to the New Edition, London, 1876. The Italian epitome by E. C[omparetti] is published in "Lucca / Tipografia Giust / 1887" (pp. 71). This includes the 1867 appendix advertising the Nightingale School, "METODO PER L'ISTRUZIONE DELLE INFERMIERE NELLO SPEDALE DI SAN TOMMASO A LONDRA (FONDAZIONE NIGHTINGALE)."

12. This is confirmed by the present-day Harrisons, a modern high-security printing company.

13. British Library MS. Add. 45751, fols. 125b–126, J. Sutherland to Nightingale, February 10, 1859. Dr. John Sutherland (1808–1891), sanitary and public health reformer, met Nightingale in the Crimea, and worked closely with her for the rest of his life.

14. British Library MS. Add. 45751, fols. 129–130b, J. Sutherland to Nightingale, February 12, 1859. The transcription of sections of this letter in Z. Cope, *Florence Nightingale and the Doctors* (London, 1958), is not entirely accurate.

15. Z. Cope, *Florence Nightingale and the Doctors*, p. 101, notes that the papers were read by a Dr. Holland.

16. British Library MS. Add. 45770, fols. 122–122v.

17. Wellcome Institute for the History of Medicine Library, MS. 5471, Nightingale to Aitken, June 8, 1859. Sir William Aitken (1825–1892) was Professor of Pathology in the Army Medical School from 1860 till shortly before his death.

18. British Library MS. Add. 45770, fols. 113–114b, Nightingale to Edwin Chadwick, December 28, 1859.

19. British Library MS. Add. 45751, fols. 151–153, Nightingale to Sutherland, [3]-4 March 1860.

20. Cook, ii. 439.

21. Cook, i. 450.

22. Cook, ii. 440.

23. British Library MS. Add. 45817, fols. 1–35.

24. *Quarterly Review* 107 (1860), pp. 392–422, citing p. 393.

25. British Library MS. Add. 45788, fol. 79b. Martineau thanks Nightingale for the first version on January 19, 1860 (fol. 59), the second on July 15 (fol. 87), and the third on May 8, 1861 (fol. 123). See V. Wheatley, *The Life and Work of Harriet Martineau* (London, 1957), p. 361.

26. See M. Cardwell, in her introduction to her edition of *Martin Chuzzlewit* (Oxford, 1982), p. xxix, and A. Summers, "The Mysterious Demise of Sarah Gamp: The Domiciliary Nurse and their Detractors, c. 1830–1860," *Victorian Studies* xxxii (1989), 365–386.

27. Dickens, *Martin Chuzzlewit*, p. 848. This is not a complaint about the few private and religious institutions that trained nurses, but rather a general comment on how, as late as 1849, the hospitals, with all their resources, had still provided nothing to ensure that the quality of their nursing improved. See also P. Smith, *Disraelian Conservatism and Social Reform* (London, 1967), p. 59.

28. British Library MS. Add. 45757, fol. 245ᵛ.

29. Claydon House MS., transcribed from the copy in the Wellcome Institute for the History of Medicine.

30. British Library MS. Add. 47716, fol. 25. The barrister Henry Bonham Carter (1827–1921) was Nightingale's cousin. In 1861 he succeeded A. H. Clough as Secretary of the Nightingale Fund.

31. Arthur Hugh Clough (1819–1861) married Nightingale's cousin Blanche Smith in 1854, and served as Secretary to the Nightingale Fund. He was a much admired poet whose short, acid satire, "The Latest Decalogue," is widely misinterpreted. The lines, "Thou shalt not kill; but needst not strive / Officiously to keep alive" are frequently cited out of context by medical professionals who support euthanasia (see *The Poems of Arthur Hugh Clough*, ed. F. L. Mulhauser, 2nd ed. [Oxford, 1974], p. 205).

32. British Library MS. Add. 47716, fol. 29.

33. British Library shelf-mark Cup.401.c.10(3), "Tracts 1860–79," containing quires A (pp. 1–16), F (pp. 65–80), G (pp. 81–96), H (pp. 97–114), and one further fragment of H (pp. 97–98 and pp. 113–114).

34. British Library MS. Add. 45817, fols. 7, 8, and 10–10v.

35. British Library MS. Add. 43400, fols. 166–167. William Farr (1807–1883) was a statistician in the office of the Registrar-General.

36. British Library MS. Add. 43400, fols 175–175v.

37. Details of the proofs are given in note 32 above. On Nightingale's relationship with King's College Hospital, see British Library MS. Add. 45752, fol. 252, about November 12, 1867; MS. Add. 47715, fol. 132, dated December 2, 1867; and MS. Add. 45753,

fol. 15, about mid-January 1868. I accept S. Goldie's conjectural dating in *A Calendar of the Letters of Florence Nightingale* (Oxford, 1983), fiche 14, C13, 919; and fiche 15, A4, 7. Puerperal fever remained a problem in hospitals for several more years. In the second edition of R. Quain's *Dictionary of Medicine*, (London, 1895), ii. 573, which reprints Nightingale's entries on nursing, C. Godson epitomizes his article on "Antiseptic Midwifery" from *The Lancet* (April 1, 1893):

> in the City of London Lying-in Hospital, where the death-rate for a long period of years had averaged over 2 per cent., it had, since the antiseptic management had been properly carried out, fallen to 0.31 per cent., the average of the last six years; and that during a period which has just reached two years upwards of 950 women had been delivered in the institution without a single death from any source whatever. No stronger evidence could be adduced to show that lying-in hospitals, formerly regarded as dangerous to enter, may now be looked upon, under proper management, as the safest places to be *confined* in.

38. These letters form part of the Nightingale-Sutherland correspondence, in British Library MS. Add. 45757, fols. 242–249.
39. This may well be the interleaved copy now in the British Library (shelf mark CUP 401.c.9).
40. C. Woodham-Smith, *Florence Nightingale* (London, 1950), p. 526, gives the date.
41. The dry earth closet is clearly described in the James Bartlett's article, "Sewerage," in *The Encyclopaedia Britannica*, 13th edition (1926), xxiv. 737:

> The dry-earth system introduced by the Rev. Henry Moule (1801–1880), and patented in 1860, takes advantage of the oxidizing effect which a porous substance such as dry earth exerts by bringing any sewage with which it is mixed into intimate contact with the air contained in its pores.
>
> . . . Numerous forms of earth-closet are sold in which a suitable quantity of earth is automatically thrown into the pan at each time of use (fig. 10), but a box filled with dry earth and a hand scoop will answer the purpose nearly as well.

42. British Library MS. Add. 45817, fols. 12–12v.
43. This is noted in Cook, *Life of Florence Nightingale*, ii. 442; the correspondence about this is recorded in S. Goldie, *A Calendar of the Letters of Florence Nightingale* (Oxford, 1983).
44. British Library MS. Add. 45788, fol. 123.
45. V. Wheatley, *Harriet Martineau*, p. 253.
46. *Beeton's Dictionary of Practical Recipes* (1870), p. 293; Isabella Beeton, *The Book of Household Management, Entirely New Edition, Five Hundred and Fifty-eighth Thousand* (London, 1892), p. 1551. The preface to this complete revision is dated November 1888.

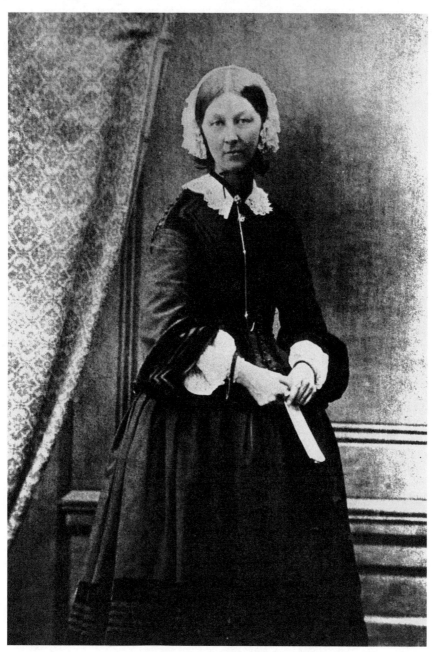

Carte de visite of Florence Nightingale, 1865.

Part
Two

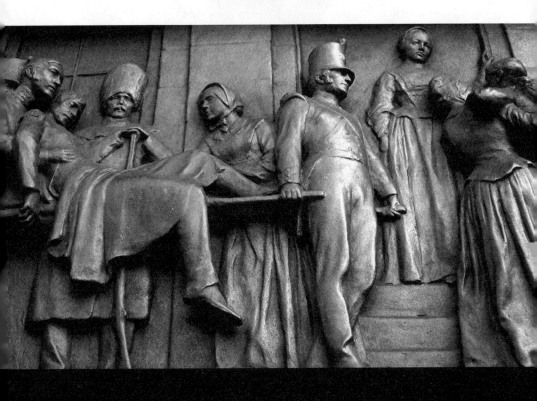

Notes on Nursing

What It Is and What It Is Not

1860 LIBRARY STANDARD EDITION

NOTES ON NURSING:

WHAT IT IS, AND WHAT IT IS NOT.

BY

FLORENCE NIGHTINGALE.

NEW EDITION, REVISED AND ENLARGED.

LONDON:

HARRISON, 59, PALL MALL,

Bookseller to the Queen

1860.

PREFACE.

THE following notes are by no means intended as a rule of thought by which nurses can teach themselves to nurse, still less as a manual to teach nurses to nurse. They are meant simply to give hints for thought to women who have personal charge of the health of others. Every woman, or at least almost every woman, in England has, at one time or another of her life, charge of the personal health of somebody, whether child or invalid,—in other words, every woman is a nurse. Every day sanitary knowledge, or the knowledge of nursing, or in other words, of how to put the constitution in such a state as that it will have no disease, or that it can recover from disease, takes a higher place. It is recognized as the knowledge which every one ought to have—distinct from medical knowledge, which only a profession can have.

If, then, every woman must, at some time or other of her life, become a nurse, *i.e.*, have charge

of somebody's health, how immense and how
valuable would be the produce of her united
experience if every woman would think how to
nurse.

I do not pretend to teach her how, I ask her to
teach herself, and for this purpose I venture to
give her some hints.

———————

DIGEST.

PAGES.

Introductory ....   1—7

I. Disease a reparative process   1
    Disease not always the cause of the sufferings supposed
        to be inherent to disease   2
    What nursing ought to do   2
    Nursing the sick, little understood   3
    Nursing ought to assist the reparative process   3
II. Nursing the well, little understood   4
    Curious deductions from an excessive death rate   4
    Child life a test of healthy conditions   6

I.—Ventilation and Warming ..   ..   8—28

First rule of nursing, to keep the air within as pure as the
    air without   8
Why are uninhabited rooms shut up?   9
A common madness   9
How to ventilate without chill   10
Open windows   12
What kind of warmth desirable   12
Bedrooms almost universally foul   12
How to open your windows   13
Schools   14
Work rooms   15
An air-test of essential consequence   16
When warmth must be most carefully looked to   18
Hot bottles   19
Cold air not ventilation, nor does fresh air necessarily chill   20
Draughts   20
Night air   22
Air from the outside. Open your windows, shut your doors   23
Smoke   23

PAGE.

Airing damp things in patient's room 24

Effluvia from excreta 25

Chamber utensils without lids 26

Don't make your sick room into a sewer 26

Abolish slop-pails 27

Fumigations 28

II.—Health of Houses .... 29—48

Five points essential 29

  1. Pure air 29

    Health of carriages 29

  2. Pure water.... 30

  3. Drainage 31

    Sinks 31

  4. Cleanliness.... 32

  5. Light 33

Three common errors in managing the health of houses 34

Head in charge must see to House Hygiene, not do it herself 35

Does God think of these things so seriously? 35

How does He carry out His laws? 36

How does He teach His laws? 37

Servants' rooms.... 38

Physical degeneration in families. Its causes 38

Consumption produced by foul air.... 39

Both in soldiers and "young ladies".... 40

Is consumption hereditary and inevitable? 41

Increase of births and of deaths in unhealthy districts 42

Don't make your sick room into a ventilating shaft for the

  whole house 45

Infection 45

Diseases are not individuals arranged in classes, like cats and

  dogs, but conditions growing out of one another 46

Why must children have measles, &c? 47

III.—Petty Management .... 49—62

Illustrations of the want of it.... 50

Strangers coming into the sick room 50

Sick-room airing the whole house 50

Uninhabited room fouling the whole house 51

Lingering smell of paint, a want of care 51

PAGE.

Delivery and non-delivery of letters and messages	51
Why let your patient ever be surprised?	51
Partial measures such as "being always in the way" yourself, increase instead of saving the patient's anxiety. Because they can be only partial	52
What is the cause of half the accidents which happen?....	54
Petty management better understood in institutions than in private houses	55
What institutions are the exception?	55
Nursing in Regimental hospitals	57
Question for persons "in charge"	58
What it is to be "in charge"	58
Why hired nurses give trouble	61
Nurses not expected to "nurse"—reason why there are few good ones	61

IV.—Noise ....   63—82

Unnecessary noise	63
Never let a patient be waked out of his first sleep	63
Noise which excites expectation	64
Whispered conversation in the room	65
Or just outside the door	66
Affectation	66
Noise of female dress	66
Patient's repulsion to nurses who rustle	67
Burning of the crinolines	68
Indecency of the crinolines	68
Patients obliged to defend themselves against their nurses	69
Hurry peculiarly hurtful to sick	70
How to visit the sick and not hurt them	70
These things not fancy	71
Interruption damaging to sick	72
And to well	72
Keeping a patient standing	72
Never speak to a patient in the act of moving	73
Patients dread surprise	73
Effects of over exertion on sick	75
Careless observation of the results of careless visits	75
Don't lean upon the sick bed....	76
Difference between real and fancy patients	76
Conciseness necessary with sick	77
And calmness	77

PAGE.

Irresolution most painful to them   77
What a patient must not have to see to   78
Reading aloud   79
(1.) Read aloud slowly, distinctly, and steadily to the sick   79
    The sick would rather be told a thing than have it read
      to them   79
(2.) Never read aloud by fits and starts to the sick   80
    People overhead   81
    Music   82

V.—Variety   ....   83—89

Variety a means of recovery   83
Colour and form means of recovery....   83
This is no fancy....   84
Flowers   84
Effect of body on mind....   85
Sick suffer to excess from mental as well as bodily pain....   86
Help the sick to vary their thoughts   86
Desperate desire in the sick to "see out of window"   87
Supply to the sick the defect of manual labour....   88
Physical effect of colour   88

VI.—Taking Food   ....   90—97

Want of attention to hours of taking food....   90
Life often hangs upon minutes in taking food   91
Chronic cases sometimes starved   92
Food never to be left by the patient's side....   92
Patient had better not see more food than his own   93
You cannot be too careful as to quality in sick diet   95
Nurse must have some rule of thought about her patient's
    diet   96
Nurse must have some rule of time about her patient's diet   96
Keep your patient's cup dry underneath   97

VII.—What Food   ....   98—110

Common errors in diet....   98
Beef tea   98
Eggs   98

PAGE.

Meat without vegetables 99
Arrowroot 99
Milk, butter, cream, &c.... 99
Intelligent cravings of particular classes of sick for particular
    articles of diet 100
Sweet things 101
Jelly 101
Beef tea 102
Observation, not chemistry, must decide sick diet 103
Home-made bread 104
Sound observation has scarcely yet been brought to bear
    upon sick diet 105
Tea and coffee 105
Cocoa 109
Bulk 109

VIII.—Bed and Bedding .... 111—119

Feverishness a symptom of bedding 111
Uncleanliness of ordinary bedding.... 111
Air not only your clean sheets, but also your dirty ones.... 112
Iron spring bedstead the best 113
Comfort and cleanliness of two beds 113
Bed not to be too wide 114
Nor too high 114
Nor in a dark place 115
Nor a four-poster with curtains 115
Scrofula often a result of disposition of bedclothes 116
Bed sores 116
Heavy and impervious bedclothes 117
Nurses often do not think the sick room any business
    of theirs but only the sick.... 117
Pillows 118
Invalid chairs 119

IX.—Light .... 120—123

Light essential both to health and to recovery.... 120
Aspect, view, and sunlight, matters of first importance to
    the sick 121
Without sunlight body and mind degenerate 123
Almost all patients lie with their faces to the light 123

PAGES.

X.—Cleanliness of Rooms and Walls .... 124—132

Cleanliness of carpets and furniture 124
Dust never removed now 124
How a room is *dusted* 125
Floors 126
Washing floors 126
Papered, plastered, oil-painted walls 128
Atmospheres of painted and papered rooms quite distinguish
 able 128
How to keep your room wall clean at the expense of
 your clothes 129
Best kind of wall for sick-rooms 129
(1.) Dirty air from without 129
 Best kind of outside wall for houses 129
(2.) Dirty air from within 130
(3.) Dirty air from the carpet.... 130
 Remedies 131

XI.—Personal Cleanliness .... 133—137

Poisoning by the skin 133
Ventilation and skin cleanliness equally essential 133
Steaming and rubbing the skin 135
Soft water 136

XII.—Chattering Hopes and Advices .... 138—149

Advising the sick 138
Chattering hopes the bane of the sick 139
Patient does not want to talk of himself 140
Absurd statistical comparisons made in common conversation
 by sensible people for the benefit of the sick 140
Absurd consolations put forth for the benefit of the
 sick 141
Wonderful presumption of the advice given to the sick 143
Advisers the same now as two hundred years ago 143
Mockery of the advice given to the sick 144
Means of giving pleasure to the sick 145
Two new classes of patients peculiar to this generation.... 149

PAGES.

XIII.—Observation of the Sick .... 150—182

What is the use of the question, Is he better? 150
Want of truth the result of want of observation.... 152
Leading questions useless or misleading 153
Means of obtaining inaccurate information 155
As to food patient takes or does not take.... 156
More important to spare the patient thought than physical
    exertion 158
Means of obtaining inaccurate information as to diarrhoea 159
Means of cultivating sound and ready observation 159
Sound and ready observation essential in a nurse 161
Englishwomen—great capacity for, little practice in, close
    observation 162
Difference of excitable and *accumulative* temperaments 163
Superstition the fruit of bad observation.... 164
Physiognomy of disease little known 165
Peculiarities of patients 167
Nurse must observe for herself, patient will not tell her 169
Accidents arising from nurse's want of observation 170
Is the faculty of observing on the decline? 171
Approach of death—paleness not invariable 172
Two misleading habits of mind:—
1. Non-observation of general conditions 173
    Observers look too much to what is palpable to their
      senses, not to what is implied by conditions.... 174
    Pulses 175
    To arrive at a sound judgement, not only what the
      patient is but what he is likely to do must be taken
      into account.... 178
2. "Average rate of mortality"tells us only that so
    many in the hundred will die. Observation must
    tell us *which* in the hundred will die 179
    What observation is for 181
    What a confidential nurse should be 181
    Observation is for practical purposes 182

Conclusion .... 183—195

Sanitary nursing as essential in surgical as in medical cases,
    but not to supersede surgical nursing.... 183
Children: their greater susceptibility 184
Summary 188

PAGE.

(1.) Reckless amateur physicking by women. Real
knowledge of the laws of health its only check   188

(2.) What pathology teaches. What observation teaches.
What medicine does. What nature does   191

(3.) What does not make a good nurse   192
The two jargons of the day   194

Supplementary Chapter   ....   196—222

What is a nurse?   196–206

"He hates to be watched"   197

What is experience?   197

A nurse must have a "calling" for her occupation   198

A nurse with a calling   199

A nurse without a calling   199

A man's definition of a nurse   200

A lady's definition of a nurse   201

What are the elements of a nurse's duty?   202

"Afraid of my nurse"   203

Observations which might be made by the sick-bed   204–206

Convalescence   206–211

Hints for the sick will not do for convalescents   206

Difference of sickness and convalescence   206

Surgical patients should not be ill   207

Restraint necessary in convalescence   207

Convalescent appetites   207

Convalescent imaginations.   209

Change of air essential   209

Convalescent institutions   210

Convalescents require nursing as well as change of air. ...   210

Children in London   211–215

To save not only sick but "delicate" children—"delicate"
from excessive nursing—chiefly in the class which can
afford too much of every thing artificial   211

Not "London air" does all the mischief but London life. ...   211

Good gained in the country lost   212

Difficult to poison a house in the country, but very little will
do it in London   212

Constant "smell of dinner test"   212

Children in town go out (when they do) like dogs in leashes
or invalids in carriages   213

All this artificial fear not necessary, though it soon creates
some foundation for itself   213

PAGE.

Well-instructed lifeless victims	213
Three injuries to children	214
Appetite-test; in country—in town	214
Tea not to be given to children as to sick	214
Summary	215
Note upon some errors propagated by Novels	215–217
1. The joys of convalescence	215
2. Marriage of cousins	216
3. Unreality of death-bed fiction....	216
4. Articles of food for sick....	216
5. Infection	216
Method of polishing floors	217
Note upon employment of women	219
Note as to the number of women employed as nurses in	
Great Britain....	220–222

NOTES ON NURSING:

WHAT IT IS, AND WHAT IT IS NOT.

NOTES ON NURSING:

WHAT IT IS, AND WHAT IT IS NOT.

———

SHALL we begin by taking it as a general prin- *Disease a reparative process.* ciple—that all disease, at some period or other of its course, is more or less a reparative process, not necessarily accompanied with suffering: an effort of nature to remedy a process of poisoning or of decay, which has taken place weeks, months, sometimes years beforehand, unnoticed, the termination of the disease being then, while the antecedent process was going on, determined?

If we accept this as a general principle we shall be immediately met with anecdotes and instances to prove the contrary. Just so if we were to take, as a principle—all the climates of the earth are meant to be made habitable for man, by the efforts of man—the objection would be immediately raised,—Will the top of Mont Blanc ever be made habitable? Our answer would be, it will be many thousands of years before we have reached the bottom of Mont Blanc in making the earth healthy. Wait till we have reached the bottom before we discuss the top.

Of the sufferings of disease, disease not always the cause.

In watching disease, both in private houses and in public hospitals, the thing which strikes the experienced observer most forcibly is this, that the symptoms or the sufferings generally considered to be inevitable and incident to the disease are very often not symptoms of the disease at all, but of something quite different—of the want of fresh air, or of light, or of warmth, or of quiet, or of cleanliness, or of punctuality and care in the administration of diet, of each or of all of these. And this quite as much in private as in hospital nursing.

The reparative process which Nature has instituted, and which we call disease, has been hindered by some want of knowledge or attention, in one or in all of these things, and pain, suffering, or interruption of the whole process sets in.

If a patient is cold, if a patient is feverish, if a patient is faint, if he is sick after taking food, if he has a bed-sore, it is generally the fault not of the disease, but of the nursing.

What nursing ought to do.

I use the word nursing for want of a better. It has been limited to signify little more than the administration of medicines and the application of poultices. It ought to signify the proper use of fresh air, light, warmth, cleanliness, quiet, and the proper selection and administration of diet—all at the least expense of vital power to the patient.

It has been said and written scores of times, that every woman makes a good nurse. I believe, on the contrary, that the very elements of nursing are all but unknown.

Nursing the sick little understood.

By this I do not mean that the nurse is always to blame. Bad sanitary, bad architectural, and bad administrative arrangements often make it impossible to nurse. But the art of nursing ought to include such arrangements as alone make what I understand by nursing possible.

To recur to the first objection. If we are asked, Is such or such a disease a reparative process? Can such an illness be unaccompanied with suffering? Will any care prevent such a patient from suffering this or that?—I humbly say, I do not know. But when you have done away with all that pain and suffering, which in patients are the symptoms not of their disease, but of the absence of one or all of the above-mentioned essentials to the success of Nature's reparative processes, we shall then know what are the symptoms of and the sufferings inseparable from the disease.

Nursing ought to assist the reparative process.

Another and the commonest exclamation which will be instantly made is—Would you do nothing, then, in cholera, fever, &c.?—so deep-rooted and universal is the conviction that to give medicine is to be doing something, or rather everything; to give air, warmth, cleanliness, &c., is to do nothing. The reply is, that in these and many other similar diseases the exact value of particular remedies and modes of treatment is by no means ascertained, while there is universal experience as to the extreme importance of careful nursing in determining the issue of the disease.

Nursing the well.

II. The very elements of what constitutes good nursing are as little understood for the well as for the sick. The same laws of health or of nursing, for they are in reality the same, obtain among the well as among the sick. The breaking of them produces only a less violent consequence among the former than among the latter,—and this sometimes, not always.

It is constantly objected,—"But how can I obtain this medical knowledge? I am not a doctor. I must leave this to doctors."

Little understood.

Oh, mothers of families! You who say this, do you know that one in every seven infants in this civilized land of England perishes before it is one year old? That, in London, two in every five die before they are five years old? And, in the other great cities of England, nearly one out of two?

Curious deductions from an excessive death rate.

Upon this fact the most wonderful deductions have been strung. For a long time an announcement something like the following has been going the round of the papers:—"More than 25,000 children die every year in London under 10 years of age; therefore we want a Children's Hospital."

Last spring there was a prospectus issued, and divers other means taken to this effect:—"There is a great want of sanitary knowledge in women; therefore we want a Women's Hospital." Now, both the above facts are too sadly true. But what is the deduction? The causes of the enormous child mortality are perfectly well known; they are chiefly want of cleanliness, want of ventilation, careless dieting and clothing, want of white-washing; in one word, defective *household* hygiene. The remedies are just as well known; and among them is certainly not the establishment of a Child's Hospital. This may be a want; just as there may be a want of hospital room for adults. But the Registrar-General would certainly never think of giving us, as a cause for the high rate of child mortality in (say) Liverpool, that there was not sufficient hospital room for children; nor would he urge upon us, as a remedy, to found a hospital for them.

Again, women, and the best women, are wofully deficient in sanitary knowledge; although it is to women that we must look, first and last, for its application, as far as *household* hygiene is concerned. But who would ever think of citing the institution of a Women's Hospital as the way to cure this want?

We have it, indeed, upon very high authority that there is some fear lest hospitals, as they have been *hitherto*, may not have generally increased, rather than diminished, the rate of mortality—especially of child mortality.

Child life a test of healthy conditions.

"The life duration of tender babies" (as some Saturn, turned analytical chemist, says) "is the most delicate test" of sanitary conditions. Is all this premature suffering and death necessary? Or did Nature intend mothers to be always accompanied by doctors? Or is it better to learn the piano-forte than to learn the laws which subserve the preservation of offspring?

Macaulay somewhere says,[1] that it is extraordinary that, whereas the laws of the motions of the heavenly bodies, far removed as they are from us, are perfectly well understood, the laws of the human mind, which are under our observation all day and every day, are no better understood than they were two thousand years ago.

But how much more extraordinary is it that, whereas what we might call the coxcombries of education—*e.g.,* the elements of astronomy—are now taught to every school-girl, neither mothers of families of any class, nor school-mistresses of any class, nor nurses of children, nor nurses of hospitals, are taught anything about those laws which God has assigned to the relations of our bodies with the world in which He has put them. In other words, the laws which make these bodies, into which He has put our minds, healthy or unhealthy organs of those minds, are all but unlearnt. Not but that these laws—the laws of life—are in a certain measure understood, but not even mothers think it worth their while to study them—to study how to give their children healthy existences. They call it medical or physiological knowledge, fit only for doctors.

Another objection.

We are constantly told,—"But the circumstances which govern our children's healths are beyond our control. What can we do with winds? There is the east wind. Most people can tell before they get up in the morning whether the wind is in the east."[2]

To this one can answer with more certainty than to the former objections. Who is it who knows when the wind is in the east? Not the Highland drover, certainly, exposed to the east wind, but the young lady who is worn out with the want of exposure to fresh air, to sunlight, &c. Put the latter under as good sanitary circumstances as the former, and she too will not know when the wind is in the east.

I.—VENTILATION AND WARMING.

THE very first canon of nursing, the first and the last thing upon which a nurse's attention must be fixed, the first essential to the patient, without which all the rest you can do for him is as nothing, with which I had almost said you may leave all the rest alone, is this: To KEEP THE AIR HE BREATHES AS PURE AS THE EXTERNAL AIR, WITHOUT CHILLING HIM. Yet what is so little attended to? Even where it is thought of at all, the most extraordinary misconceptions reign about it. Even in admitting air into the patient's room or ward, few people ever think where that air comes from. It may come from a corridor into which other wards are ventilated, from a hall, always unaired, always full of the fumes of gas, dinner, of various kinds of mustiness; from an underground kitchen, sink, wash-house, water-closet, or even, as I myself have had sorrowful experience, from open sewers loaded with filth; and with this the patient's room or ward is aired, as it is called—poisoned, it should rather be said. Always air from the air without, and that, too, through those windows, through which the air comes freshest. From a closed court, especially if the wind do not blow that way, air may come as stagnant as any from a hall or corridor.

Again, a thing I have often seen both in private houses and institutions. A room remains uninhabited; the fire-place is carefully fastened up with a board; the windows are never opened; probably the shutters are kept always shut; perhaps some kind of stores are kept in the room: no breath of fresh air can by possibility enter into that room, nor any ray of sun. The air is as stagnant, musty, and corrupt as it can by possibility be made. It is quite ripe to breed small-pox, scarlet fever, diphtheria, or anything else you please.

Yet the nursery, ward, or sick room adjoining will positively be aired (?) by having the door opened into that room. Or children will be put into that room, without previous preparation, to sleep.

The common idea as to uninhabited rooms is that they may safely be left with doors, windows, shutters, and chimney board, all closed—hermetically sealed if possible—to keep out the dust, it is said; and that no harm will happen if the room is but opened a short hour before the inmates are put in. The question has often been asked for uninhabited rooms—But when ought the windows to be opened? The answer is—When ought they to be shut?

Why are uninhabited rooms shut up?

A short time ago a man walked into a back-kitchen in Queen's-square, and cut the throat of a poor consumptive creature, sitting by the fire.

A common madness.

The murderer did not deny the act, but simply said,"It's all right." Of course he was mad.

But in our case, the extraordinary thing is that the victim says, "It's all right," and that we are not mad. Yet, although we "nose" the murderers in the musty, unaired, unsunned room, the scarlet fever which is behind the door, or the fever and hospital gangrene which are stalking among the crowded beds of a hospital ward, we say, "It's all right."

How to venti- late without chill.

With a proper supply of windows, and a proper supply of fuel in open fire places, fresh air is com- paratively easy to secure when your patient or patients are in bed. Never be afraid of open windows then. People don't catch cold in bed. This is a popular fallacy. With proper bed-clothes and hot bottles, if necessary, you can always keep a patient warm in bed, and well ventilate him at the same time.

But a careless nurse, be her rank and education what it may, will stop up every cranny, and keep a hot-house heat when her patient is in bed,—and, if he is able to get up, leave him comparatively unpro- tected. The time when people take cold (and there are many ways of taking cold, besides a cold in the nose,) is when they first get up after the two- fold exhaustion of dressing and of having had the skin relaxed by many hours, perhaps days, in bed, and thereby rendered more incapable of re-action. Then the same temperature which refreshes the patient in bed may destroy the patient just risen. And common sense will point out that, while purity of air is essential, a temperature must be secured which shall not chill the patient. Otherwise, the best that can be expected will be a feverish reaction.

To have the air within as pure as the air without, it is not necessary, as often appears to be thought, to make it as cold.

In the afternoon again, without care, the patient whose vital powers have then risen often finds the room as close and oppressive as he found it cold in the morning. Yet the nurse will be terrified if a window is opened.

It is very desirable that the windows in a sick room should be such as that the patient shall, if he can move about, be able to open and shut them easily himself.* In fact, the sick room is very seldom kept aired if this is not the case—so very few people have any perception of what is a healthy atmosphere for the sick. The sick man often says, "This room, where I spend twenty-two hours out of the twenty-four is fresher than the other where I only spend two. Because here I can manage the windows myself." And it is true.

---

* NOTE.—Delirious fever cases, where there is any danger of the patient jumping out of window, are, of course, exceptions. It is absolutely necessary that such cases should be kept cool and well aired. I would undertake, with four gimlets, to save all risk of accidents, by merely preventing the sashes, both upper and lower, from being opened more than a few inches.

Open windows.

I know an intelligent humane house surgeon who makes a practice of keeping the ward windows open. The physicians and surgeons invariably close them while going their rounds; and the house surgeon, very properly, as invariably opens them whenever the doctors have turned their backs.

In a little book on nursing, published a short time ago, we are told, that "with proper care it is very seldom that the windows cannot be opened for a few minutes twice in the day to admit fresh air from without." I should think not; nor twice in the hour either. It only shows how little the subject has been considered.

What kind of warmth desirable

Of all methods of keeping patients warm the very worst certainly is to depend for heat on the breath and bodies of the sick. I have known a medical officer keep his ward windows hermetically closed, thus exposing the sick to all the dangers of an infected atmosphere, because he was afraid that, by admitting fresh air, the temperature of the ward would be too much lowered. This is a destructive fallacy.

To attempt to keep a ward warm at the expense of making the sick repeatedly breathe their own hot, humid, putrescing atmosphere is a certain way to delay recovery or to destroy life.

Bedrooms almost universally foul.

Do you ever go into the bed-rooms of any persons of any class, whether they contain one, two, or twenty people, whether they hold sick or well, at night, or before the windows are opened in the morning, and ever find the air anything but unwholesomely close and foul? And why should it be so? And of how much importance is it that it should not be so? During sleep, the human body, even when in health, is far more injured by the influence of foul air than when awake. Why can't you keep the air all night, then, as pure as the air without in the rooms you sleep in? But for this, you must have sufficient outlet for the impure air you make yourself to go out; sufficient inlet for the pure air from without to come in. You must have open chimneys, open windows, or ventilators; no close curtains round your beds; no shutters or curtains to your windows, none of the contrivances by which you undermine your own health or destroy the chances of recovery of your sick.

Open the window above, not below. If your windows do not open above, the sooner they are made to do so the better. An inch or two will be enough for two people in a moderately-sized bed-room in winter. In a children's nursery or bed-room more will be required, according to the number. The worst place to admit air either into sick room or hospital ward, is at or near the level of the floor. Air admitted in this situation cools the floor and the lower strata of air; and if the patient is able to step out of bed, the cold air may give him a dangerous chill. During mild weather and summer time your windows may be wide open. In this, as in other things, common

How to open your windows.

sense must be used. Ventilation of a bedroom or a sick room does not mean throwing the window up to the top, or drawing it down as far as it will come; still less does it mean opening the windows at intervals and keeping them shut between times, thereby subjecting the patient to the risk of frequent and violent alternations of temperature. It means simply keeping the air fresh.

The true criterion of this is to step out of the bedroom or sick room, in the morning, into the open air. If, on returning to it, you feel the least sensation of closeness, the ventilation has not been enough, and that room has been unfit for either sick or well to sleep in.

Schools.

Of all places, public or private schools, where a number of children or young persons sleep in the same dormitory, require this test of freshness to be constantly applied. If it be hazardous for two children to sleep together in an unventilated bedroom, it is more than doubly so to have four, and much more than trebly so to have six under the same circumstances. People rarely remember this; yet, if parents were as solicitous about the air of school bedrooms as they are about the food the children are to eat, and the kind of education they are to receive, at school, depend upon it due attention would be bestowed on this vitally important matter, and they would cease to have their children sent home either ill, or because scarlet fever or some other "current contagion" had broken out in the school. There are schools where attention is paid to these things, and where "children's epidemics" are unknown.

How much sickness, death, and misery are produced by the present state of many factories, warehouses, workshops, and workrooms! The places where poor dressmakers, tailors, letter-press printers, and other similar trades have to work for their living, are generally in a worse sanitary condition than any other portion of our worst towns. Many of these places of work were never constructed for such an object. They are badly adapted garrets, sitting-rooms, or bedrooms, generally of an inferior class of house. No attention is paid to cubic space or ventilation. The poor workers are crowded on the floor to a greater extent than occurs with any other kind of overcrowding. In many cases 100 cubic feet would be considered by employers an extravagant extent of space for a worker. The constant breathing of foul air, saturated with moisture, and the action of such air upon the skin renders the inmates peculiarly susceptible of the impression of cold, which is an index indeed of the danger of pulmonary disease to which they are exposed. The result is, that they make bad worse, by over-heating the air and closing up every cranny through which ventilation could be obtained. In such places, and under such circumstances of constrained posture, want of exercise, hurried and insufficient meals,

Work-rooms.

long exhausting labour and foul air—is it wonderful that a great majority of them die early of chest disease, generally of consumption? Intemperance is a common evil of these workshops. The men can only complete their work under the influence of stimulants, which help to undermine their health and destroy their morals, while hurrying them to premature graves. Employers rarely consider these things. Healthy workrooms are no part of the bond into which they enter with their work-people. They pay their money, which they reckon their part of the bargain. And for this wage the workman or workwoman has to give work, health, and life.

Do men and women who employ fashionable tailors and milliners ever think of these things?

An air-test of essential consequence.

And yet the master is no gainer. His goods are spoiled by foul air and gas fumes, his own health and that of his family suffers, and his work is not so well done as it would be, were his people in health. It is now admitted to be cheaper for all manufacturing purposes to have pure soft water than hard water. And the time will come when it will be found cheaper to supply shops, warehouses, and work-rooms with pure air than with foul air.

Dr. Angus Smith's air-test,[3] if it could be made of simple application, would be invaluable to use in every sleeping and sick room. Just as without the use of a thermometer no nurse should ever put a patient into a bath, so, if this air-test were made

in some equally simple form, should no nurse, or
mother, or superintendent, be without it in any ward,
nursery, or sleeping-room. But to be used, the air-
test must be made as simple a little instrument as
the thermometer, and both should be self-registering.
The sense of nurses and mothers become so dulled
to foul air that they are perfectly unconscious of
what an atmosphere they have let their children,
patients, or charges sleep in. But if the tell-tale
air-test were to exhibit in the morning, both to
nurses and patient and to the superior officer going
round, what the atmosphere has been during the
night, I question if any greater security could be
afforded against a recurrence of the misdemeanour.

And, oh! the crowded national school! where
so many children's epidemics have their origin;
and the crowded, unventilated work-room, which
sends so many consumptive men and women to the
grave; what a tale its air-test would tell! We
should have parents saying, and saying rightly,
"I will not send my child to that school. I will
not trust my son or my daughter in that tailor's or
milliner's workshop, the air-test stands at 'Horrid.'"
And the dormitories of our great boarding schools!
Scarlet fever would be no more ascribed to contagion but to its right cause, the air-test standing at
"Foul."

We would hear no longer of "mysterious dispensations," nor of "plague and pestilence" being
"in God's hands," when, so far as we know, He has

put them into our own. The little air-test would both betray the cause of these "mysterious pestilences," and call upon us to remedy it.

When warmth must be most carefully looked to.

A careful nurse will keep a constant watch over her sick, especially weak, protracted, and collapsed cases, to guard against the effects of the loss of vital heat by the patient himself. In certain diseased states much less heat is produced than in health; and there is a constant tendency to the decline and ultimate extinction of the vital powers by the call made upon them to sustain the heat of the body. Cases where this occurs should be watched with the greatest care from hour to hour, I had almost said from minute to minute. The feet and legs should be examined by the hand from time to time, and whenever a tendency to chilling is discovered, hot bottles, hot bricks, or warm flannels, with some warm drink, should be made use of until the temperature is restored. The fire should be, if necessary, replenished. Patients are frequently lost in the latter stages of disease from want of attention to such simple precautions. The nurse may be trusting to the patient's diet, or to his medicine, or to the occasional dose of stimulant which she is directed to give him, while the patient is all the while sinking from want of a little external warmth. Such cases happen at all times, even during the height of summer. This fatal chill is most apt to occur towards early morning at the period of the lowest temperature of the twenty-four hours, and at the time when the effect of the preceding day's diets is exhausted.

Generally speaking, you may expect that weak patients will suffer cold much more in the morning than in the evening. The vital powers are much lower. If they are feverish at night, with burning hands and feet, they are almost sure to be chilly and shivering in the morning. But nurses are very fond of heating the foot-warmer at night, and of neglecting it in the morning, when they are busy. I should reverse the matter.

What can nurses be thinking of who put a **Hot bottles.** bottle of boiling water to the patient's feet, hoping that it will keep warm all the twenty-four hours? Of course, every time he touches it, it wakes him. It sends the blood to the head. It makes his feet tender. And then the nurse leaves it in the bed after it has become quite cold. A hot bottle should never be hotter than it can be comfortably touched with the naked hand. It should not be expected to keep warm longer than eight hours. Tin foot-warmers are too hot and too cold. Stone bottles are the best, or India-rubber. But careless nurses make sad havoc with the latter, by putting in water too hot, or by letting the screw get out of order, and the patient be deluged in his bed.

All these things require common sense and care. Yet perhaps in no one single thing is so little common sense shown, in all ranks, as in nursing.

The art of nursing, as now practised, seems to be expressly constituted to unmake what God had made disease to be, viz., a reparative process.[4]

Cold air not ventilation, nor fresh air a method of chill.

The extraordinary confusion between cold and ventilation, in the minds of even well educated people, illustrates this. To make a room cold is by no means necessarily to ventilate it. Nor is it at all necessary, in order to ventilate a room, to chill it. Yet, if a nurse finds a room close, she will let out the fire, thereby making it closer, or she will open the door into a cold room, without a fire, or an open window in it, by way of improving the ventilation. The safest atmosphere of all for a patient is a good fire and an open window, excepting in extremes of temperature. (Yet no nurse can ever be made to understand this.) To ventilate a small room without draughts of course requires more care than to ventilate a large one.

With private sick, I think, but certainly with hospital sick, the nurse should never be satisfied as to the freshness of their atmosphere, unless she can feel the air gently moving over her face, when still.

Draughts.

But it is often observed that nurses who make the greatest outcry against open windows are those who take the least pains to prevent dangerous draughts. The door of the patients' room or ward *must* sometimes stand open to allow of persons passing in and out, or heavy things being carried in and out. The careful nurse will keep the door shut while she shuts the windows, and then, and not before, set the door open, so that a patient may not be left sitting up in bed, perhaps in a profuse perspiration, directly in the draught between the open door and window. Neither, of course, should a patient, while being washed or in any way exposed, remain in the draught of an open window or door.

It is truly provoking to see stupid women bring into disrepute the life-spring of the patient, viz., fresh air, by their stupidity. Chest and throat attacks may undoubtedly be brought on by the nurse letting her sick run about without slippers, flannel or dressing-gowns,[5] in a room where she has left the wintry wind blowing in upon them, without taking any precaution if they should leave their beds. Certain beds are sometimes pointed out in certain wards, in a kind of helpless way, as being predestined to bronchitis, because of the "draught from the door." Why should there be a draught from the door? If there be, why should the draught fall on a patient? Is there no such thing as a screen to be had; or if the bed space be in a draught which cannot be prevented, why not remove the bed? The same thing happens frequently in private sick rooms. A careless nurse will leave a window open on one side of a patient, and a door on the other. It never seems to occur to her that window-sashes can be put down while there is occasion for opening the door.

She will come into the sick room and leave the door open till she goes out again, for no reason that any body can discover but her own blindness. And she will leave the window open over her patient who is washing or sitting up in a night-dress, and then say, "He has taken cold from the open window." He has taken cold from your own thoughtlessness. Neither leaving doors open nor drawing down windows over your patients when the surface is exposed is ventilation. It is simply carelessness.

Night air.   Another extraordinary fallacy is the dread of night air. What air can we breathe at night but night air? The choice is between pure night air from without, and foul night air from within. Most people prefer the latter. An unaccountable choice. What will they say if it is proved to be true that fully one-half of all the disease we suffer from is occasioned by people sleeping with their windows shut? An open window most nights in the year can never hurt any one. This is not to say that light is not necessary for recovery. In great cities, night air is often the best and purest air to be had in the twenty-four hours. I could better understand in towns shutting the windows during the day than during the night, for the sake of the sick. The absence of smoke, the quiet, all tend to making night the best time for airing the patients. One of our highest medical authorities on Consumption and Climate has told me that the air in London is never so good as after ten o'clock at night.

The only time when it can be unsafe to open the window at night is when the air is more foul without than within. This may be the case in close back courts, and in malarial countries, or at hours when there is a sudden fall of temperature. But even in malarial districts it is found that thin gauze curtains, while admitting the air, are a protection from malaria.

Always air your room, then, from the outside air, if possible. Windows are made to open; doors are made to shut—a truth which seems extremely difficult of apprehension. I have seen a careful nurse airing her patient's room through the door near to which were two gaslights (each of which consumes as much air as eleven men), a kitchen, a corridor, the composition of the atmosphere in which consisted of gas, paint, foul air, never changed, full of effluvia, including a current of sewer air from an ill-placed sink, ascending in a continual stream by a well-staircase, and discharging themselves constantly into the patient's room. The window of the said room, if opened, was all that was desirable to air it. Every room must be aired from without—every passage from without— But the fewer passages there are in a hospital the better.

Air from the outside.

Open your windows, shut your doors.

If we are to preserve the air within as pure as the air without, it is needless to say that the

Smoke.

chimney must not smoke. Almost all smoky chimneys can be cured—from the bottom, not *from* the top. Often it is only necessary to have an inlet for air to supply the fire, which is feeding itself, for want of this, from its own chimney. On the other hand, almost all chimneys can be made to smoke by a careless nurse, who lets the fire get low, and then overwhelms it with coal; not, as we verily believe, in order to spare herself trouble (for very rare is unkindness to the sick), but from not thinking what she is about.

Airing damp things in a patient's room.

In laying down the principle that the first object of the nurse must be to keep the air breathed by her patient as pure as the air without, it must not be forgotten that everything in the room which can give off effluvia, besides the patient, evaporates itself into his air. And it follows that there ought to be nothing in the room, excepting him, which can give off effluvia or moisture. Out of all damp towels, &c., which become dry in the room, the damp, of course, goes into the patient's air. Yet this "of course" seems as little thought of as if it were an obsolete fiction. How very seldom you see a nurse who acknowledges by her practice that nothing at all ought to be aired in the patient's room, that nothing at all ought to be cooked at the patient's fire! Indeed the arrangements often make this rule impossible to observe.

If the nurse be a very careful one, she will,

when the patient leaves his bed, but not his room, open the sheets wide, and throw the bed clothes back, in order to air his bed. And she will spread the wet towels or flannels carefully out upon a horse, in order to dry them. Now either these bed clothes and towels are not dried and aired, or they dry and air themselves into the patient's air. And whether the damp and effluvia do him most harm in his air or in his bed, I leave to you to determine, for I cannot.

Even in health people cannot repeatedly breathe air in which they live with impunity, on account of its becoming charged with unwholesome matter from the lungs and skin. In disease, where everything given off from the body is highly noxious and dangerous, not only must there be plenty of ventilation to carry off the effluvia, but everything which the patient passes must be instantly removed away, as being more noxious than even the emanations from the sick.

Effluvia from excreta.

Of the fatal effects of the effluvia from the excreta it would seem unnecessary to speak, were they not so constantly neglected. Concealing the utensil behind the vallance to the bed seems all the precaution which is thought necessary for safety in private nursing. Did you but think for one moment of the atmosphere under that bed, the saturation of the under side of the mattress with the warm evaporations, you would be startled and frightened too!

Chamber uten-
sils without
lids.

The use of any chamber utensil *without a lid* should be utterly abolished, whether among sick or well. You can easily convince yourself of the necessity of this absolute rule, by taking one with a lid, and examining the under side of that lid. It will be found always covered, whenever the utensil is not empty, by condensed offensive moisture. Where does that go, when there is no lid?

Don't make
your sick-room
into a sewer.

But never, never should the possession of this indispensable lid confirm you in the abominable practice of letting the chamber utensil remain in a patient's room unemptied, except once in the twenty-four hours, *i.e.*, when the bed is made. Yes, impossible as it may appear, I have known the best and most attentive nurses guilty of this; aye, and have known, too, a patient afflicted with severe diarrhoea for ten days, and the nurse (a very good one) not know of it, because the chamber utensil (one with a lid) was emptied only once in the twenty-four hours, and that by the housemaid who came in and made the patient's bed every evening. As well might you have a sewer under the room, or think that in a water-closet the plug need be pulled up but once a day. Also take care that your *lid*, as well as your utensil, be always thoroughly rinsed.

If a nurse declines to do these kinds of things for her patient, "because it is not her business," I should say that nursing was not her calling. I have seen surgical "sisters," women whose hands were worth to them two or three guineas a-week, down upon their knees scouring a room or hut, because they thought it otherwise not fit for their patients to go into. I am far from wishing nurses to scour. It is a waste of power. But I do say that these women had the true nurse-calling—the good of their sick first, and second only the consideration what it was their "place" to do—and that women who wait for the housemaid to do this, or for the charwoman to do that,[6] when their patients are suffering, have not the *making* of a in them.

Earthenware, or if there is any wood, highly polished and varnished wood, are the only materials fit for patients' utensils. The very lid of the old abominable close-stool is enough to breed a pestilence. It becomes saturated with offensive matter, which scouring is only wanted to bring out. I prefer an earthenware lid as being always cleaner. But there are various good new-fashioned arrangements.

A slop-pail should never be brought into a sick room. It should be a rule invariable, rather more important in the private house than elsewhere, that the utensil should be carried directly to the water-closet, emptied there, rinsed there, and brought back. There should always be water and a cock in every water-closet for rinsing. But even if there is not, you must carry water there to rinse with.

Abolish slop-pails.

I have actually seen, in the private sick room, the utensils emptied into the foot-pan, and put back, unrinsed, under the bed. I can hardly say which is most abominable, whether to do this or to rinse the utensil *in* the sick room. In the best hospitals it is now a rule that no slop-pail shall ever be brought into the wards, but that the utensils shall be carried direct to be emptied and rinsed at the proper place. I would it were so in the private house.

Fumigations. Let no one ever depend upon fumigations, "disinfectants," and the like, for purifying the air. The offensive thing, not its smell, must be removed. A celebrated medical lecturer began one day, "Fumigations, gentlemen, are of essential importance. They make such an abominable smell that they compel you to open the window." I wish all disinfecting fluids invented made such an "abominable smell" that they forced you to admit fresh air. That would be a useful invention.

II.—HEALTH OF HOUSES.*

THERE are five essential points in securing the health of houses:— Health of houses. Five points essential.

1. Pure air.
2. Pure water.
3. Efficient drainage.
4. Cleanliness.
5. Light.

Without these, no house can be healthy. And it will be unhealthy just in proportion as they are deficient.

1. To have pure air, your house must be so constructed as that the outer atmosphere shall find Pure air.

---

* The health of carriages, especially close carriages, is not of sufficient universal importance to mention here, otherwise than cursorily. Children, who are always the most delicate test of sanitary conditions, generally cannot enter a close carriage without being sick—and very lucky for them that it is so. A close carriage, with the horse-hair cushions and linings always saturated with organic matter, and unaired from the musty foulness of the coach-house, if to this be added the windows up, is one of the most unhealthy of human receptacles. The idea of taking an *airing* in it is something preposterous. Dr. Angus Smith has shown that a crowded railway carriage, which goes at the rate of 30 miles an hour, is as unwholesome as the strong smell of a sewer, or as a back yard in one of the most unhealthy courts off one of the most unhealthy streets in Manchester. Health of carriages.

its way with ease to every corner of it. House architects hardly ever consider this. The object in building a house is to obtain the largest interest for the money, not to save doctor's bills to the tenants. But, if tenants should ever become so wise as to refuse to occupy unhealthily constructed houses, and if Insurance Companies should ever come to understand their interest so thoroughly as to pay a Sanitary Surveyor to look after the houses where their clients live, speculative architects would speedily be brought to their senses. As it is, they build what pays best. And there are always people foolish enough to take the houses they build. And if in the course of time the families die off, as is so often the case, nobody every thinks of blaming any but Providence for the result. Ill-informed medical men aid in sustaining the delusion, by laying the blame on "current contagions." Badly constructed houses do for the healthy what badly constructed hospitals do for the sick. Once insure that the air in a house is stagnant, and sickness is certain to follow.

Pure water.

2. Pure water is more generally introduced into houses than it used to be, thanks to the exertions of the sanitary reformers. Within the last few years, a large part of London was in the daily habit of using water polluted by the drainage of its sewers and water closets. This has happily been remedied. But, in many parts of the country, well water of a very impure kind is used for

domestic purposes. And when epidemic disease shows itself, persons using such water are almost sure to suffer.

3. It would be curious to ascertain by inspec- Drainage tion, how many houses in London are really well drained. Many people would say, surely all or most of them. But many people have no idea in what good drainage consists. They think that a sewer in the street, and a pipe leading to it from the house is good drainage. All the while the sewer may be nothing but a laboratory from which epidemic disease and ill health is being distilled into the house. No house with any untrapped unventilated drain pipe communicating imme- diately with an unventilated sewer, whether it be from water closet, sink, or gully-grate, can ever be healthy. An untrapped sink may at any time spread fever or pyaemia among the inmates of a palace.

The ordinary oblong sink is an abomination. Sinks. That great surface of stone, which is always left wet, is always exhaling into the air. I have known whole houses and hospitals smell of the sink. I have met just as strong a stream of sewer air coming up the back staircase of a grand London house from the sink, as I have ever met at Scutari; and I have seen the rooms in that house all venti- lated by the open doors, and the passages all *un*ventilated by the closed windows, in order that as much of the sewer air as possible might be conducted into and retained in the bed-rooms. It is wonderful!

Another great evil in house construction is carrying drains underneath the house. Such drains are never safe. All house drains should begin and end outside the walls. Many people will readily admit, as a theory, the importance of these things. But how few are there who can intelligently trace disease in their households to such causes! Is it not a fact, that when scarlet fever, measles, or small-pox appear among the children, the very first thought which occurs is "where" the children can have "caught" the disease? And the parents immediately run over in their minds all the families with whom they may have been. They never think of looking at home for the source of the mischief. If a neighbour's child is seized with small-pox, the first question which occurs is whether it had been vaccinated. No one would undervalue vaccination; but it becomes of doubtful benefit to society when it leads people to look abroad for the source of evils which exist at home.

Cleanliness.   4. Without cleanliness, within and without your house, ventilation is comparatively useless. In certain foul districts of London, poor people used to object to open their windows and doors because of the foul smells that came in. Rich people like to have their stables and dunghill near their houses. But does it ever occur to them that with many arrangements of this kind it would be safer to keep the windows shut than open? You cannot have the air of the house pure with dung heaps under the windows. These are common all over London. And yet people are surprised that their children, brought up in large "well-aired" nurseries and bed-rooms suffer from children's epidemics.[7] If they studied Nature's laws in the matter of children's health, they would not be so surprised.

There are other ways of having filth inside a house besides having dirt in heaps. Old papered walls of years' standing, dirty carpets, uncleaned furniture, are just as ready sources of impurity to the air as if there were a dung-heap in the basement. People are so unaccustomed from education and habits to consider how to make a home healthy, that they either never think of it at all, and take every disease as a matter of course, to be "resigned to" when it comes "as from the hand of Providence;" or if they ever entertain the idea of preserving the health of their household as a duty, they are very apt to commit all kinds of "negligences and ignorances" in performing it.

5. A dark house is always an unhealthy house, Light. always an ill-aired house, always a dirty house. Want of light stops growth, and promotes scrofula, rickets, &c., among the children.

People lose their health in a dark house, and if they get ill they cannot get well again in it. More will be said about this farther on.

Three common
errors in
managing the
health of
houses.

Three out of many "negligences and igno-rances" in managing the health of houses gene-rally, I will here mention as specimens—1. That the female head in charge of any building does not think it necessary to visit every hole and corner of it every day. How can she expect those who are under her to be more careful to maintain her house in a healthy condition than she who is in charge of it?—2. That it is not considered essential to air, to sun, and to clean rooms while uninhabited; which is simply ignoring the first elementary notion of sanitary things, and laying the ground ready for all kinds of diseases.—3. That the win-dow, and one window, is considered enough to air a room. Have you never observed that any room without a fire-place is always close? And, if you have a fire-place, would you cram it up not only with a chimney-board, but perhaps with a great wisp of brown paper, in the throat of the chimney —to prevent the soot from coming down, you say? If your chimney is foul, sweep it; but don't expect that you can ever air a room with only one aperture; don't suppose that to shut up a room is the way to keep it clean. It is the best way to foul the room and all that is in it. Don't imagine that if you, who are in charge, don't look to all these things yourself, those under you will be more careful than you are. It appears as if the part of a mistress now is to complain of her servants, and to accept their excuses—not to show them how there need be neither complaints made nor excuses.

But again, to look to all these things yourself, does not mean to do them yourself. "I always open the windows," the head in charge often says. If you do it, it is by so much the better, certainly, than if it were not done at all. But can you not insure that it is done when not done by yourself? Can you insure that it is not undone when your back is turned? This is what being "in charge" means. And a very important meaning it is, too. The former only implies that just what you can do with your own hands is done. The latter, that what ought to be done is always done.

Head in charge must see to House Hygiene, not do it herself.

And now, you think these things trifles, or at least exaggerated. But what you "think" or what I "think," matters little. Let us see what God thinks of them. God always justifies His ways. While we are "thinking," He has been teaching. I have known cases of hospital pyaemia quite as severe in handsome private houses as in any of the worst hospitals, and from the same cause, viz., foul air. Yet nobody learnt the lesson. Nobody learnt *anything* at all from it. They went on *thinking*—thinking that the sufferer had scratched his thumb, or that it was singular that "all the servants" had "whitlows," or that something was "much about this year; there is always sickness in our house." This is a favourite mode of thought—leading *not* to inquire what is the

Does God think of these things so seriously?

uniform cause of these general "whitlows," but to stifle all inquiry. In what sense is "sickness" being "always there," a justification of its being "there" at all?

How does He carry out His laws?

What was the cause of hospital pyaemia being in that large private house? It was that the sewer air from an ill-placed sink was carefully conducted into all the rooms by sedulously opening all the doors, and closing all the passage windows. It was that the slops were emptied into the foot pans;—it was that the utensils were never properly rinsed;—it was that the chamber crockery was rinsed with dirty water;—it was that the beds were never properly shaken, aired, picked to pieces, or changed. It was that the carpets and curtains were always musty;—it was that the furniture was always dusty;—it was that the papered walls were saturated with dirt;—it was that the floors were never cleaned;—it was that the uninhabited rooms were never sunned, or cleaned, or aired;—it was that the cupboards were always reservoirs of foul air;—it was that the windows were always tight shut up at night;—it was that no window was ever systematically opened, even in the day, or that the right window was not opened. A person gasping for air might open a window for himself. But the servants were not taught to open the windows, to shut the doors; or they opened the windows upon a dank well between high walls, not upon the airier court; or they opened the room doors into the unaired halls and passages, by way of airing the rooms. Now all this is not fancy, but fact. In that handsome house there have been in one summer three cases of hospital pyaemia, one of phlebitis, two of consumptive cough:[8] all the *immediate* products of foul air. When, in temperate climates, a house is more unhealthy in summer than in winter, it is a certain sign of something wrong. Yet nobody learns the lesson. Yes, God always justifies His ways. He is teaching while you are not learning. This poor body loses his finger, that one loses his life. And all from the most easily preventible causes.

How does He teach His laws?

God lays down certain physical laws. Upon His carrying out such laws depends our responsibility (that much abused word), for how could we have any responsibility for actions, the results of which we could not foresee—which would be the case if the carrying out of His laws were *not* certain. Yet we seem to be continually expecting that He will work a miracle—*i.e.*, break His own laws expressly to relieve us of responsibility.

"With God's Blessing he will recover," is a common form of parlance. But "with God's blessing" also, it is, if he does *not* recover; and "with God's blessing" that he fell ill; and "with God's blessing" that he dies, if he does die. In other words, *all* these things happen by God's laws, which *are* His blessings, that is, which are all to contribute to teach us the way to our best happiness. Cholera is just as much His "blessing" as the exemption from it. It is to teach us how to obey His laws, which are at once our means and our inducements to advance towards perfection. "With God's blessing he will recover," is a common form of speech with people who, all the while, are neglecting the means on which God has made health or recovery to depend.

Servants' rooms.

I must say a word about servants' bed-rooms. From the way they are built, but oftener from the way they are kept, and from no intelligent inspection whatever being exercised over them, they are almost invariably dens of foul air, and the "servants' health" suffers in an "unaccountable" (?) way, even in the country. For I am by no means speaking only of London houses, where too often servants are put to live under the ground and over the roof. But in a country *"mansion,"* which was really a "mansion," (not after the fashion of advertisements), I have known three maids who slept in the same room ill of scarlet fever. "How catching it is!" was of course the remark. One look at the room, one smell of the room, was quite enough. It was no longer "unaccountable." The room was not a small one; it was up stairs, and it had two large windows—but nearly every one of the neglects enumerated above was there.

Physical degeneration in families. Its causes.

The houses of the grandmothers and great grandmothers of this generation, at least the country houses, with front door and back door always standing open, winter and summer, and a thorough draught always blowing through—with all the scrubbing, and cleaning, and polishing, and scouring which used to go on, the grandmothers, and still more the great grandmothers, always out of doors and never with a bonnet on except to go to church, these things, when contrasted with our present "civilized" habits, entirely account for the fact so often seen of a great grandmother, who was a tower of physical vigour descending into a grandmother perhaps a little less vigorous but still sound as a bell and healthy to the core, into a mother languid and confined to her carriage and house, and lastly into a daughter sickly and confined to her bed. For, remember, even with a general decrease of mortality you may often find a race thus degenerating and still oftener a family. You may see poor little feeble washed-out rags, children of a noble stock, suffering morally and physically, throughout their useless, degenerate lives, and yet people who are going to marry and to bring more such into the world, will consult nothing but their own convenience as to where they are to live, or how they are to live.

That consumption is induced by the foul air of houses, *i.e.*, by air fouled by human bodies, more than by all other causes put together, is now certain. It is often alleged, even by physicians, as throwing doubt upon this fact, that "young ladies," who do not, it is supposed, live in a "vitiated

Consumption produced by foul air.

atmosphere," yet die of consumption. But do these people know the up-stair habits of this class?

Both in soldiers and "young ladies."

—I do, or did. And of all classes there are two, viz., "young ladies," and soldiers, who are the most exposed to the influences which produce consumption. Both sleep, and partly live, in foul air. How many a time a young lady, advised to open her window and her curtains at night, says that "it would spoil her complexion." From this close, foul air both "young ladies" and soldiers go out at night in all weathers,—the one to "parties," the other to sentry duty; both enter into more foul air,—the one in crowded ball-rooms, the other in guard-rooms; both go home in damp night air after the skin and lungs have been oppressed in their functions by over crowding and want of ventilation, and both suffer from chest diseases, especially from consumption.

Insufficient and unwholesome food is an auxiliary in some people to the work of consumption. For the "fashion" of not eating is still in vogue among "young ladies," and they make up for it, not unfrequently, in their own rooms, by tea and pound cake.[9]

The object of spoiling her digestion is still further forwarded by many a young lady by the practice of taking continual and powerful aperients —still "to improve her complexion;" or, if the process of exhaustion is far advanced, by taking eau-de-Cologne, sal-volatile, or ether. It is little known how far this practice prevails.[10]

Could we devise a course more likely first to ruin the general health and sow the seeds, and then act as a forcing-house to consumption?

Again, people often point to the frequency of consumption in some families to prove its "hereditary nature." Therefore it is inevitable. It is, indeed, extremely likely that if one or two deaths occur from consumption in a family there will be many more. For the whole family has been so mismanaged, that it is very unlikely that it should *not* attack other members in succession, just as children's epidemics do. But because seventeen persons, who eat poisoned sugar-plums at Bradford, several out of the same family, all die, is it a reason for supposing their poisoning "hereditary," "contagious," or the result of a "family predisposition?"

Is consumption hereditary and inevitable?

Again, some people say, we admit that two and a half times the number die of consumption in the army as die in civil life. But it is a mistake to suppose the cause of consumption in the army to be foul air, *for* the disease is "hereditary" in civil life.

Therefore, Army surgeons select consumptive men for service, and "pass" two and a half times the number of recruits into the Army "predisposed" to consumption that exist in the civil population generally, and who would be rejected in the civil assurance offices? Is this the *Q.E.D.*?[11]

Once more; it is indeed to be feared that

weakness of digestion, or bad health *is* becoming "hereditary"in women of the upper classes, which also "predisposes" to consumption, and which, more than anything else, tends to the degeneracy of a family or race. Weakness of digestion depends upon habits; primarily and directly upon want of fresh air; secondarily and indirectly upon idleness or unhealthy excitement, unwholesome food, abuse of stimulants and aperients, and other exhausting habits.

Increase of births and of deaths in unhealthy districts.

Neglect of sanitary precautions is now generally admitted to be a cause of disease in individuals and communities; but it is not so much known as it ought to be that the same neglect when continued in families tends to degrade the stock, and finally to destroy it. It has been often stated that intermarriage is a fruitful source of family degradation; but is it considered that other habits descending from parents to offspring, such, for instance, as intemperance, breathing foul air, living in gloomy unhealthy localities and the like, also tend to degeneration? We have important indirect statistical proof of the operation of this law on comparing the proportion of births to the proportion of deaths in "registration" districts, under opposite sanitary conditions.

In healthy "registration" districts, the mortality is low and the annual proportion of births is also low, but in unhealthy districts the mortality rises, while at the same time the proportion of births increases, showing that in such districts the circuit of life is shortened.

The table of deaths and births in the 10 years, 1841–50, in six of the most healthy and in six of the least healthy districts in England, given below, illustrates the law.*

It would appear from this table that a double mortality is attended by an increase of births to the extent of 20 per cent.

The Registrar-General showed in his fifth annual report (1843) that a similar law prevails

*TABLE OF DEATHS AND BIRTHS IN HEALTHY AND UNHEALTHY DISTRICTS.		
Districts.	To 1000 persons living.	
	Deaths.	Births.
Rothbury (Northumberland)	15	24
Glendale Do.	15	31
Eastbourne (Sussex)	15	30
Holsworthy (Devon)	16	30
Battle (Sussex)	16	33
Reigate (Surrey)	16	31
Mean	15 ¼	30
Liverpool (Lancashire)	36	40
Manchester Do.	33	37
St. Saviour's, Southwark	33	37
Hull (York)	31	30
St. George's, Southwark	30	35
Leeds (York)	30	36
Mean	32	36

for the healthy and unhealthy districts of the Metropolis. In the unhealthiest sub-districts, the deaths per 1,000 were 29.9, and the births per 1,000 were 35.2, while in the healthiest sub-districts the deaths per 1,000 were 18 and the births per 1,000 were 24. This increase of births among unhealthy populations has been long known to sanitary observers, and has been thought to point to another law, namely that of a constant endeavour to preserve the race or family, the existence of which has been endangered by man's neglect of the laws on which its existence depends.

Now as to these children ushered into existence in the midst of such excessive mortality?

Has not every one had the opportunity of comparing the full healthy development of a child born in these healthy country districts with the thin, ill fed, undeveloped or ill-developed frame of the child born in unhealthy towns? And is not the conclusion irresistible that the unhealthy town child belongs to a lower family type than the healthy country child? A process of physical degradation has been going on notwithstanding the increase of births, and of these two classes of children about a third of the country children die before they reach the age of five years, while of the town children a half die before that period, and a large proportion of those who survive their fifth year are puny sickly people whose early deaths go to swell the local mortality.

These are momentous facts, if people would only ponder them, and act on the lessons they are teaching.

With regard to the health of houses where there is a sick person, it often happens that the sick room is made a ventilating shaft for the rest of the house. For while the house is kept as close, unaired, and dirty as usual, the window of the sick room is kept a little open always, and the door occasionally. Now, there are certain sacrifices which a house with one sick person in it does make to that sick person: it ties up its knocker; it lays straw before it in the street.[12] Why can't it keep itself thoroughly clean and unusually well aired, in deference to the sick person?

Don't make your sick-room into a ventilating shaft for the whole house.

We must not forget what, in ordinary language, is called "Infection;"—a thing of which people are generally so afraid that they frequently follow the very practice in regard to it which they ought to avoid. Nothing used to be considered so infectious or contagious as small pox; and people, not very long ago, used to cover up patients with heavy bed clothes, while they kept up large fires and shut the windows. Small pox, of course, under this *régime*, was very "infectious." People are somewhat wiser now in their management of this disease. They have ventured to cover the patients lightly and to keep the windows open; and we hear much less of the "infection" of small pox than we used to do. But do people in our days act with more

Infection[13]

wisdom on the subject of "infection" in fevers—
scarlet fever, measles, &c.—than their forefathers
did with small pox? Does not the popular idea of
"infection" involve that people should take greater
care of themselves than of the patient? that, for
instance, it is safer not to be too much with the
patient, not to attend too much to his wants?
Perhaps the best illustration of the utter absurdity
of this view of duty in attending on "infectious"
diseases is afforded by what was very recently the
practice, if it is not so even now, in some of the
European lazarets—in which the plague-patient
used to be condemned to the horrors of filth, over-
crowding, and want of ventilation, while the medical
attendant was ordered to examine the patient's
tongue through an opera-glass and to toss him a
lancet to open his abscesses with!

True nursing ignores infection, except to prevent it. Cleanliness and fresh air from open
windows, with unremitting attention to the patient,
are the only defence a true nurse either asks or
needs.

Wise and humane management of the patient
is the best safeguard against infection.

Diseases are not individuals arranged in classes, like cats and dogs, but conditions growing out of one another.

Is it not living in a continual mistake to look
upon diseases, as we do now, as separate entities,
which *must* exist, like cats and dogs? instead of
looking upon them as conditions, like a dirty and a
clean condition, and just as much under our own
control; or rather as the reactions of a kindly

nature, against the conditions in which we have placed ourselves.

I was brought up, both by scientific men and ignorant women, distinctly to believe that small pox, for instance, was a thing of which there was once a first specimen in the world, which went on propagating itself, in a perpetual chain of descent, just as much as that there was a first dog, (or a first pair of dogs), and that small pox would not begin itself any more than a new dog would begin without there having been a parent dog.

Since then I have seen with my eyes and smelt with my nose small pox growing up in first specimens, either in close rooms or in overcrowded wards, where it could not by any possibility have been "caught," but must have begun.

Nay, more, I have seen diseases begin, grow up, and pass into one another. Now, dogs do not pass into cats.

I have seen, for instance, with a little over-crowding, continued fever grow up; and with a little more, typhoid fever; and with a little more, typhus, and all in the same ward or hut.

Would it not be far better, truer, and more practical if we looked upon disease in this light?

For diseases, as all experience shows, are adjectives, not noun substantives.

There are not a few popular opinions, in regard to which it is useful at times to ask a question or two. For example, it is commonly thought that

Why must children have measles, &c.?

children must have what are commonly called "children's epidemics," "current contagions," &c.; in other words, that they are born to have measles, hooping-cough,[14] perhaps even scarlet fever, just as they are born to cut their teeth, if they live.

Now, do tell us, why must a child have measles?

Oh, because, you say, we cannot keep it from infection—other children have measles—and it must take them—and it is safer that it should.

But why must other children have measles? And if they have, why must yours have them too?

If you believed in and observed the laws for preserving the health of houses which inculcate cleanliness, ventilation, white-washing, and other means, and which, by the way, *are laws*, as implicitly as you believe in the popular opinion, for it is nothing more than an opinion, that your child must have children's epidemics, don't you think that, upon the whole, your child would be more likely to escape altogether?

——————

III.—PETTY MANAGEMENT.

———

ALL the results of good nursing, as detailed in these notes, may be spoiled or utterly negatived by one defect, viz.: in petty management, or, in other words, by not knowing how to manage, that what you do when you are there shall be done when you are not there. The most devoted friend or nurse cannot be always *there*. Nor is it desirable that she should. And she may give up her health, all her other duties, and yet, for want of a little management, be not one-half so efficient as another who is not one-half so devoted, but who has this art of multiplying herself—that is to say, the patient of the first will not really be so well cared for as the patient of the second.

It is as impossible in a book to teach a person in charge of sick how to *manage*, as it is to teach her how to nurse. Circumstances must vary with each different case. But it *is* possible to press upon her to think for herself:—Now, what does happen during my absence? I am obliged to be away on Tuesday. But fresh air, or punctuality, is not less important to my patient on Tuesday than it was on Monday. Or: At 10 P.M. I am never with my patient; but quiet is of no less consequence to him at 10 than it was at 5 minutes to 10.

Curious as it may seem, this very obvious consideration occurs comparatively to few, or, if it does occur, it is only to cause the devoted friend or nurse to be absent fewer hours or fewer minutes from her patient—not to arrange so as that no minute and no hour shall be for her patient without the essentials of her nursing.

Illustrations of the want of it.

A very few instances will be sufficient, not as precepts, but as illustrations.

Strangers coming into the sick room.

A strange washerwoman, coming late at night for the "things," will burst in by mistake to the patient's sick-room, after he has fallen into his first doze, giving him a shock, the effects of which are irremediable, though he himself laughs at the cause, and probably never even mentions it. The nurse who is, and is quite right to be, at her supper, has not provided that the washerwoman shall not lose her way and go into the wrong room.

Sick room airing the whole house.

The patient's room may always have the window open. But the passage outside the patient's room, though provided with several large windows, may never have one open. Because it is not understood that the charge of the sick-room extends to the charge of the passage. And thus, as often happens, the nurse makes it her business to turn the patient's room into a ventilating shaft for the foul air of the whole house.

An uninhabited room, a newly painted room, an uncleaned closet or cupboard, may often become a reservoir of foul air for the whole house, because the person in charge never thinks of arranging that these places shall be always aired, always cleaned; she merely opens the window herself "when she goes in."

That excellent paper, the *Builder*,[15] mentions the lingering of the smell of paint for a month about a house as a proof of want of ventilation. Certainly—and, where there are ample windows to open, and these are never opened to get rid of the smell of paint, it is a proof of want of management in using the means of ventilation. Of course the smell will then remain for months. Why should it go?

An agitating letter or message may be delivered, or an important letter or message *not* delivered; a visitor whom it was of consequence to see, may be refused, or one whom it was of still more consequence *not* to see may be admitted—because the person in charge has never asked herself this question:—What is done when I am not there?

Why should you let your patient ever be surprised, except by thieves? I do not know. In England, people do not come down the chimney, or through the window, unless they are thieves. They come in by the door, and somebody must open the door to them. The "somebody" charged with opening the door is one of two, three, or at most four persons. Why cannot these, at most, four persons be put in charge as to what is to be done when there is a ring at the door bell?

The sentry at a post is changed much oftener than any servant at a private house or institution can possibly be. But what should we think of such an excuse as this: that the enemy had entered such a post because A and not B had been on guard? Yet such an excuse is constantly heard in the private house or institution and accepted: viz., that such a person had been "let in" or *not* "let in," and such a parcel had been wrongly delivered or lost because A and not B had opened the door!

At all events, one may safely say, a nurse cannot be with the patient, open the door, eat her meals, take a message, all at one and the same time. Nevertheless the person in charge never seems to look the impossibility in the face.

Add to this that the *attempting* this impossibility does more to increase the poor patient's hurry and nervousness than anything else.

It is never thought that the patient remembers these things if you do not. He has not only to think whether the visit or letter may arrive, but whether you will be in the way at the particular day and hour when it may arrive. So that your *partial* measures for "being in the way" yourself, only increase the necessity for this thought.

Partial measures such as "being always in the way" yourself, increase instead of saving the patient's anxiety. Because they must be only partial.

Whereas, if you could but arrange that the thing should always be done whether you are there or not, he need never think at all about it.

For the above reasons, whatever a patient *can* do for himself, it is better, *i.e.*, less anxiety, for him to do for himself, unless the person in charge has the spirit of management.

It is evidently much less exertion for a patient to answer a letter for himself by return of post, than to have four conversations, wait five days, have six anxieties before it is off his mind, before the person who is to answer it has done so.

Apprehension, uncertainty, waiting, expectation, fear of surprise, do a patient more harm than any exertion. Remember, he is face to face with his enemy all the time, internally wrestling with him, having long imaginary conversations with him. You are thinking of something else. "Rid him of his adversary quickly," is a first rule with the sick.

There are many physical operations where *caeteris paribus* the danger is in a direct ratio to the time the operation lasts; and *caeteris paribus* the operator's success will be in direct ratio to his quickness.[16] Now there are many mental operations where exactly the same rule holds good with the sick; *caeteris paribus* their capability of bearing such operations depends directly on the quickness, *without hurry*, with which they can be got through.

For the same reasons, always tell a patient and

tell him beforehand when you are going out and when you will be back, whether it is for a day, an hour, or ten minutes. You fancy perhaps that it is better for him if he does not find out your going at all, better for him if you do not make yourself "of too much importance" to him; or else you cannot bear to give him the pain or the anxiety of the temporary separation.

No such thing. You *ought* to go, we will suppose. Health or duty requires it. Then say so to the patient openly. If you go without his knowing it, and he finds it out, he never will feel secure again that the things which depend upon you will be done when you are away, and in nine cases out of ten he will be right. If you go out without telling him when you will be back, he can take no measures nor precautions as to the things which concern you both, or which you do for him.

What is the cause of half the accidents which happen?

If you look into the reports of trials or accidents, and especially of suicides, or into the medical history of fatal cases, it is almost incredible how often the whole thing turns upon something which has happened because "he," or still oftener "she," "was not there." But it is still more incredible how often, how almost always this is accepted as a sufficient reason, a justification; why, the very fact of the thing having happened is the proof of its not being a justification. The person in charge was quite right not to be *"there,"* he was called away for quite sufficient reason, or he was away for a daily recurring and unavoidable cause: yet no provision was made to supply his absence. The fault was not in his "being away," but in there being no management to supplement his "being away." When the sun is under a total eclipse, or during the nightly absence, we light candles. But it would seem as if it did not occur to us that we must also supplement the person in charge of sick or of children, whether under an occasional eclipse or during a regular absence.

In institutions where many lives would be lost, and the effect of such want of management would be terrible and patent, there is less of it than in the private house.

So true is this, that I could mention two cases of women of very high position, both of whom died in the same way of the consequences of a surgical operation. And in both cases I was told by the highest authority that the fatal result would not have happened in a London hospital.

Petty management better understood in institutions than in private houses.

But, as far as regards the art of petty management in hospitals, all the military hospitals I know must be excluded. Upon my own experience I stand, and I solemnly declare that I have seen or known of fatal accidents, such as suicides in *delirium tremens*,* bleedings to death, dying patients

What institutions are the exception?

---

* NOTE.—The simple precaution of removing cords by which a patient can hang himself, razors by which he can cut his throat, out of his way, when inclined to do such things, is much neglected, especially in private nursing. Many inquests

dragged out of bed by drunken Medical Staff Corps men, and many other things less patent and striking, which would not have happened in London civil hospitals nursed by women. The medical officers should be absolved from all blame in these accidents. How can a medical officer mount guard all day and all night over a patient (say) in *delirium tremens?* The fault lies in there being no organized system of attendance. Were a trustworthy *man* in charge of each ward, or set of wards, not as office clerk, but as head nurse (and head nurse the best hospital serjeant, or ward master, is not now and cannot be, from default of the proper regulations), the thing would not, in all probability, have happened. But were a trust-worthy *woman* in charge of the ward, or set of wards, the thing would not, in all certainty, have happened. In other words, it does not happen where a trustworthy woman is really in charge. And, in these remarks, I by no means refer only to exceptional times of great emergency in war hospitals, but also, and quite as much, to the ordinary run of military hospitals at home, in time of peace; or to a time in war when our army was actually more healthy than at home in peace,

---

upon suicides shew this, and the friends are invariably absolved by the verdict. In a Military Hospital, an officer of rank cut his own throat, in *delirium tremens,* with a razor which no one ever thought of removing. Who among us has not some melancholy experience similar, although not identical?

and the pressure on our hospitals consequently much less.

It is often said that, in regimental hospitals, patients ought to "nurse each other," because the number of sick altogether being, say, but thirty, and out of these one only perhaps being seriously ill, and the other twenty-nine having little the matter with them, and nothing to do, they should be set to nurse the one; also, that soldiers are so trained to obey, that they will be the most obedient, and therefore the best of nurses, add to which they are always kind to their comrades.

Nursing in Regimental Hospitals.

Now, have those who say this, considered that, in order to obey, you must know *how* to obey, and that these soldiers certainly do not know how to obey in nursing. I have seen these "kind" fellows (and how kind they are no one knows so well as myself) move a comrade so that, in one case at least, the man died in the act. I have seen the comrades' "kindness" produce abundance of spirits, to be drunk in secret. Let no one understand by this that female nurses ought to, or could be introduced in regimental hospitals. It would be most undesirable, even were it not impossible. But the head nurseship of a hospital serjeant is the more essential, the more inexperienced the "orderlies." Undoubtedly, a London hospital "sister" does sometimes set relays of patients to watch a critical case; but, undoubtedly also, always under her own superintendence; and she is called to whenever there is something to be done, and she knows how to do it. The patients are not left to do it of their own unassisted genius, however "kind" and willing they may be.

Question for persons "in charge."

In both, the institution and the private house, let whoever is in charge keep this simple question in her head (*not*, how can I always do this right thing myself? but), how can I provide for this right thing to be always done?

Then, when anything wrong has actually happened in consequence of her absence, which absence we will suppose to have been quite right, let her question still be (*not*, how can I provide against any of such absences? which is neither possible nor desirable, but), how can I provide against any thing wrong arising out of my absence?

Many people seem to think that the world stands still while they are away, or at dinner, or ill. If the sick have an accident during that time, is it their fault, not yours? I once heard an official justly told, "Patients, Sir, will not stop dying, while we are in church."

It is the invariable sign of a bad nurse and manager when her excuse that such a person was neglected or such a thing was left undone, is, that she was "out of the way." What does that signify? The thing that signifies is that the neglect should not happen.

What it is to be "in charge."

How few men, or even women, understand, either in great or in little things, what it is the being "in charge"—I mean, know how to carry out a "charge." From the most colossal calamities, down to the most trifling accidents, results are often traced (or rather *not* traced) to such want of some one "in charge" or of his knowing how to be "in charge." A short time ago the bursting of a funnel-casing on board the finest and strongest ship that ever was built, on her trial trip, destroyed several lives, and put several hundreds in jeopardy—not from any undetected flaw in her new and untried works—but from a tap being closed which ought not to have been closed —from what every child knows would make its mother's tea-kettle burst. And this simply because no one seemed to know what it is to be "in charge," or *who* was in charge. Nay more, the jury at the inquest actually altogether ignored the same, and apparently considered the tap "in charge," for they gave as a verdict "accidental death."

This is the meaning of the word, on a large scale. On a much smaller scale, it happened, a short time ago, that an insane person burnt herself slowly and intentionally to death, while in her doctor's charge, and almost in her nurse's presence.[17] Yet neither was considered "at all to blame." The very fact of the accident happening proves its own case. There is nothing more to be said. Either they did not know their business, or they did not know how to perform it.

To be "in charge" is certainly not only to

carry out the proper measures yourself but to see that every one else does so too; to see that no one either wilfully or ignorantly thwarts or prevents such measures. It is neither to do everything yourself, nor to appoint a number of people to each duty, but to ensure that each does that duty to which he is appointed. This is the meaning which must be attached to the word by (above all) those "in charge" of sick, whether of numbers or of individuals, (and indeed I think it is with individual sick that it is least understood. One sick person is often waited on by four with less precision, and is really less cared for than ten who are waited on by one; or at least than forty who are waited on by four; and all for want of this one person "in charge.")

It is often said that there are few good servants now: I say there are few good mistresses now. As the jury seems to have thought the tap was in charge of the ship's safety, so mistresses now seem to think the house is in charge of itself. They neither know how to give orders, nor how to teach servants to obey orders—*i.e.*, to obey intelligently, which is the real meaning of all discipline.

Again, people who are in charge often seem to have a pride in feeling that they will be "missed," that no one can understand or carry on their arrangements, their system, books, accounts, &c., but themselves. It seems to me that the pride is rather in carrying on a system, in keeping stores, closets, books, accounts, &c., so that anybody can understand and carry them on—so that, in case of absence or illness, one can deliver everything up to others and know that all will go on as usual, and one shall never be missed.

It is often complained, that professional nurses, brought into private families, in case of sickness, make themselves intolerable by "ordering about" the other servants, under plea of not neglecting the patient. Both things are true; the patient is often neglected, and the servants are often unfairly "put upon." But the fault is generally in the want of management of the head in charge. It is surely for her to arrange both that the nurse's place is, when necessary, supplemented, and that the patient is never neglected—things with a little management quite compatible, and, indeed, only attainable together. It is certainly not for the nurse to "order about" the servants.

Why hired nurses give trouble.

In being asked to recommend a sick-nurse, what is it one is asked for? To send a nurse to save the patient's friends from "sitting up;" to save the servant from "running up and down stairs;" not to ensure the patient being better nursed. Physicians of large practice have assured me that their experience was the same.

Surely here is the root of the whole matter. People's object in having a nurse is *not* that she should "nurse,"—they do not know what "nursing" is,—they want a drudge. The "running up and

Nurses not expected to "nurse"— reason why there are few good ones.

down stairs," the "sitting up," are indeed unmercifully exacted of the poor individual called a nurse. I should call her a *lift*.

No wonder there is little or no good nursing in private families.

A nurse should do nothing but nurse. If you want a charwoman, have one. Nursing is a specialty. Army doctors used to be asked to sit in judgment on stores and accounts, and to overlook washing bills. Happily for the sick, army doctors are now set free for their professional duties. Are the duties of the nurse, though subordinate, less important?

How to be ill is certainly an essential complement of *how to nurse*. One part of the subject is not complete without the other. But on the whole the first duty is generally better performed than the second.

There is one point, however, on the other side, in which, according to the experience of all people and institutions who send out nurses, the sick, or perhaps oftener the friends of the sick, lamentably fail. And this is in expecting nurses to "sit up" night after night without any proper provision for ensuring to them quiet and regular sleep during the day. In sending out a nurse a precise bargain must always be made for her sleep.

———————

IV.—NOISE.

UNNECESSARY noise, or noise that creates an expectation in the mind, is that which hurts a patient. It is rarely the loudness of the noise, the effect upon the organ of the ear itself, which appears to affect the sick. How well a patient will generally bear, *e.g.*, the putting up of a scaffolding close to the house, when he cannot bear the talking still less the whispering, especially if it be of a familiar voice, outside his door. Unnecessary noise.

There are certain patients, no doubt, especially where there is slight concussion or other disturbance of the brain, who are affected by mere noise. But intermittent noise, or sudden and sharp noise, in these as in all other cases, affects far more than continuous noise—noise with jar far more than noise without. Of one thing you may be certain, that anything which wakes a patient suddenly out of his sleep will invariably put him into a state of greater excitement, do him more serious, aye, and lasting mischief, than any continuous noise, however loud.

Never to allow a patient to be waked, intentionally or accidentally, is a *sine qua non* of all good nursing.[18] If he is roused out of his first sleep, Never let a patient be waked out of his first sleep.

he is almost certain to have no more sleep. It is a curious but quite intelligible fact that, if a patient is waked after a few hours' instead of a few minutes' sleep, he is much more likely to sleep again. Because pain, like irritability of brain, perpetuates and intensifies itself. If you have gained a respite of either in sleep you have gained more than the mere respite. Both the probability of recurrence and of the same intensity will be diminished, whereas both will be terribly increased by want of sleep. This is the reason why sleep is so all-important. This is the reason why a patient, waked in the early part of his sleep, loses, not only his sleep, but his power to sleep. A healthy person who allows himself to sleep during the day will lose his sleep at night. But it is exactly the reverse with the sick generally; the more they sleep the better will they be able to sleep.

A good nurse can apply hot bottles to the feet, or give the nourishment ordered, hour by hour, without disturbing, but rather composing the patient. I have seen one of the (would-be) careful nurses neglect to warm the legs of a patient, invariably cold in the early morning, because "she did not like to disturb him." Such an excuse stamps a woman at once as incapable of her trust.

Noise which excites expectation.

I have often been surprised at the thoughtlessness, (resulting in cruelty, quite unintentional), of friend or of doctor who will hold a long conversation just in the room or passage adjoining to the room of the patient, who is either every moment expecting them to come in, or who has just seen them, and knows they are talking about him. If he is an amiable patient, he will try to occupy his attention elsewhere and not to listen—and this makes matters worse—for the strain upon his attention and the effort he makes are so great that it is well if he is not worse for hours after. If it is a whispered conversation in the same room, then it is absolutely cruel; for it is impossible that the patient's attention should not be involuntarily strained to hear. Walking on tip-toe, doing anything in the room very slowly, are injurious, for exactly the same reasons. A firm light quick step, a steady quick hand are the desiderata; not the slow, lingering, shuffling foot, the timid, uncertain touch. Slowness is not gentleness, though it is often mistaken for such; quickness, lightness, and gentleness are quite compatible. Again, if friends and doctors did but watch, as nurses can and should watch, the features sharpening, the eyes growing almost wild, of fever patients who are listening for the entrance from the corridor of the persons whose voices they are hearing there, these would never run the risk again of creating such expectation, or irritation of mind. Such unnecessary noise has undoubtedly induced or aggravated delirium in many cases. I have known such. In one case death ensued. It is but fair to say that this death was attributed to fright. It was the result of a

Whispered conversation in the room.

127

long whispered conversation, within sight of the patient, about an impending operation; but any one who has known the more than stoicism, the cheerful coolness, with which the certainty of an operation will be accepted by any patient, capable of bearing an operation at all, if it is properly communicated to him, will hesitate to believe that it was mere fear which produced, as was averred, the fatal result in this instance. It was rather the uncertainty, the strained expectation as to what was to be decided upon.

Or just outside the door.

I need hardly say that the other common course, namely, for a doctor or friend to leave the patient and communicate his opinion on the result of his visit to the friends just outside the patient's door, or inside the adjoining room, after the visit, but within hearing or knowledge of the patient is, if possible, worst of all.

Affectation.

Affectation, like whispering or walking on tiptoe, is peculiarly painful to the sick. An affectedly quiet voice, an affectedly sympathising voice, like an undertaker's at a funeral, sets all their nerves on edge. Advice, such as what I have been giving, does more harm than good, if it only makes people *affect* composure and quiet, when with the sick. Better almost make your natural noise.

Noise of female dress.

It is, I think, alarming, peculiarly at this time, when the female ink-bottles are perpetually impressing upon us "woman's" "particular worth and general missionariness,"[19] to see that the dress of woman is daily more and more unfitting them for any "mission," or usefulness at all. It is equally unfitted for all poetic and all domestic purposes. A man is now a more handy and far less objectionable being in a sick room than a woman. Compelled by her dress, every woman now either shuffles or waddles—only a man can cross the floor of a sick room without shaking it! What is become of woman's light step?—the firm, light, quick step we have been asked for?

Lord Melbourne said "I would rather have men about me when I am ill; I think it requires very strong health to put up with women." I am quite of his opinion.[20]

Unnecessary noise, then, is the most cruel absence of care which can be inflicted either on sick or well. For, in all these remarks, the sick are only mentioned as suffering in a greater proportion than the well from precisely the same causes.

Unnecessary (although slight) noise injures a sick person much more than necessary noise (of a much greater amount).

All doctrines about mysterious affinities and aversions will be found to resolve themselves very much,[21] if not entirely, into presence or absence of care in these things.

A nurse who rustles (I am speaking of nurses professional and unprofessional) is the horror of a patient, though perhaps he does not know why.

Patient's repulsion to nurses who rustle.

The fidget of silk and of crinoline,[22] the crackling of starched petticoats, the rattling of keys, the creaking of stays and of shoes, will do a patient more harm than all the medicines in the world will do him good.

The noiseless step of woman, the noiseless drapery of woman, are mere figures of speech in this day. Her skirts (and well if they do not throw down some piece of furniture) will at least brush against every article in the room as she moves.

Burning of the crinolines.

Fortunate it is if her skirts do not catch fire— and if the nurse does not give herself up a sacrifice together with her patient, to be burnt in her own petticoats. I wish the Registrar-General would tell us the exact number of deaths by burning occasioned by this absurd and hideous custom. But if people will be stupid, let them take measures to protect themselves from their own stupidity—measures which every chemist knows, such as putting alum into starch, which prevents starched articles of dress from blazing up.

Indecency of the crinolines.

I wish too that people who wear crinoline could see the indecency of their own dress as other people see it. A respectable elderly woman stooping forward, invested in crinoline, exposes quite as much of her own person to the patient lying in the room as any opera dancer does on the stage. But no one will ever tell her this unpleasant truth.

Again, one nurse cannot open the door without making everything rattle. Or she opens the door unnecessarily often, for want of remembering all the articles that might be brought in at once.

I have seen an expression of real terror pass across a patient's face, whenever a nurse came into the room who stumbled over the fire irons, &c.

I have seen patients, scarcely able to crawl, get out of bed before such a nurse came in and put out of her way everything she could throw down,— shut the window, sure that she would leave the door open—hide everything they were likely to want, (not because they had no right to have it, but because she would inadvertently put it out of their reach).

A good nurse will always make sure that no door or window in her patient's room shall rattle or creak; that no blind or curtain shall, by any change of wind through the open window, be made to flap—especially will she be careful of all this before she leaves her patients for the night. If you wait till your patients tell you, or remind you of these things, where is the use of their having a nurse? There are more shy than exacting patients, in all classes; and many a patient passes a bad night, time after time, rather than remind his nurse every night of all the things she has forgotten.

If there are blinds to your windows always take care to have them well up, when they are not being used. A little piece slipping down, and flapping with every draught, will distract a patient.

Hurry pecu-
liarly hurtful
to sick.

All hurry or bustle is peculiarly painful to the sick. And when a patient has compulsory occupations to engage him, instead of having simply to amuse himself, it becomes doubly injurious. The friend who remains standing and fidgeting about while a patient is talking business to him, or the friend who sits and proses, the one from an idea of not letting the patient talk, the other from an idea of amusing him,—each is equally inconsiderate. Always sit down when a sick person is talking business to you, show no signs of hurry, give complete attention and full consideration if your advice is wanted, and go away the moment the subject is ended.

How to visit
the sick and
not hurt them.

Always sit within the patient's view, so that when you speak to him he has not painfully to turn his head round in order to look at you. Everybody involuntarily looks at the person speaking. If you make this act a wearisome one on the part of the patient you are doing him harm. So also if by continuing to stand you make him continuously raise his eyes to see you. Be as motionless as possible, and never gesticulate in speaking to the sick.

Never make a patient repeat a message or request, especially if it be some time after. Occupied patients are often accused of doing too much of their own business. They are instinctively right.

How often you hear the person, charged with the request of giving the message or writing the letter, say half an hour afterwards to the patient, "Did you appoint 12 o'clock?" or "What did you say was the address?" or ask perhaps some much more agitating question—thus causing the patient the effort of memory, or worse still, of decision, all over again. It is really less exertion to him to write his letters himself. This is the almost universal experience of occupied invalids.

This brings us to another caution. Never speak to an invalid from behind, nor from the door, nor from any distance from him, nor when he is doing anything.

The official politeness of servants in these things is so grateful to invalids, that many prefer, without knowing why, having none but servants about them.

These things are not fancy.[23] If we consider that, with sick as with well, every thought decomposes some nervous matter,—that decomposition as well as recomposition of nervous matter is always going on, and more quickly with the sick than with the well,—that to obtrude abruptly another thought upon the brain while it is in the act of destroying nervous matter by thinking, is calling upon it to make a new exertion,—if we consider these things, which are facts, not fancies, we shall remember that we are doing positive injury by interrupting, by "startling a fanciful" person, as it is called. Alas! it is no fancy.

These things not fancy.

Interruption damaging to sick.

If the invalid is forced, by his avocations, to continue occupations requiring much thinking, the injury is doubly great. In feeding a patient suffering under delirium or stupor you may suffocate him, by giving him his food suddenly; but if you rub his lips gently with a spoon, and thus attract his attention, he will swallow the food unconsciously, but with perfect safety. Thus it is with the brain. If you offer it a thought, especially one requiring a decision, abruptly, you do it a real not fanciful injury. Never speak to a sick person suddenly; but, at the same time, do not keep his expectation on the tip-toe.

And to well.

This rule, indeed, applies to the well quite as much as to the sick. I have never known persons who exposed themselves for years to constant interruption who did not muddle away their intellects by it at last. The process with them may be accomplished without pain. With the sick, pain gives warning of the injury.

Keeping a patient standing.

Do not meet or overtake a patient who is moving about in order to speak to him, or to give him any message or letter. You might just as well give him a box on the ear. I have seen a patient fall flat on the ground who was standing when his nurse came into the room. This was an accident which might have happened to the most careful nurse. But the other is done with intention. A patient in such a state is not going to the East Indies. If you would wait ten seconds, or walk ten yards further, any promenade he could make would be over. You do not know the effort it is to a patient to remain standing for even a quarter of a minute to listen to you. If I had not seen the thing done by the kindest nurses and friends, I should have thought this caution quite superfluous.

It is absolutely essential then that a nurse should lay this down as a positive rule to herself, never to speak to any patient who is standing or moving, as long as she exercises so little observation as not to know when a patient cannot bear it. Many of the accidents which happen from feeble patients tumbling down stairs, fainting after getting up, &c., happen solely from the nurse popping out of a door to speak to the patient just at that moment; or from his fearing that she will do so. And that if the patient were even left to himself, till he can sit down, such accidents would much seldomer occur. If the nurse accompanies the patient let her not call upon him to speak. It is incredible that nurses cannot picture to themselves the strain upon the heart, the lungs, and the brain which the act of moving is to any feeble patient.

Never speak to a patient in the act of moving.

Patients are often accused of being able to "do much more when nobody is by." It is quite true that they can. Unless nurses can be brought to attend to considerations of the kind of which we have given here but a few specimens, a very weak

Patients dread surprise.

patient finds it really much less exertion to do things for himself than to ask for them. And he will, in order to do them, (very innocently and from instinct) calculate the time his nurse is likely to be absent, from a fear of her "coming in upon" him or speaking to him, just at the moment when he finds it quite as much as he can do to crawl from his bed to his chair, or from one room to another, or down stairs, or out of doors for a few minutes. Some extra call made upon his attention at that moment will quite upset him. In these cases you may be sure that a patient in the state we have described does not make such exertions more than once or twice a-day, and probably much about the same hour every day. And it is hard, indeed, if nurse and friends cannot calculate so as to let him make them undisturbed.[24] Remember, that many patients can walk who cannot stand or even sit up. Standing is, of all positions, the most trying to a weak patient.

Everything you do in a patient's room, after he is "put up" for the night, increases tenfold the risk of his having a bad night. But, if you rouse him up after he has fallen asleep, you do not risk, you secure him a bad night.

One hint I would give to all who attend or visit the sick, to all who have to pronounce an opinion upon sickness or its progress. Come back and look at your patient *after* he has had an hour's animated conversation with you. It is the best test of his real state we know. But never pronounce upon him from merely seeing what he does, or how he looks, during such a conversation. Learn also carefully and exactly, if you can, how he passed the night after it.

People rarely, if ever, faint while making an exertion. It is after it is over. Indeed, almost every effect of over-exertion appears after, not during such exertion. It is the highest folly to judge of the sick, as is so often done, when you see them merely during a period of excitement. People have very often died of that which, it has been proclaimed at the time, has "done them no harm."

Effects of over-exertion on sick.

As an old experienced nurse, I do most earnestly deprecate all such careless words.[25] I have known patients delirious all night, after seeing a visitor who called them "better," thought they "only wanted a little amusement," and who came again, saying, "I hope you were not the worse for my visit," neither waiting for an answer, nor even looking at the case. No real patient will ever say, "Yes, but I was a great deal the worse."

Careless observation of the results of careless visits.

It is not, however, either death or delirium of which, in these cases, there is most danger to the patient. Unperceived consequences are far more likely to ensue. *You* will have impunity—the poor patient will *not*. That is, the patient will suffer, although neither he nor the inflictor of the injury will attribute it to its real cause. It will not be directly traceable,[26] except by a very careful observant nurse. The patient will often not even mention what has done him most harm.

Don't lean upon the sick-bed.

Remember never to lean against, sit upon, or unnecessarily shake, or even touch the bed in which a patient lies. This is invariably a painful annoyance. If you shake the chair on which he sits, he has a point by which to steady himself, in his feet. But on a bed or sofa, he is entirely at your mercy, and he feels every jar you give him all through him.

Difference between real and fancy patients.[27]

In all that we have said, both here and elsewhere, let it be distinctly understood that we are not speaking of hypochondriacs. To distinguish between real and fancied disease forms an important branch of education of a nurse.[28] To manage fancy patients forms an important branch of her duties. But the nursing which real and that which fancied patients require is of different, or rather of opposite, character. And the latter will not be spoken of here. Indeed, many of the symptoms which are here mentioned are those which distinguish real from fancied disease.

It is true that hypochondriacs very often do that behind a nurse's back which they would not do before her face. Many such I have had as patients who scarcely ate anything at their regular meals; but if you concealed food for them in a drawer, they would take it at night or in secret. But this is from quite a different motive. They do it from the wish to conceal. Whereas the real patient will often boast to his nurse or doctor, if these do not shake their heads at him, of how much he has done, or eaten, or walked. To return to real disease.

Conciseness and decision are, above all things, necessary with the sick. Let your thought expressed to them be concisely and decidedly expressed. What doubt and hesitation there may be in your own mind must never be communicated to theirs, not even (I would rather say especially not) in little things. Let your doubt be to yourself, your decision to them. People who think outside their heads, the whole process of whose thought appears, like Homer's,[29] in the act of secretion, who tell everything that led them towards this conclusion and away from that, ought never to be with the sick.

Conciseness necessary with sick.

I have been told by women who had difficult confinements, that their strength depended upon the firmness of doctor and nurse. If either had betrayed that there was anything unusual or doubtful in the case, they felt it would have been "all over" with them.

And calmness.

I have observed the same thing in acute cases, when the scale was trembling between life and death. If the doctor betrayed any want of decision, if the nurse lost any portion of her calmness or self-possession, it just turned the scale in favour of death.

Irresolution is what all patients most dread. Rather than meet this in others, they will collect

Irresolution most painful to them.

all their data, and make up their minds for themselves. A change of mind in others, whether it is regarding an operation, or re-writing a letter, always injures the patient more than the being called upon to make up his mind to the most dreaded or difficult decision. Farther than this, in very many cases, the imagination in disease is far more active and vivid than it is in health. If you propose to the patient change of air to one place one hour, and to another the next, he has, in each case, immediately constituted himself in imagination the tenant of the place, gone over the whole premises in idea, and you have tired him as much by displacing his imagination, as if you had actually carried him over both places.

Above all leave the sick room quickly and come into it quickly, not suddenly, not with a rush. But don't let the patient be wearily waiting for when you will be out of the room or when you will be in it. Conciseness and decision in your movements, as well as your words, are necessary in the sick room, as necessary as absence of hurry and bustle. To possess yourself entirely will ensure you from either failing—either loitering or hurrying.

What a patient must not have to see to.

If a patient has to see, not only to his own but also to his nurse's punctuality, or perseverance, or readiness, or calmness, to any or all of these things, he is far better without that nurse than with her—however valuable and handy her services may otherwise be to him, and however incapable he may be of rendering them to himself.

With regard to reading aloud in the sick room, my experience is, that when the sick are too ill to read to themselves, they can seldom bear to be read to. Children, eye-patients, and uneducated persons are exceptions, or where there is any mechanical difficulty in reading. People who like to be read to, have generally not much the matter with them; while in fevers, or where there is much irritability of brain, the effort of listening to reading aloud has often brought on delirium. I speak with great diffidence; because there is an almost universal impression that it is *sparing* the sick to read aloud to them. But two things are certain:—

Reading aloud.

(1.) If there is some matter which *must* be read to a sick person, do it slowly. People often think that the way to get it over with least fatigue to him is to get it over in least time. They gabble; they plunge and gallop through the reading. There never was a greater mistake. Houdin, the conjuror, says that the way to make a story seem short is to tell it slowly.[30] So it is with reading to the sick. I have often heard a patient say to such a mistaken reader, "Don't read it to me; tell it me."* Unconsciously he is aware that this will

Read aloud slowly, distinctly, and steadily to the sick.

* Sick children, if not too shy to speak, will always express this wish. They invariably prefer a story to be *told* to them, rather than read to them.

The sick would rather be told a thing than have it read to them.

regulate the plunging, the reading with unequal paces, slurring over one part, instead of leaving it out altogether, if it is unimportant, and mumbling another. If the reader lets his own attention wander, and then stops to read up to himself, or finds he has read the wrong bit, then it is all over with the poor patient's chance of not suffering. Very few people know how to read to the sick; very few read aloud as pleasantly even as they speak. In reading they sing, they hesitate, they stammer, they hurry, they mumble; when in speaking they do none of these things. Reading aloud to the sick ought always to be rather slow, and exceedingly distinct, but not mouthing— rather monotonous, but not sing song—rather loud, but not noisy—and above all, not too long. Be very sure of what your patient can bear.

Never read aloud by fits and starts to the sick.

(2.) The extraordinary habit of reading to one's-self in a sick room, and reading aloud to the patient any bits which will amuse him, or more often the reader, is unaccountably thoughtless. What *do* you think the patient is thinking of during your gaps of non-reading? Do you think that he amuses himself upon what you have read for precisely the time it pleases you to go on read-ing to yourself, and that his attention his ready for something else at precisely the time it pleases you to begin reading again? Whether the person thus read to be sick or well, whether he be doing nothing or doing something else while being thus read to, the self-absorption and want of observation of the person who does it, is equally difficult to understand—although very often the read*ee* is too amiable to say how much it disturbs him.

One thing more:—From the flimsy manner in which most modern houses are built, where every step on the stairs, and along the floors, is felt all over the house; the higher the story, the greater the vibration. It is inconceivable how much the sick suffer by having anybody overhead. In the solidly built old houses, which, fortunately, most hospitals are, the noise and shaking is comparatively trifling. But it is a serious cause of suffering, in lightly built houses, and with the irritability peculiar to some diseases. Better far put such patients at the top of the house, even with the additional fatigue of stairs, if you cannot secure the room above them being untenanted; you may otherwise bring on a state of restlessness which no opium will subdue.[31] Do not neglect the warning, when a patient tells you that he "feels every step above him to cross his heart." Remember that every noise a patient cannot *see* partakes of the character of suddenness to him;[32] and I am persuaded that patients with these peculiarly irritable nerves, are positively less injured by having persons in the same room with them than overhead, or separated by only a thin compartment. Any sacrifice to secure silence for

People overhead.

these cases is worth while, because no air, however good, no attendance, however careful, will do anything for such cases without quiet.

Music.

The effect of music upon the sick has been scarcely at all noticed. In fact, its expensiveness, as it is now, makes any general application of it quite out of the question. I will only remark here, that wind instruments, including the human voice, and stringed instruments, capable of continuous sound, have generally a beneficent effect— while the piano-forte, with such instruments as have *no* continuity of sound, has just the reverse. The finest piano-forte playing will damage the sick, while an air, like "Home, sweet home,"[33] or "Assisa a piè d'un salice,"[34] on the most ordinary grinding organ will sensibly soothe them—and this quite independent of association.

Music, to the well, who *ought* to be active, gives the enjoyment of active life, without their having earned it. Music to the sick, who *cannot* be active, gives the enjoyment and takes away the nervous irritation of their incapacity.

V.—VARIETY.

To any but an old nurse, or an old patient, the degree would be quite inconceivable to which the nerves of the sick suffer from seeing the same walls, the same ceiling, the same surroundings during a long confinement to one or two rooms.

Variety a means of recovery.

The superior cheerfulness of persons suffering severe paroxysms of pain over that of persons suffering from nervous debility has often been remarked upon,[35] and attributed to the enjoyment of the former of their intervals of respite. I incline to think that the majority of cheerful cases is to be found among those patients who are not confined to one room, whatever their suffering, and that the majority of depressed cases will be seen among those subjected to a long monotony of objects about them.

The nervous frame really suffers as much from this as the digestive organs from long monotony of diet, as *e.g.*, the soldier from his twenty-one years' "boiled beef."

The effect in sickness of beautiful objects, of variety of objects, and especially of brilliancy of colour, is hardly at all appreciated.

Colour and form means of recovery.

Such cravings are usually called the "fancies" of

patients. And often, doubtless, patients have "fancies," as, *e.g.*, when they desire two contradictions. But much more often, their (so-called) "fancies" are the most valuable indications of what is necessary for their recovery. And it would be well if nurses would watch these (so-called) "fancies" closely.

I have seen, in fevers (and felt, when I was a fever patient myself)[36] the most acute suffering produced from the patient (in a hut) not being able to see out of window, and the knots in the wood being the only view. I shall never forget the rapture of fever patients over a bunch of bright-coloured flowers. I remember (in my own case) a nosegay of wild flowers being sent me, and from that moment recovery becoming more rapid.

This is no fancy.

People say the effect is only on the mind. It is no such thing. The effect is on the body, too. Little as we know about the way in which we are affected by form, by colour, and light, we do know this, that they have an actual physical effect.

Variety of form and brilliancy of colour in the objects presented to patients are actual means of recovery.

But it must be *slow* variety, *e.g.*, if you show a patient ten or twelve engravings successively, ten-to-one that he does not become cold and faint, or feverish, or even sick; but hang one up opposite him, one on each successive day, or week, or month, and he will revel in the variety.

Flowers.

The folly and ignorance which reign too often

supreme over the sick room, cannot be better exemplified than by this. While the nurse will leave the patient stewing in a corrupting atmosphere, the best ingredient of which is carbonic acid; she will deny him, on the plea of unhealthiness, a glass of cut-flowers, or a growing plant. Now, no one ever saw "over-crowding" by plants in a room or ward. And the carbonic acid they give off at nights would not poison a fly. Nay, in overcrowded rooms, they actually absorb carbonic acid and give off oxygen. Cut-flowers also decompose water and produce oxygen gas. It is true there are certain flowers, *e.g.,* lilies, the smell of which is said to depress the nervous system. These are easily known by the smell, and can be avoided.

Volumes are now written and spoken upon the effect of the mind upon the body. Much of it is true. But I wish a little more was thought of the effect of the body on the mind. You who believe yourselves overwhelmed with anxieties, but are able every day to walk up Regent-street, or out in the country, to take your meals with others in other rooms, &c., &c., you little know how much your anxieties are thereby lightened; you little know how intensified they become to those who can have no change; how the very walls of their sick rooms seem hung with their cares; how the ghosts of their troubles haunt their beds; how impossible it is for them to escape from a pursuing thought without some help from variety.

Effect of body on mind.

Sick suffer to
excess from
mental as well
as bodily pain.

It is a matter of painful wonder to the sick themselves how much painful ideas predominate over pleasurable ones in their impressions; they reason with themselves; they think themselves ungrateful; it is all of no use. The fact is, that these painful impressions are far better dismissed by a real laugh, if you can excite one by books or conversation, than by any direct reasoning; or if the patient is too weak to laugh, some impression from nature is what he wants.[37] I have mentioned the cruelty of letting him stare at a dead wall. In many diseases, especially in convalescence from fever, that wall will appear to make all sorts of faces at him; now flowers never do this. Form, colour, will free your patient from his painful ideas better than any argument.

A patient can just as much move his leg when it is fractured as change his thoughts when no external help from variety is given him. This is, indeed, one of the main sufferings of sickness; just as the fixed posture is one of the main sufferings of the broken limb.

Help the sick
to vary their
thoughts.

It is an ever recurring wonder to see educated people, who call themselves nurses, acting thus. They vary their own objects, their own employments, many times a day; and while nursing (!) some bed-ridden sufferer, they let him lie there staring at a dead wall, without any change of object to enable him to vary his thoughts; and it never even occurs to them, at least to move his bed so that he can look out of window. No, the bed is to be always left in the darkest, dullest, remotest part of the room.

I remember a case in point. A man received an injury to the spine, from an accident, which after a long confinement ended in death. He was a workman—had not in his composition a single grain of what is called "enthusiasm for nature"— but he was desperate to "see once more out of window." His nurse actually got him on her back, and managed to perch him up at the window for an instant, "to see out." The consequence to the poor nurse was a serious illness, which nearly proved fatal. The man never knew it; but a great many other people did. Yet the consequence in none of their minds, so far as I know, was the conviction that the craving for variety in the starving eye is just as desperate as that for food in the starving stomach, and tempts the famishing creature in either case to steal for its satisfaction. No other word will express it but "desperation." And it sets the seal of ignorance and stupidity just as much on the governors and attendants of the sick if they do not provide the sick-bed with a "view," or with variety of some kind, as if they did not provide the hospital with a kitchen.

Desperate desire in the sick to "see out of window."

And in no case does consideration of these matters meet with the same success as it does for the sick. Poets rave about the "charms of nature." I question whether the intensest pleasure ever felt in nature is not that of the sick man raising a forest tree, six inches high, from an acorn or a horse-chestnut, in a London back-court. Europe perhaps never gives such during a life-long travel.

It is a very common error among the well to think that "with a little more self-control" the sick might, if they choose, "dismiss painful thoughts" which "aggravate their disease," &c. Believe me, almost *any* sick person, who behaves decently well, exercises more self-control every moment of his day than you will ever know till you are sick yourself. Almost every step that crosses his room is painful to him; almost every thought that crosses his brain is painful to him; and if he can speak without being savage, and look without being unpleasant, he is exercising self-control.

Suppose you have been up all night, and instead of being allowed to have your cup of tea, you were to be told that you ought to "exercise self-control," what should you say? Now, the nerves of the sick are always in the state that yours are in after you have been up all night.

Supply to the sick the defect of manual labour.

We will suppose the diet of the sick to be cared for. Then, this state of nerves is most frequently to be relieved by care in affording them a pleasant view, a judicious variety as to flowers,* and pretty things. Light by itself will often

Physical effect of colour.

* No one who has watched the sick can doubt the fact, that some feel stimulus from looking at scarlet flowers, exhaustion from looking at deep blue, &c.

relieve it. The craving for "the return of day," which the sick so constantly evince, is generally nothing but the desire for light, the remembrance of the relief which a variety of objects before the eye affords to the harassed sick mind.

Again, every man and every woman has some amount of manual employment, excepting a few fine ladies, who do not even dress themselves, and who are virtually in the same category, as to nerves, as the sick. Now, you can have no idea of the relief which manual labour is to you—of the degree to which the deprivation of manual employment increases the peculiar irritability from which many sick suffer.

A little needle-work, a little writing, a little cleaning, would be the greatest relief the sick could have, if they could do it; these *are* the greatest relief to you, though you do not know it. Reading, though it is often the only thing the sick can do, is not this relief. Bearing this in mind, bearing in mind that you have all these varieties of employment which the sick cannot have, bear also in mind to obtain for them all the varieties which they can enjoy.

I need hardly say that excess in needle-work, in writing, in any other continuous employment, will produce the same irritability that defect in manual employment (as one cause) produces in the sick.

———

VI.—TAKING FOOD.

EVERY careful observer of the sick will agree in this, that thousands of patients are annually starved in the midst of plenty, from want of attention to the ways which alone make it possible for them to take food. This want of attention is as remarkable in those who urge upon the sick to do what is quite impossible to them, as in the sick themselves who will not make the effort to do what is perfectly possible to them.

For instance, to the large majority of very weak patients it is quite impossible to take any solid food before 11 A.M., nor then, if their strength is still further exhausted by fasting till that hour. For weak patients have generally feverish nights and, in the morning, dry mouths; and, if they could eat with those dry mouths, it would be the worse for them. A spoonful of beef-tea, of arrow-root and wine, of egg flip, every hour, will give them the requisite nourishment, and prevent them from being too much exhausted to take at a later hour the solid food, which is necessary for their recovery. And every patient who can swallow at all can swallow these liquid things, if he chooses.

But how often do we hear a mutton-chop, an egg, a bit of bacon, ordered to a patient for breakfast, to whom (as a moment's consideration would show us) it must be quite impossible to masticate such things at that hour.

Again, a nurse is ordered to give a patient a tea-cup full of some article of food every three hours. The patient's stomach rejects it. If so, try a table-spoon full every hour; if this will not do, a tea-spoon full every quarter of an hour.

I am bound to say, that I think more patients are lost by want of care and ingenuity in these momentous minutiae in private nursing than in public hospitals. And I think there is more of the *entente cordiale* to assist one another's hands between the doctor and his head nurse in the latter institutions, than between the doctor and the patient's friends in the private house.[38]

If we did but know the consequences which may ensue, in very weak patients, from ten minutes' fasting or repletion (I call it repletion when they are obliged to let too small an interval elapse between taking food and some other exertion, owing to the nurse's unpunctuality), we should be more careful never to let this occur. In very weak patients there is often a nervous difficulty of swallowing, which is so much increased by any other call upon their strength that, unless they have their food punctually at the minute, which minute again must be arranged so as to fall

Life often hangs upon minutes in taking food.

in with no other minute's occupation, they can take nothing till the next respite occurs—so that an unpunctuality or delay of ten minutes may very well turn out to be one of two or three hours. And why is it not as easy to be punctual to a minute? Life often literally hangs upon these minutes.

In acute cases, where life or death is to be determined in a few hours, these matters are very generally attended to, especially in Hospitals; and the number of cases is large where the patient is, as it were, brought back to life by exceeding care on the part of the Doctor or Nurse, or both, in ordering and giving nourishment with minute selection and punctuality.

Patients often starved in chronic cases.

But, in chronic cases, lasting over months and years, where the fatal issue is often determined at last by mere protracted starvation, I had rather not enumerate the instances which I have known where a little ingenuity, and a great deal of perseverance, might, in all probability, have averted the result. The consulting the hours when the patient can take food, the observation of the times, often varying, when he is most faint, the altering seasons of taking food, in order to anticipate and prevent such times—all this, which requires observation, ingenuity, and perseverance (and these really constitute the good Nurse), might save more lives than we wot of.

Food never to be left by the patient's side.

To leave the patient's untasted food by his side, from meal to meal, in hopes that he will eat it in the interval, is simply to prevent him from taking any food at all. Patients have been literally incapacitated from taking one article of food after another, by this piece of ignorance. Let the food come at the right time, and be taken away, eaten or uneaten, at the right time; but never let a patient have "something always standing" by him, if you don't wish to disgust him of everything.

On the other hand, a patient's life has been saved (he was sinking for want of food) by the simple question, put to him by the doctor, "But is there no hour when you feel you could eat?" "Oh, yes," he said, "I could always take something at — o'clock and — o'clock." The thing was tried and succeeded. Patients very seldom, however, can tell this; it is for you to watch and find it out.

A patient should, if possible, not see or smell either the food of others, or a greater amount of food than he himself can consume at one time, or even hear food talked about or see it in the raw state. I know of no exception to the above rule. The breaking of it always induces a greater or less incapacity of taking food.[39]

Patient had better not see more food than his own.

In hospital wards it is of course impossible to observe all this; and in single wards, where a patient must be continuously and closely watched, it is frequently impossible to relieve the attendant, so that his or her own meals can be taken out of the ward. But it is not the less true that, in such cases, even where the patient is not himself aware of it, his possibility of taking food is limited by seeing the attendant eating meals under his observation. In some cases the sick are aware of it, and complain. A case where the patient was supposed to be insensible, but complained as soon as able to speak, is now present to my recollection.

Remember, however, that the extreme punctuality in well-ordered hospitals, the rule that nothing shall be done in the ward while the patients are having their meals, go far to counterbalance what unavoidable evil there is in having patients together. The private nurse may be often seen dusting or fidgeting about in a sick room all the while the patient is eating, or trying to eat.

That the more alone an invalid can be when taking food, the better, is unquestionable; and, even if he must be fed, the nurse should not allow him to talk, or talk to him, especially about food, while eating.

When a person is compelled, by the pressure of occupation, to continue his business while sick, it ought to be a rule WITHOUT ANY EXCEPTION WHATEVER, that no one shall bring business to him or talk to him while he is taking food, nor go on talking to him on interesting subjects up to the last moment before his meals, nor make an engagement with him immediately after, so that there be any hurry of mind while taking them.

Upon the observance of these rules, especially the first, often depends the patient's capability of taking food at all, or, if he is amiable and forces himself to take food, of deriving any nourishment from it.

A nurse should never put before a patient milk that is sour, meat or soup that is turned, an egg that is bad, or vegetables underdone. Yet often these things are brought in to the sick in a state perfectly perceptible to every nose or eye except the nurse's.[40] It is here that the clever nurse appears; she will not bring in the peccant article, but, not to disappoint the patient, she will whip up something else in a few minutes. Remember that sick cookery should half do the work of your poor patient's weak digestion. But if you further impair it with your bad articles, I know not what is to become of him or of it.

You cannot be too careful as to quality in sick diet.

If the nurse is an intelligent being, and not a mere carrier of diets to and from the patient, let her exercise her intelligence in these things. How often have we known a patient eat nothing at all in the day, because one meal was left untasted (at that time he was incapable of eating), at another the milk was sour, the third was spoiled by some other accident. And it never occurred to the nurse to extemporize some expedient,—it never occurred to her that as he had had no solid food that day, he might eat a bit of toast (say) with his tea in the evening, or he might have some meal an hour earlier. A patient who cannot touch his dinner at two, will often accept it gladly, if brought to him at seven. But somehow nurses never "think of these things." One would imagine they did not consider themselves bound to exercise their judgment; they leave it to the patient. Now I am quite sure that it is better for a patient rather to suffer these neglects than to try to teach his nurse to nurse him, if she does not know how. It ruffles him, and if he is ill he is in no condition to teach, especially upon himself. The above remarks apply much more to private nursing than to hospitals.

Nurse must have some rule of thought about her patient's diet.

I would say to the nurse, have a rule of thought about your patient's diet; consider, remember how much he has had, and how much he ought to have to-day. Generally, the only rule of the private patient's diet is what the nurse has to give. It is true she cannot give him what she has not got; but his stomach does not wait for her convenience, or even her necessity. If it is used to having its stimulus at one hour to-day, and to-morrow it does not have it, because she has failed in getting it, he will suffer. She must be always exercising her ingenuity to supply defects, and to remedy accidents which will happen among the best contrivers, but from which the patient does not suffer the less, because "they cannot be helped."

Nurse must have some rule of time about the patient's diet.

Why, because the nurse has not got some food to-day which the patient takes, can the patient wait four hours for it to-day, who could not wait two hours yesterday? Yet this is the only logic one generally hears. On the other hand, the opposite course, viz., of the nurse giving the patient a thing because she *has* got it, is equally fatal. If she happens to have fresh jelly, or fresh fruit, she will frequently give it to the patient half-an-hour after his dinner, or at his dinner, when he cannot possibly eat that and the broth too—or, worse still, leave it by his bed-side till he is so sickened with the sight of it, that he cannot eat it at all.

One very minute caution,—take care not to spill into your patient's saucer, in other words, take care that the outside bottom rim of his cup is quite dry and clean; if, every time he lifts his cup to his lips, he has to carry the saucer with it, or else to drop the liquid upon and to soil his sheet, or his bed-gown, or pillow, or, if he is sitting up, his dress, you have no idea what a difference this minute want of care on your part makes to his comfort and even to his willingness for food.

Keep your patient's cup dry underneath.

VII.—WHAT FOOD?

Common errors in diet.

I will mention one or two of the most common errors among women in charge of sick respecting

Beef tea.

sick diet. One is the belief that beef tea is the most nutritive of all articles. Now, just try and boil down a lb. of beef into beef tea, evaporate your beef tea, and see what is left of your beef. You will find that there is barely a teaspoonful of solid nourishment to half-a-pint of water in beef tea;— nevertheless there is a certain reparative quality in it, we do not know what, as there is in tea;—but it may safely be given in almost any inflammatory disease, and is as little to be depended upon with the healthy or convalescent as where much nourish-

Eggs.

ment is required. Again, it is an ever ready saw that an egg is equivalent to a lb. of meat,—whereas it is not at all so. Also, it is seldom noticed with how many patients, particularly of nervous or bilious temperament, eggs disagree. All puddings made with eggs, are distasteful to them in consequence. An egg, whipped up with wine, is often the only form in which they can take this kind of nourishment. Again, if the patient has attained to eating meat, it is supposed that to give him meat is the only thing needful for his recovery; whereas scorbutic sores have been actually known to appear among sick persons living in the midst of plenty in England, which could be traced to no other source than this, viz.: that the nurse, depending on meat alone, had allowed the patient to be without vegetables for a considerable time, these latter being so badly cooked that he always left them untouched. Arrowroot is another grand dependence of the nurse. As a vehicle for wine, and as a restorative quickly prepared, it is all very well. But it is nothing but starch and water. Flour is both more nutritive, and less liable to ferment, and is preferable wherever it can be used.

Meat without vegetables.

Arrowroot.

Again, milk and the preparations from milk, are a most important article of food for the sick. Butter is the lightest kind of animal fat, and though it wants the sugar and some of the other elements which there are in milk, yet it is most valuable both in itself and in enabling the patient to eat more bread. Flour, oats, groats, barley, and their kind, are, as we have already said, preferable in all their preparations to all the preparations of arrowroot, sago, tapioca, and their kind. Cream, in many long chronic diseases, is quite irreplaceable by any other article whatever. It seems to act in the same manner as beef tea, and to most it is much easier of digestion than milk. In fact, it seldom disagrees. Cheese is not usually digestible by the sick, but it is pure nourishment for repairing waste;

Milk, butter, cream, &c.

and I have seen sick, and not a few either, whose craving for cheese showed how much it was needed by them.*

But, if fresh milk is so valuable a food for the sick, the least change or sourness in it, makes it of all articles, perhaps, the most injurious; diarrhoea is a common result of fresh milk allowed to become at all sour. The nurse therefore ought to exercise her utmost care in this. In large institutions for the sick, even the poorest, the utmost care is exercised. Wenham Lake ice is used for this express purpose every summer, while the private patient, perhaps, never tastes a drop of milk that is not sour, all through the hot weather, so little does the private nurse understand the necessity of such care. Yet, if you consider that the only drop of real nourishment in your patient's tea is the drop of milk, and how much almost all English patients depend upon their tea, you will see the great importance of not

Intelligent cravings of particular sick for particular articles of diet.

* In the diseases produced by bad food, such as scorbutic dysentery and diarrhoea, the patient's stomach often craves for and digests things, some of which certainly would be laid down in no dietary that ever was invented for sick, and especially not for such sick. These are fruit, pickles, jams, gingerbread, fat of ham or of bacon, suet, cheese, butter, milk. These cases I have seen not by ones, nor by tens, but by hundreds. And the patient's stomach was right and the book was wrong. The articles craved for, in these cases, might have been principally arranged under the two heads of fat and vegetable acids.

There is often a marked difference between men and women in this matter of sick feeding. Women's digestion is generally slower.

depriving your patient of this drop of milk. Buttermilk, a totally different thing, is often very useful, especially in fevers.

In laying down rules of diet, by the amounts of "solid nutriment" in different kinds of food, it is constantly lost sight of what the patient requires to repair his waste, what he can take and what he can't. You cannot diet a patient from a book, you cannot make up the human body as you would make up a prescription,—so many parts "carboniferous," so many parts "nitrogenous" will constitute a perfect diet for the patient. The nurse's observation here will materially assist the doctor— the patient's "fancies" will materially assist the nurse. For instance, sugar is one of the most nutritive of all articles, being pure carbon, and is particularly recommended in some books. But the vast majority of all patients in England, young and old, male and female, rich and poor, hospital and private, dislike sweet things,—and while I have never known a person take to sweets when he was ill who disliked them when he was well, I have known many fond of them when in health, who in sickness would leave off anything sweet, even to sugar in tea,—sweet puddings, sweet drinks, are their aversion; the furred tongue almost always likes what is sharp or pungent. Scorbutic patients are an exception, they often crave for sweetmeats and jams.

Jelly is another article of diet in great favour

Sweet things.

Jelly.

163

with nurses and friends of the sick; even if it could be eaten solid, it would not nourish, but it is simply the height of folly to take ⅛ oz. of gelatine and make it into a certain bulk by dissolving it in water and then to give it to the sick, as if the mere bulk represented nourishment. It is now known that jelly does not nourish, that it has a tendency to produce diarrhoea,—and to trust to it to repair the waste of a diseased constitution is simply to starve the sick under the guise of feeding them. If one hundred spoonfuls of jelly were given in the course of the day, you would have given one spoonful of gelatine, which spoonful has no nutritive power whatever.

And, nevertheless, gelatine contains a large quantity of nitrogen, which is one of the most powerful elements in nutrition; on the other hand, beef tea may be chosen as an illustration of great nutrient power in sickness, co-existing with a very small amount of solid nitrogenous matter.

Beef tea.

Dr. Christison says that "every one will be struck with the readiness with which" certain classes of "patients will often take diluted meat juice or beef tea repeatedly, when they refuse all other kinds of food."[41] This is particularly remarkable in "cases of gastric fever, in which," he says, "little or nothing else besides beef tea or diluted meat juice" has been taken for weeks or even months; "and yet a pint of beef tea contains scarcely ¼ oz. of anything but water."—The result is so striking that he asks what is its mode of action? "Not simply nutrient—¼ oz. of the most nutritive material cannot nearly replace the daily wear and tear of the tissues in any circumstances. Possibly," he says, "it belongs to a new denomination of remedies."

It has been observed that a small quantity of beef tea added to other articles of nutrition augments their power out of all proportion to the additional amount of solid matter.

The reason why jelly should be innutritious and beef tea nutritious to the sick, is a secret yet undiscovered, but it clearly shows that careful observation of the sick is the only clue to the best dietary.

Chemistry has as yet afforded little insight into the dieting of the sick. All that chemistry can tell us is the amount of "carboniferous" or "nitrogenous" elements discoverable in different dietetic articles. It has given us lists of dietetic substances, arranged in the order of their richness in one or other of these principles; but that is all. In the great majority of cases, the stomach of the patient is guided by other principles of selection than merely the amount of carbon or nitrogen in the diet. No doubt, in this as in other things, nature has very definite rules for her guidance, but these rules can only be ascertained by the most careful observation at the bed-side. She there teaches us that living chemistry, the chemistry of reparation, is something different from the

Observation not chemistry, must decide sick diet.

chemistry of the laboratory. Organic chemistry is useful, as all knowledge is, when we come face to face with nature; but it by no means follows that we should learn in the laboratory any one of the reparative processes going on in disease.

Again, the nutritive power of milk and of the preparations from milk, is very much undervalued; there is nearly as much nourishment in half a pint of milk as there is in a quarter of a lb. of meat. But this is not the whole question or nearly the whole. The main question is, what the patient's stomach can assimilate or derive nourishment from, and of this the patient's stomach is the sole judge. Chemistry cannot tell this. The patient's stomach must be its own chemist. The diet which will keep the healthy man healthy, will kill the sick one. The same beef which is the most nutritive of all meat, and which nourishes the healthy man, is the least nourishing of all food to the sick man, whose half-dead stomach can *assimilate* no part of it, that is, make no food out of it. On a diet of beef tea healthy men on the other hand speedily lose their strength.

Home made bread.

I have known patients live for many months without touching bread, because they could not eat baker's bread. These were mostly country patients, but not all. Home-made bread or brown bread is a most important article of diet for many patients. The use of aperients may be entirely superseded by it. Oat cake is another.

To watch for the opinions, then, which the patient's stomach gives, rather than to read "analyses of foods," is the business of all those who have to settle what the patient is to eat— perhaps the most important thing to be provided for him after the air he is to breathe.[42]

Now the medical man who sees the patient only once a day, or even only once or twice a week, cannot possibly tell this without the assistance of the patient himself, or of those who are in constant observation of the patient. The utmost the medical man can tell is whether the patient is weaker or stronger at this visit than he was at the last visit. I should therefore say that incomparably the most important office of the nurse, after she has taken care of the patient's air, is to take care to observe the effect of his food, and report it to the medical attendant.

It is quite incalculable the good that would certainly come from such *sound* and close observation in this almost neglected branch of nursing, or the help it would give to the medical man.

A great deal too much against tea is said by wise people, and a great deal too much of tea is given to the sick by foolish people. When you see the natural and almost universal craving in English sick for their "tea," you cannot but feel that nature knows what she is about. But a little tea or coffee restores them quite as much as a great deal, and a great deal of tea and especially of coffee

Tea and coffee.

167

impairs the little power of digestion they have. Yet a nurse, because she sees how one or two cups of tea or coffee restores her patient, thinks that three or four cups will do twice as much. This is not the case at all; it is however certain that there is nothing yet discovered which is a substitute to the English patient for his cup of tea; he can take it when he can take nothing else, and he often can't take anything else if he has it not.[43] I should be very glad if any of the abusers of tea would point out what to give to an English patient after a sleepless night, instead of tea. If you give it at five or six o'clock in the morning, he may even sometimes fall asleep after it, and get perhaps his only two or three hours' sleep during the twenty-four. At the same time you never should give tea or coffee to the sick, as a rule, after five o'clock in the afternoon. Sleeplessness in the early night is from excitement generally, and is increased by tea or coffee; sleeplessness which continues to the early morning is from exhaustion often, and is relieved by tea. The only English patients I have ever known refuse tea, have been typhus cases, and the first sign of their getting better was their craving again for tea. In general, the dry and dirty tongue always prefers tea to coffee, and will quite decline milk, unless with tea. Coffee is a better restorative than tea, but a greater impairer of the digestion. Let the patient's taste decide. You will say that, in cases of great thirst, the patient's craving decides that it will drink a *great deal* of tea, and that you cannot help it. But in these cases be sure that the patient requires diluents for quite other purposes than quenching the thirst;[44] he wants a great deal of some drink, not only of tea, and the doctor will order what he is to have, barley water or lemonade, or soda water and milk, as the case may be.

It is made a frequent recommendation to persons about to incur great exhaustion, either from the nature of the service or from their being not in a state fit for it,[45] to eat a piece of bread before they go. I wish the recommenders would themselves try the experiment of substituting a piece of bread for a cup of tea or coffee or beef tea as a refresher. They would find it a very poor comfort. When soldiers have to set out fasting on fatiguing duty, when nurses have to go fasting in to their patients, it is a hot restorative they want, and ought to have, before they go, not a cold bit of bread. And dreadful have been the consequences of neglecting this. If they can take a bit of bread *with* the hot cup of tea, so much the better, but not *instead* of it. The fact that there is more nourishment in bread than in almost anything else has probably induced the mistake. That it is a fatal mistake there is no doubt. It seems, though very little is known on the subject, that what "assimilates" itself directly and with the least trouble of digestion with the human body is the best for the above circumstances. Bread requires two or three processes of assimilation, before it becomes like the human body.

The almost universal testimony of English men and women who have undergone great fatigue, such as riding long journeys without stopping, or sitting up for several nights in succession, is that they could do it best upon an occasional cup of tea —and nothing else.

Let experience, not theory, decide upon this as upon all other things.

Lehmann, quoted by Dr. Christison, says that, among the well and active "the infusion of 1 oz. of roasted coffee daily will diminish the waste" going on in the body "by one-fourth," and Dr. Christison adds that tea has the same property. Now this is actual experiment. Lehmann weighs the man and finds the fact from his weight. It is not deduced from any "analysis" of food.[46] All experience among the sick shows the same thing.

In making coffee for the sick, it is absolutely necessary to buy it in the berry and grind it at home. Otherwise you may reckon upon its containing a certain amount of chicory, *at least*. This is not a question of the taste or of the wholesomeness of chicory. It is that chicory has nothing at all of the properties for which you give coffee. And therefore you may as well not give it.

Again, all laundresses, mistresses of dairy-farms, head nurses (I speak of the good old sort only—

women who unite a good deal of hard manual labour with the head-work necessary for arranging the day's business, so that none of it shall tread upon the heels of something else) set great value, I have observed, upon having a high-priced tea. This is called extravagant. But these women are "extravagant" in nothing else. And they are right in this. Real tea-leaf tea alone contains the restorative they want; which is not to be found in sloe-leaf tea.[47]

The mistresses of houses, who cannot even go over their own house once a-day, are incapable of judging for these women. For they are incapable themselves, to all appearance, of the spirit of arrangement (no small task) necessary for managing a large ward or dairy.

Cocoa is often recommended to the sick in lieu of tea or coffee. But independently of the fact that English sick very generally dislike cocoa, it has quite a different effect from tea or coffee. It is an oily starchy nut, having no restorative power at all, but simply increasing fat. It is pure mockery of the sick, therefore, to call it a substitute for tea. For any renovating stimulus it has, you might just as well offer them chestnuts instead of tea. *Cocoa.*

An almost universal error among nurses is in the bulk of the food, and especially the drinks, they offer to their patients. Suppose a patient ordered four oz. brandy during the day, how is he to take this if you make it into four pints with diluting it? *Bulk.*

The same with tea and beef tea, with arrowroot, milk, &c. You have not increased the nourishment, you have not increased the renovating power of these articles, by increasing their bulk,—you have very likely diminished both by giving the patient's digestion more to do, and, most likely of all, the patient will leave half of what he has been ordered to take, because he cannot swallow the bulk with which you have been pleased to invest it. It requires very nice observation and care (and meets with hardly any) to determine what will not be too thick or strong for the patient to take, while giving him no more than the bulk which he is able to swallow.

———————

VIII.—BED AND BEDDING.

A few words upon bedsteads and bedding; and principally as regards patients who are entirely, or almost entirely, confined to bed. Feverishness a symptom of bedding.

Feverishness is generally supposed to be a symptom of fever—in nine cases out of ten it is a symptom of bedding.

The patient has had re-introduced into the body the emanations from himself which day after day and week after week saturate his unaired bedding. How can it be otherwise? Look at the ordinary bed in which a patient lies.

If I were looking out for an example in order to show what *not* to do, I should take the specimen of an ordinary bed in a private house: a wooden bedstead, two or even three mattresses up to above the height of a table; a vallance attached to the frame—nothing but a miracle could ever thoroughly dry or air such a bed and bedding. The patient must inevitably alternate between cold damp after his bed is made, and warm damp before, both saturated with organic matter,[48] and this from the time the mattresses are put under him till the time they are picked to pieces, if this is ever done. Uncleanliness of ordinary bedding.

For the same reason, if, after washing a patient, you must put the same night-dress on him again, always give it a preliminary warm at the fire. The night-gown he has worn must be, to a certain extent, damp. It has now got cold from having been off him for a few minutes. The fire will dry and at the same time air it. This is much more important than with clean things.

If you consider that an adult in health exhales by the lungs and skin in the twenty-four hours three pints at least of moisture,[49] loaded with organic matter ready to enter into putrefaction; that in sickness the quantity is often greatly increased, the quality is always more noxious—just ask yourself next where does all this moisture go to? Chiefly into the bedding, because it cannot go anywhere else. And it stays there; because, except perhaps a weekly change of sheets, scarcely any other airing is attempted. A nurse will be careful to fidgetiness about airing the clean sheets from clean damp, but airing the dirty sheets from noxious damp will never even occur to her. Besides this, the most dangerous effluvia we know of are from the excreta of the sick—these are placed, at least temporarily, where they must throw their effluvia into the under side of the bed, and the space under the bed is never aired; it cannot be, with our arrangements. Must not such a bed be always saturated, and be always the means of re-introducing into the system of the unfortunate

Air your dirty sheets, not only your clean ones

patient who lies in it, that excrementitious matter to eliminate which from the body nature had expressly appointed the disease?

My heart always sinks within me when I hear the good housewife, of every class, say, "I assure you the bed has been well slept in," and one can only hope it is not true. What? is the bed already saturated with somebody else's damp before my patient comes to exhale into it his own damp? Has it not had a single chance to be aired? No, not one. "It has been slept in every night."

The only way of really nursing a real patient is to have an *iron* bedstead, with rheocline springs,[50] which are permeable by the air up to the very mattress (no vallance, of course), the mattress to be a thin hair one; the bed to be not above 3 ½ feet wide. If the patient be entirely confined to his bed, there should be *two* such bedsteads; each bed to be "made" with mattress, sheets, blankets, &c., complete—the patient to pass twelve hours in each bed; on no account to carry his sheets with him. The whole of the bedding to be hung up to air for each intermediate twelve hours. Of course there are many cases where this cannot be done at all— many more where only an approach to it can be made. I am indicating the ideal of nursing, and what has actually been done. But about the kind of bedstead there can be no doubt, whether there be one or two provided.

Iron spring bedstead the best.

Comfort and cleanliness of *two* beds.

Bed not to be
too wide.

There is a prejudice in favour of a wide bed—I believe it to be a prejudice. All the refreshment of moving a patient from one side to the other of his bed is far more effectually secured by putting him into a fresh bed; and a patient who is really very ill does not stray far in bed. But it is said there is no room to put a tray down on a narrow bed. No good nurse will ever put a tray on a bed at all. If the patient can turn on his side, he will eat more comfortably from a bed-side table; and on no account whatever should a bed ever be higher than a sofa. Otherwise the patient feels himself "out of humanity's reach"; he can get at nothing for himself: he can move nothing for himself. If the patient cannot turn, a table over the bed is a better thing. I need hardly say that a patient's bed should never have its side against the wall. The nurse must be able to get easily to both sides of the bed, and to reach easily every part of the patient without stretching—a thing impossible if the bed be either too wide or too high.

Bed not to be
too high.

When I see a patient in a room nine or ten feet high upon a bed between four and five feet high, with his head, when he is sitting up in bed, actually within two or three feet of the ceiling,[51] I ask myself, is this expressly planned to produce that peculiarly distressing feeling common to the sick, viz., as if the walls and ceiling were closing in upon them, and they becoming sandwiches between floor and ceiling, which imagination is not, indeed, here so far from the truth? If, over and above this, the window stops short of the ceiling, then the patient's head may literally be raised above the stratum of fresh air, even when the window is open. Can human perversity any farther go, in unmaking the process of restoration which God has made? The fact is, that the heads of sleepers or of sick should never be higher than the throat of the chimney, which ensures their being in the current of best air. And we will not suppose it possible that you have closed your chimney with a chimney-board.

If a bed is higher than a sofa, the difference of the fatigue of getting in and out of bed will just make the difference, very often, to the patient (who can get in and out of bed at all) of being able to take a few minutes' exercise, either in the open air or in another room. It is so very odd that people never think of this, or of how many more times a patient who is in bed for the twenty-four hours is obliged to get in and out of bed than they are, who only, it is to be hoped, get into bed once and out of bed once during the twenty-four hours.

A patient's bed should always be in the lightest spot in the room; and he should be able to see out of window. *Nor in a dark place.*

I need scarcely say that the old four-post bed with curtains is utterly inadmissible, whether for sick or well. Hospital bedsteads are in many respects very much less objectionable than private ones. *Nor a four poster with curtains.*

Scrofula often a result of disposition of bedclothes.

There is reason to believe that not a few of the apparently unaccountable cases of scrofula among children proceed from the habit of sleeping with the head under the bed clothes, and so inhaling air already breathed, which is farther contaminated by exhalations from the skin. Patients are sometimes given to a similar habit, and it often happens that the bed clothes are so disposed that the patient must necessarily breathe air more or less contaminated by exhalations from his skin.[52] A good nurse will be careful to attend to this. It is an important part, so to speak, of ventilation.

Consumptive patients often put their heads under the bed clothes, because it relieves a paroxysm of coughing, brought on by a change of temperature or of moisture in our changeable atmosphere.[53] Of all places to take warm air from, one's own body is certainly the worst. And perhaps, if nurses do encourage this practice, we need no longer wonder at the "rapid decline" of some consumptive patients. A folded silk handkerchief, lightly laid over the mouth, a respirator, medicated inhalations, or merely inhaling the steam from a basin of boiling water, will relieve the paroxysm of coughing without such danger. But inhalations must be carefully managed, so as not to make the patient damp.

Bed sores.

It may be worth while to remark, that where there is any danger of bed-sores a blanket should never be placed *under* the patient. It retains damp and acts like a poultice.

Never use anything but light Witney blankets as bed covering for the sick.[54] The heavy cotton impervious counterpane is bad, for the very reason that it keeps in the emanations from the sick person, while the blanket allows them to pass through. Weak patients are invariably distressed by a great weight of bed-clothes, which often prevents their getting any sound sleep whatever. *Heavy and impervious bed-clothes.*

I once told a "very good nurse" that the way in which her patient's room was kept was quite enough to account for his sleeplessness; and she answered with perfect good-humour that she was not at all surprised at it—as if the state of the room were, like the state of the weather, entirely out of her power. Now in what sense was this woman to be called a "nurse?" *Nurses often do not think the sick-room any business of theirs, but only the sick.*

A true nurse will always make her patient's bed herself, not leave it to the housemaid. In well-managed hospital wards, the head nurse (or "sister") makes the beds of the worst cases herself, and is always the best bed-maker in the ward. If you consider the importance of sleep to the sick, the necessity of a well-made bed to procure them sleep, you will not leave this essential part of your functions to *any* one. But a careless nurse doubles the blankets over the patient's chest, instead of leaving the lightest weight there—she puts a thick warm blanket under him—she does not turn his mattress *every* way every day; and the patient would rather than not that his bed were made by anybody else.

One word about pillows. Every weak patient, be his illness what it may, suffers more or less, from difficulty in breathing. (1.) To take the weight of the body off the poor chest, which is hardly up to its work as it is, ought therefore to be the object of the nurse in arranging his pillows. Now what does she do and what are the consequences? She piles the pillows one a-top of the other like a wall of bricks. The head is thrown upon the chest. And the shoulders are pushed forward, so as not to allow the lungs room to expand. The pillows, in fact, lean upon the patient, not the patient upon the pillows. It is impossible to give a rule for this, because it must vary with the figure of the patient. But the object is to support, with the pillows, the back *below* the breathing apparatus, to allow the shoulders room to fall back, and to support the head, without throwing it forward. The suffering of dying patients is immensely increased by neglect of these points. And many an invalid, too weak to drag about his pillows himself, slips his book or anything at hand behind the lower part of his back to support it. (2.) Tall patients suffer much more than short ones, because of the *drag* of the long limbs upon the waist. Something to press the feet against is a relief to all.

Having said this about the two principles to be observed for giving ease to patients in bed, I must add that they apply equally to them when up. I scarcely ever saw an invalid chair which was not constructed in express violation of both—which did not, that is, *increase* the drag of the limbs upon the waist, and throw too much of the weight upon the axis of the spine, thereby preventing any relief to the chest. An ordinary *low* well-stuffed arm-chair with pillows and a footstool is generally far better than any of the elaborate invalid chairs. The very idea of mounting into one of them terrifies a patient. They are all too high, too deep in the seat, and they do not support the legs and feet so as to raise the knees, generally a great relief to invalids sitting up. To support the patient's frame, at as many points as possible, is essential. And this is what invalid chairs do *not* do; and when the patient is in, he cannot get out.

IX.—LIGHT.[55]

Light essential
to both health
and recovery.

IT is the unqualified result of all my experience with the sick, that second only to their need of fresh air is their need of light;[56] that, after a close room, what hurts them most is a dark room, and that it is not only light but direct sun-light they want. You had better carry your patient about after the sun, according to the aspect of the rooms, if circumstances permit, than let him linger in a room when the sun is off. People think the effect is upon the spirits only. This is by no means the case. The sun is not only a painter but a sculptor. You admit that he does the photograph. Without going into any scientific exposition, we must admit that light has quite as real and tangible effects upon the human body. But this is not all. Who has not observed the purifying effect of light, and especially of direct sun-light, upon the air of a room? Here is an observation within everybody's experience. Go into a room where the shutters are always shut, (in a sick room or a bedroom there should never be shutters shut), and though the room be uninhabited, though the air has never been polluted by the breathing of human beings, you will observe a close, musty smell of corrupt air, of air, *i.e.,* unpurified by the effect of the sun's rays. The mustiness of dark rooms and corners, indeed, is proverbial. The cheerfulness of a room, the usefulness of light, in treating disease is all-important.

A very high authority in hospital construction has said that people do not enough consider the difference between wards and dormitories in planning their buildings. But I go farther, and say, that healthy people never remember the difference between *bed*-rooms and *sick*-rooms, in making arrangements for the sick. To a sleeper in health it does not signify what the view is from his bed. He ought never to be in it excepting when asleep, and at night. Aspect does not very much signify either (provided the sun reach his bed-room some time in every day, to purify the air), because he ought never to be his in bed-room except during the hours when there is no sun. But the case is exactly reversed with the sick, even should they be as many hours out of their beds as you are in yours, which probably they are not. Therefore, that they should be able, without raising themselves or turning in bed, to see out of a window from their beds, to see sky and sun-light at least, if you can show them nothing else, I assert to be, if not of the very first importance for recovery, at least something very near it. And you should therefore look to the position of the beds of your sick one of

Aspect, view, and sunlight, matters of first importance to the sick.

the very first things. If they can see out of two windows instead of one, so much the better. Again, the morning sun and the mid-day sun—the hours when they are quite certain not to be up, are of more importance to them, if a choice must be made, than the afternoon sun. Perhaps you can take them out of bed in the afternoon and set them by the window, where they can see the sun. But the best rule is, if possible, to give them direct sunlight from the moment he rises till the moment he sets.

Another great difference between the *bed*-room and the *sick*-room is, that the *sleeper* has a very large balance of fresh air to begin with, when he begins the night, if his room has been open all day as it ought to be; the *sick* man has not, because all day he has been breathing the air in the same room, and dirtying it by the emanations from himself. Far more care is therefore necessary to keep up a constant change of air in the sick room.

It is hardly necessary to add that there are acute cases, (particularly a few ophthalmic cases, and diseases where the eye is morbidly sensitive), where a subdued light is necessary. But a dark north room is inadmissible even for these. You can always moderate the light by blinds and curtains.

Heavy, thick, dark window or bed curtains should, however, hardly ever be used for any kind of sick in this country. A light white curtain at the head of the bed is, in general, all that is necessary, and a green blind to the window, to be drawn down only when necessary.

One of the greatest observers of human things (not physiological), says, in another language, "Where there is sun there is thought." All physiology goes to confirm this. Where is the shady side of deep valleys, there is cretinism. Where are cellars and the unsunned sides of narrow streets, there is the degeneracy and weakliness of the human race—mind and body equally degenerating.[57] Put the pale withering plant and human being into the sun,[58] and, if not too far gone, each will recover health and spirit.

Without sunlight we degenerate body and mind.

It is a curious thing to observe how almost all patients lie with their faces turned to the light, exactly as plants always make their way towards the light; a patient will even complain that it gives him pain "lying on that side." "Then why *do* you lie on that side?" He does not know,— but we do. It is because it is the side towards the window. A fashionable physician has recently published in a government report that he always turns his patients' faces from the light. Yes, but nature is stronger than fashionable physicians, and depend upon it she turns the faces back and *towards* such light as she can get. Walk through the wards of a hospital, remember the bed sides of private patients you have seen,[59] and count how many sick you ever saw lying with their faces towards the wall.

Almost all patients lie with their faces to the light.

X.—CLEANLINESS OF ROOMS AND WALLS.

Cleanliness of carpets and furniture.

IT cannot be necessary to tell a nurse that she should be clean or that she should keep her patient clean,—seeing that the greater part of nursing consists in preserving cleanliness. No ventilation can freshen a room or ward where the most scrupulous cleanliness is not observed. Unless the wind be blowing through the windows at the rate of twenty miles an hour, dusty carpets, dirty wainscots, musty curtains and furniture, will infallibly produce a close smell. I have lived in a large and expensively furnished London house, where the only constant inmate in two very lofty rooms, with opposite windows, was myself, and yet, owing to the above-mentioned dirty circumstances, no opening of windows could ever keep those rooms free from closeness; but the carpet and curtains having been turned out of the rooms altogether, they became instantly as fresh as could be wished. It is pure nonsense to say that in London a room cannot be kept clean. Many of our hospitals show the exact reverse.

Dust never removed now.

But no particle of dust is ever or can ever be removed or really got rid of by the present system of dusting. Dusting in these days means nothing but flapping the dust from one part of a room on to another with doors and windows closed. What you do it for, I cannot think. You had much better leave the dust alone, if you are not going to take it away altogether. For from the time a room begins to be a room, up to the time when it ceases to be one, no one atom of dust ever actually leaves its precincts. Tidying a room means nothing now but removing a thing from one place, which it has kept clean for itself, on to another and a dirtier one. Flapping by way of cleaning is only admissible in the case of pictures, or anything made of paper. The only way I know to *remove* dust, the plague of all lovers of fresh air, is to wipe everything with a damp cloth. And all furniture ought to be so made as that it may be wiped with a damp cloth without injury to itself, and so polished as that it may be damped without injury to others. To "dust," as it is now practised, truly means to distribute dust more equally over a room.

If you like to clean your furniture by laying out your clean clothes upon your dirty chairs or sofa, this is one way certainly of doing it. Having witnessed the morning process called "tidying the room," for many years, and with ever increasing astonishment, I can describe what it is. From the chairs, tables, or sofa, upon which the "things" have lain during the night, and which are therefore comparatively clean from dust or blacks,[60] the

How a room is dusted.

poor *"things"* having "caught" it, they are removed to other chairs, tables, sofas, upon which you could write your name with your finger in the dust or blacks. The *other* side of the "things" is therefore now evenly dirtied or dusted. The house-maid then flaps every thing, or some things, not out of her reach, with a thing called a duster—the dust flies up, then re-settles more equally than it lay before the operation. The room has now been "put to rights."[61]

Floors.

As to floors, the only really clean floor I know is the Berlin *lackered* floor,[62] which is wet rubbed and dry rubbed every morning to remove the dust. The French *parquet* is always more or less dusty, although infinitely superior in point of cleanliness and healthiness to our absorbent floor.

For a sick room, a carpet is perhaps the worst expedient which could by any possibility have been invented. If you must have a carpet, the only safety is to take it up two or three times a year, instead of once. A dirty carpet literally infects the room. And if you consider the enormous quantity of organic matter from the feet of people coming in, which must saturate it, this is by no means surprising.

Washing floors.

Washing floors of sick rooms is most objection-able, for this reason. In any school-room or ward, much inhabited, a smell, while the floor is being scoured, quite different from that of soap and water, is very perceptible. It is the exhalation from the organic matter which has saturated the absorbing floor from the feet and breath of the inhabitants.

This is one cause of erysipelas in hospitals.

Dry dirt is comparatively safe dirt. Wet dirt becomes dangerous.

Uncleansed towns in dry climates have been made pestilential by having a water-supply.

Doctors have proscribed scrubbing in hospitals. And nurses have done it in the earliest morning, so as not to be detected.

What is to be done?

In the sick room, the doctor should always be asked whether and at what hour he chooses the floor to be washed. If a patient can be moved, it will probably be best to wash the floor only when he can be taken into another room, and his own room dried by fire and opened windows before he returns. A dry day and not a damp one is, therefore, necessary.

But a private sick room (where there is not the same going to and fro as in a hospital ward) has been kept perfectly clean by wiping the floor with a damp cloth and drying it with a floor-brush.

All the furniture was wiped in the same way with a cloth wrung out of hot water—thus freeing the room from dust.

This was in an operation case.

In more than one hospital the purpose has been answered by planing the floors, saturating them with "drying" linseed oil, well rubbed in, staining them (for the sake of appearance merely), and using beeswax and turpentine.

The floor was cleaned by using a brush with a cloth tied over it. And if anything offensive was spilt, it was washed off immediately with soap and water and the place dried.

I hope the day will come in England when absorbent floors will cease to be ever used, whether in school-rooms, lunatic asylums, hospitals, or houses.

Papered, plastered, oil-painted walls.

As for walls, the worst is the papered wall; the next worst is plaster. But the plaster can be redeemed by frequent lime-washing; the paper requires frequent renewing. A glazed paper gets rid of a good deal of the danger. But the ordinary bed-room paper is all that it ought *not* to be.

Atmosphere in painted and papered rooms quite distin-guishable.

A person who has accustomed her senses to compare atmospheres proper and improper, for the sick and for children, could tell, blind-fold, the difference of the air in old painted and in old papered rooms, *caeteris paribus*. The latter will always be musty, even with all the windows open.

The close connection between ventilation and cleanliness is shown in this. An ordinary light paper will last clean much longer if there is an Arnott's ventilator in the chimney than it other-wise would.[63]

The best wall now extant is oil paint. From this you can wash the animal exuviae.*

These are what make a room musty.

The best wall for a sick-room or ward that could be made is pure white non-absorbent cement or glass, or glazed tiles, if they were made sightly enough. *Best kind of wall for a sick-room.*

Air can be soiled just like water. If you blow into water you will soil it with the animal matter from your breath. So it is with air. Air is always soiled in a room where walls and carpets are saturated with animal exhalations.

Want of cleanliness, then, in rooms and wards, which you have to guard against, may arise in three ways.

1. Dirty air coming in from without, soiled by sewer emanations, the evaporation from dirty streets, smoke, bits of unburnt fuel, bits of straw, bits of horse dung. *Dirty air from without.*

If people would but cover the outside walls of their houses with plain or encaustic tiles, what an incalculable improvement would there be in light, cleanliness, dryness, warmth, and consequently economy. The play of a fire-engine would then effectually wash the outside of a house. This kind *Best kind of wall for a house.*

---

* If you like to wipe your dirty door, or some portion of your dirty wall, by hanging up your clean gown or shawl against it on a peg, this is one way certainly, and the most usual way, and generally the only way of cleaning either door or wall in a bed-room. *How to keep your wall clean at the expense of your clothes.*

of *walling* would stand next to paving in improving the health of towns.

Dirty air from within. 2. Dirty air coming from within, from dust, which you often displace, but never remove. And this recalls what ought to be a *sine qua non*. Have as few ledges in your room or ward as possible. And under no pretence have any ledge whatever out of sight. Dust accumulates there, and will never be wiped off. This is a certain way to soil the air. Besides this, the animal exhalations from your inmates saturate your furniture. And if you never clean your furniture properly, how can your rooms or wards be anything but musty? Ventilate as you please, the rooms will never be sweet. Besides this, there is a constant *degradation*, as it is called, taking place from everything except polished or glazed articles—*e.g.*, in colouring certain green papers arsenic is used. Now in the very dust even, which is lying about in rooms hung with this kind of green paper, arsenic has been distinctly detected. You see your dust is anything but harmless; yet you will let such dust lie about your ledges for months, your rooms for ever.

Again, the fire fills the room with coal-dust.

Dirty air from the carpet. 3. Dirty air coming from the carpet. Above all, take care of the carpets, that the animal dirt left there by the feet of visitors does not stay there. Floors, unless the grain is filled up and polished, are just as bad. The smell, already mentioned, from the floor of a school-room or ward, when any moisture brings out the organic matter by which it is saturated, might alone be enough to warn us of the mischief that is going on.

The outer air, then, can only be kept clean by sanitary improvements, and by consuming smoke. The expense in soap, which this single improvement would save, is quite incalculable. Remedies.

The inside air can only be kept clean by excessive care in the ways mentioned above—to rid the walls, carpets, furniture, ledges, &c., of the organic matter and dust—dust consisting greatly of this organic matter—with which they become saturated, and which is what really makes the room musty.

Without cleanliness, you cannot have all the effect of ventilation; without ventilation, you can have no thorough cleanliness.

Very few people, be they of what class they may, have any idea of the exquisite cleanliness required in the sick-room. For much of what is here said applies less to the hospital than to the private sick-room. The smoky chimney, the dusty furniture, the utensils emptied but once a day, often keep the air of the sick constantly dirty in the best private houses.

The well have a curious habit of forgetting that what is to them but a trifling inconvenience, to be patiently "put up" with, is to the sick a source of suffering, delaying recovery, if not actually hastening death. The well are scarcely ever more than eight hours, at most, in the same room. Some change they can always make, if only for a few minutes. Even during the supposed eight hours, they can change their posture or their position in the room. But the sick man, who never leaves his bed, who cannot change by any movement of his own his air, or his light, or his warmth; who cannot obtain quiet, or get out of the smoke, or the smell, or the dust; he is really poisoned or depressed by what is to you the merest trifle.

"What can't be cured must be endured," is the very worst and most dangerous maxim for a nurse which ever was made. Patience and resignation in her are but other words for carelessness or indifference—contemptible, if in regard to herself; culpable, if in regard to her sick.

XI.—PERSONAL CLEANLINESS.

IN almost all diseases, the function of the skin Poisoning by the skin. is, more or less, disordered; and in many most important diseases nature relieves herself almost entirely by the skin. This is particularly the case with children. But the excretion, which comes from the skin, is left there, unless removed by washing or by the clothes. Every nurse should keep this fact constantly in mind,—for, if she allow her sick to remain unwashed, or their clothing to remain on them after being saturated with perspiration or other excretion, she is interfering injuriously with the natural processes of health just as effectually as if she were to give the patient a dose of slow poison by the mouth. Poisoning by the skin is no less certain than poisoning by the mouth—only it is slower in its operation.

The amount of relief and comfort experienced Ventilation and skin-cleanliness equally essential. by sick after the skin has been carefully washed and dried, is one of the commonest observations made at a sick bed. But it must not be forgotten that the comfort and relief so obtained are not all. They are, in fact, nothing more than a sign that the vital powers have been relieved by removing something that was oppressing them. The nurse, therefore, must never put off attending to the personal cleanliness of her patient under the plea that all that is to be gained is a little relief, which can be quite as well given later.

In all well-regulated hospitals this ought to be, and generally is, attended to. But it is very generally neglected with private sick.

Just as it is necessary to renew the air round a sick person frequently, to carry off morbid effluvia from the lungs and skin, by maintaining free ventilation, so is it necessary to keep the pores of the skin free from all obstructing excretions. The object, both of ventilation and of skin-cleanliness, is pretty much the same,—to wit, removing noxious matter from the system as rapidly as possible.

Care should be taken in all these operations of sponging, washing, and cleansing the skin, not to expose too great a surface at once, so as to check the perspiration, which would renew the evil in another form.

The various ways of washing the sick need not here be specified,—the less so as the doctors ought to say which is to be used.

In several forms of diarrhoea, dysentery, &c., where the skin is hard and harsh, the relief afforded by washing with a great deal of soft soap is incalculable. In other cases, sponging with tepid soap and water, then with tepid water, and drying with a hot towel will be ordered.

Every nurse ought to be careful to wash her hands very frequently during the day. If her face, too, so much the better.

One word as to cleanliness merely as cleanliness.

Compare the dirtiness of the water in which you have washed when it is cold without soap, cold with soap, hot with soap. You will find the first has hardly removed any dirt at all, the second a little more, the third a great deal more. But hold your hand over a cup of hot water for a minute or two, and then, by merely rubbing with the finger, you will bring off flakes of dirt or dirty skin. After a vapour bath you may peel your whole self clean in this way. What I mean is, that by simply washing or sponging with water you do not really clean your skin. Take a rough towel, dip one corner in very hot water,—if a little spirit be added to it it will be more effectual,—and then rub as if you were rubbing the towel into your skin with your finger. The black flakes which will come off will convince you that you were not clean before, however much soap and water you have used. These flakes are what require removing. And you can really keep yourself cleaner with a tumbler of hot water and a rough towel and rubbing, than with a whole apparatus of bath and soap and sponge, without rubbing. It is quite nonsense to say that anybody need be dirty. Patients have been kept as clean by these means on a long

Steaming and rubbing the skin.

voyage, when a basin full of water could not be afforded, and when they could not be moved out of their berths, as if all the appurtenances of home had been at hand.

Washing, however, with a large quantity of water has quite other effects than those of mere cleanliness. The skin absorbs the water and becomes softer and more perspirable. To wash with soap and soft water is, therefore, desirable from other points of view than that of cleanliness.

Soft Water. But the water must be soft. People very little think of this. They think mainly of hard water as chapping their hands, not as being a promoter of drunkenness, uncleanliness, indigestion. It is very little observed that "water-dressings," every day more used by surgeons, have absolutely the opposite effect, viz., poisoning the sore, when made with very hard water, to what they have, viz. cleansing and healing the sore, when the water is soft. When water is hard, it is worth while to have distilled water for every water-dressing. For all washing of the sick, it is worth while to collect rain-water, or condense steam from a boiler, or to boil water, which will often remove from one-half to three-fourths of the hardness. Soap and *hard* water actually dirty your patient's skin. The oil in the soap, the exudations from the skin, and the lime in the water, unite to form a kind of varnish upon the skin, which comes off in the above-mentioned black flakes when rubbed.

The use of soft or filtered water for making tea or drinks, boiling vegetables, or mixing medicines, is very important. A careless nurse sometimes takes the water from the wash-hand stand for this last purpose. She had often as well not give the medicine at all.

———————

XII.—CHATTERING HOPES AND ADVICES.

THE sick man to his advisers.

"My advisers! Their name is Legion.[64] * * * Somehow or other, it seems a provision of the universal destinies, that every man, woman, and child should consider him, her, or itself privileged especially to advise me. Why? That is precisely what I want to know." And this is what I have to say to them. I have been advised to go to every place extant in and out of England—to take every kind of exercise by every kind of cart, carriage—yes, and even swing (!) and dumb-bell (!) in existence; to imbibe every different kind of stimulus that ever has been invented. And this when those *best* fitted to know, viz., medical men, after long and close attendance, had declared any journey out of the question, had prohibited any kind of motion whatever, had closely laid down the diet and drink. What would my advisers say, were they the medical attendants, and I, the patient, left their advice, and took the casual adviser's? But the singularity in Legion's mind is this: it never occurs to him that everybody else is doing the same thing, and that I, the patient, *must* perforce say, in sheer self-defence, like Rosalind, "I could not do with all."[65]

"Chattering Hopes" may seem an odd heading. But I really believe there is scarcely a greater worry which invalids have to endure than the incurable hopes of their friends. There is no one practice against which I can speak more strongly from actual personal experience, wide and long, of its effects during sickness observed both upon others and upon myself.[66] I would appeal most seriously to all friends, visitors, and attendants of the sick to leave off this practice of attempting to "cheer" the sick by making light of their danger and by exaggerating their probabilities of recovery.

Far more now than formerly does the medical attendant tell the truth to the sick who are really desirous to hear it about their own state.

How intense is the folly, then, to say the least of it, of the friend, be he even a medical man, who thinks that his opinion, given after a cursory observation, will weigh with the patient, against the opinion of the medical attendant, given, perhaps after years of observation, after using every help to diagnosis afforded by the stethoscope, the examination of pulse, tongue, &c.; and certainly after much more observation than the friend can possibly have had.

Supposing the patient to be possessed of common sense,—how can the "favourable" opinion, if

Chattering hopes the bane of the sick.

it is to be called an opinion at all, of the casual visitor "cheer" him,—when different from that of the experienced attendants. Unquestionably the latter may, and often does, turn out to be wrong. But which is most likely to be wrong?

Patient does not want to talk of himself. The fact is, that the patient is not "cheered" at all by these well-meaning, most tiresome friends.[67]

Absurd statistical comparisons made in common conversation by sensible people for the benefit of the sick. *There are, of course, cases, as in first confinements, when an assurance from the doctor or experienced nurse to the frightened suffering woman that there is nothing unusual in her case, that she has nothing to fear but a few hours' pain, may cheer her most effectually. This is advice of quite another order. It is the advice of experience to utter inexperience. But the advice we have been referring to is the advice of inexperience to bitter experience; and, in general, amounts to nothing more than this, that *you* think *I* shall recover from consumption, because somebody knows somebody somewhere who has recovered from fever.

I have heard a doctor condemned whose patient did not, alas! recover, because another doctor's patient of a *different* sex, of a *different* age, recovered from a *different disease*, in a *different* place. Yes, this is really true. If people who make these comparisons did but know (only they do not care to know), the care and preciseness with which such comparisons require to be made, (and are made), in order to be of any value whatever, they would spare their tongues. In comparing the deaths of one hospital with those of another, any statistics are justly considered absolutely valueless which do not give the ages, the sexes, and the diseases of all the cases. It does not seem necessary to mention this. It does not seem necessary to say that there can be no comparison between old men with dropsies and young women with consumptions. Yet the cleverest men and the cleverest women are often heard making such comparisons, ignoring entirely sex, age, disease, place—in fact, *all* the conditions essential to the question. It is the merest *gossip*.

On the contrary, he is depressed and wearied. If, on the one hand, he exerts himself to tell each successive member of this too numerous conspiracy, whose name is Legion, why he does not think as they do,—in what respect he is worse,—what symptoms exist that they know nothing of,—he is fatigued instead of "cheered," and his attention is fixed upon himself. In general, patients who! are really ill, do not want to talk about themselves. Hypochondriacs do, but again I say we are not on the subject of hypochondriacs.

If, on the other hand, and which is much more frequently the case, the patient says nothing, but the Shakesperian "Oh!" "Ah!" "Go to!" and "In good sooth!"[68] in order to escape from the conversation about himself the sooner, he is depressed by want of sympathy. He feels isolated in the midst of friends. He feels what a convenience it would be, if there were any single person to whom he could speak simply and openly, without pulling the string upon himself of this shower-bath of silly hopes and encouragements; to whom he could express his wishes and directions without that person persisting in saying, "I hope that it will please God yet to give you twenty years," or, "You have a long life of activity before you." How often we see at the end of biographies, or of cases recorded in medical papers, "after a long illness A. died rather suddenly," or, "unexpectedly, both to himself and to others." "Unexpectedly" to others,

Absurd consolations put forth for the benefit of the sick.

perhaps, who did not see, because they did not look; but by no means "unexpectedly to himself," as I feel entitled to believe, both from the internal evidence in such stories, and from watching similar cases: there was every reason to expect that A. would die, and he knew it; but he found it useless to insist upon his knowledge to his friends.

In these remarks I am alluding neither to acute cases which terminate rapidly nor to "nervous" cases.

By the first much interest in their own danger is very rarely felt. In writings of fiction, whether novels or biographies, these death-beds are generally depicted as almost seraphic in lucidity of intelligence. Sadly large has been my experience in death-beds, and I can only say that I have seldom or never seen such. Indifference, excepting with regard to bodily suffering, or to some duty the dying man desires to perform, is the far more usual state.

The "nervous case," on the other hand, delights in figuring to himself and others a fictitious danger.

But the long chronic case, who knows too well himself, and who has been told by his physician that he will never enter active life again, who feels that every month he has to give up something he could do the month before—oh! spare such sufferers your chattering hopes. You do not know how you worry and weary them. Such real sufferers cannot bear to talk of themselves, still less to hope for what they cannot at all expect.

So also as to all the advice showered so profusely upon such sick, to leave off some occupation, to try some other doctor, some other house, climate, pill, powder, or specific; I say nothing of the inconsistency, for these advisers are sure to be the same persons who exhorted the sick man not to believe his own doctor's prognostics, because "doctors are always mistaken," but to believe some other doctor, because "this doctor is always right." Sure also are these advisers to be the persons to bring the sick man fresh occupation, while exhorting him to leave his own.

Wonderful is the face with which friends, lay and medical, will come in and worry the patient with recommendations to do something or other, having just as little knowledge as to its being feasible, or even safe for him, as if they were to recommend a man to take exercise, not knowing he had broken his leg. What would the friend say, if *he* were the medical attendant, and if the patient, because some *other* friend had come in, because somebody, anybody, nobody, had recommended something, anything, nothing, were to disregard *his* orders, and take that other body's recommendation? But people never think of this.

Wonderful presumption of the advisers of the sick.

A celebrated historical personage has related the common-places which, when on the eve of executing a remarkable resolution, were showered

Advisers the same now as two hundred years ago.

in nearly the same words by every one around successively for a period of six months. To these the personage states that it was found least trouble always to reply the same thing, viz., that it could not be supposed that such a resolution had been taken without sufficient previous consideration. To patients enduring every day for years from every friend or acquaintance, either by letter or *vivâ voce*, some torment of this kind, I would suggest the same answer. It would indeed be spared, if such friends and acquaintances would but consider for one moment, that it is probable the patient has heard such advice at least fifty times before, and that, had it been practicable, it would have been practised long ago. But of such consideration there appears to be no chance. Strange, though true, that people should be just the same in these things as they were a few hundred years ago!

To me these commonplaces, leaving their smear upon the cheerful, single-hearted, constant devotion to duty, which is so often seen in the decline of such sufferers, recall the slimy trail left by the snail on the sunny southern garden-wall loaded with fruit.

Mockery of the advice given to sick.

No mockery in the world is so hollow as the advice showered upon the sick. It is of no use for the sick to say anything, for what the adviser wants is, *not* to know the truth about the state of the patient, but to turn whatever the sick may say to the support of his own argument, set forth, it must be repeated, without any inquiry whatever into the patient's real condition. "But it would be impertinent or indecent in me to make such an inquiry," says the adviser. True; and how much more impertinent is it to give your advice when you can know nothing about the truth, and admit you could not inquire into it.

To nurses I say—these are the visitors who do your patient harm. When you hear him told:—1. That he has nothing the matter with him, and that he wants cheering. 2. That he is committing suicide, and that he wants preventing. 3. That he is the tool of somebody who makes use of him for a purpose. 4. That he will listen to nobody, but is obstinately bent upon his own way; and 5. That he ought to be called to the sense of duty, and is flying in the face of Providence;—then know that your patient is receiving all the injury that he can receive from a visitor.

How little the real sufferings of illness are known or understood. How little does any one in good health fancy him or even *her*self into the life of a sick person.[69]

Do, you who are about the sick or who visit the sick, try and give them pleasure, remember to tell them what will do so. How often in such visits the sick person has to do the whole conversation, exerting his own imagination and memory,

Means of giving pleasure to the sick.

207

while you would take the visitor, absorbed in his own anxieties, making no effort of memory or imagination, for the sick person. "Oh! my dear, I have so much to think of, I really quite forgot to tell him that; besides, I thought he would know it," says the visitor to another friend. How could "he know it"? Depend upon it, the people who say this are really those who have little "to think of." There are many burthened with business who always manage to keep a pigeon-hole in their minds, full of things to tell the "invalid."

I do not say, don't tell him your anxieties— I believe it to be good for him and good for you too; but if you tell him what is anxious, surely you can remember to tell him what is pleasant too.

A sick person does so enjoy hearing good news: —for instance, of a love and courtship, while in progress to a good ending. If you tell him only when the marriage takes place, he loses half the pleasure, which Gods knows he has little enough of; and ten to one but you have told him of some love-making with a bad ending.

A sick person also intensely enjoys hearing of any *material* good, any positive or practical success of the right. He has so much of books and fiction, of principles, and precepts, and theories; do, instead of advising him with advice he has heard at least fifty times before, tell him of one benevolent act which has really succeeded practically,—it is like a day's health to him.*

You have no idea what the craving of sick with undiminished power of thinking, but little power of doing, is to hear of good practical action, when they can no longer partake in it.

Do observe these things, especially with invalids. Do remember how their life is to them disappointed and incomplete. You see them lying there with miserable disappointments, from which they can have no escape but death, and you can't remember to tell them of what would give them so much pleasure, or at least an hour's variety.

They don't want you to be lachrymose and whining with them, they like you to be fresh and active and interested, but they cannot bear absence of mind, and they are so tired of the advice and preaching they receive from every body, no matter whom it is, they see.

There is no better society than babies and sick people for one another. Of course you must manage this so that neither shall suffer from it, which is perfectly possible. If you think the "air

---

* A small pet animal is often an excellent companion for the sick, for long chronic cases especially. A bird in a cage is sometimes the only pleasure of an invalid confined for years to the same room. If he can feed and clean the animal himself, he ought always to be encouraged and assisted to do so. An invalid, in giving an account of his nursing by a nurse and a dog, infinitely preferred that of the dog: "above all, it did not *talk*."

of the sick room" bad for the baby, why it is bad for the invalid too, and, therefore, you will of course correct it for both. It freshens up a sick person's whole mental atmosphere to see "the baby." And a very young child, if unspoiled, will generally adapt itself wonderfully to the ways of a sick person, if the time they spend together is not too long.

If you knew how unreasonably sick people suffer from reasonable causes of distress, you would take more pains about all these things. An infant laid upon the sick bed will do the sick person, thus suffering, more good than all your eloquence. A piece of good news will do the same. Perhaps you are afraid of "disturbing" him. You say there is no comfort for his present cause of affliction. It is perfectly reasonable. The distinction is this, if he is obliged to act, do not "disturb" him with another subject of thought just yet; help him to do what he wants to do: but, if he *has* done this, or if nothing *can* be done, then "disturb" him by all means. You will relieve, more effectually, unreasonable suffering from reasonable causes by telling him "the news," showing him "the baby," or giving him something new to think of or to look at than by all the logic in the world.

It has been very justly said that sick and invalids are like children in this, there is no *proportion* in events to them. Now it is your business as their visitor to restore this right proportion for them—

to show them what the rest of the world is doing. How can they find it out otherwise? You will find them far more open to conviction than children in this. And you will find that their unreasonable intensity of suffering from unkindness, from want of sympathy, &c., will disappear with their freshened interest in the big world's events. But then you must be able to give them real interests, not gossip.*

* NOTE.—There are two classes of patients which are unfortunately becoming more common every day, especially among women of the richer orders, to whom all these remarks are pre-eminently inapplicable. 1. Those who make health an excuse for doing nothing, and at the same time allege that the being able to do nothing is their only grief. 2. Those who have brought upon themselves ill-health by over pursuit of amusement, which they and their friends have most unhappily called intellectual activity. I scarcely know a greater injury that can be inflicted than the advice too often given to the first class "to vegetate"—or than the admiration too often bestowed on the latter class for "pluck."

Two new classes of patients peculiar to this generation.

XIII. OBSERVATION OF THE SICK.

THERE is no more silly or universal question scarcely asked than this, "Is he better?" Ask it of the medical attendant, if you please. But of whom else, if you wish for a real answer to your question, would you ask it? Certainly not of the casual visitor; certainly not of the nurse, while the nurse's observation is so little exercised as it is now. What you want are facts, not opinions—for who can have any opinion of any value as to whether the patient is better or worse, excepting the constant medical attendant, or the really observing nurse?

The most important practical lesson that can be given to nurses is to teach them what to observe—how to observe—what symptoms indicate improvement—what the reverse—which are of importance—which are of none—which are the evidence of neglect—and of what kind of neglect.

All this is what ought to make part, and an essential part, of the training of every nurse. At present how few there are, either professional or unprofessional, who really know at all whether any sick person they may be with is better or worse.

The vagueness and looseness of the information one receives in answer to that much abused question, "Is he better?" would be ludicrous, if it were not painful. The only sensible answer (in the present state of knowledge about sickness) would be "How can I know? I cannot tell how he was when I was not with him."

I can record but a very few specimens of the answers which I have heard made by friends and nurses, and accepted by physicians and surgeons at the very bed-side of the patient, who could have contradicted every word but did not—sometimes from amiability, often from shyness, oftenest from languor!

"How often have the bowels acted, nurse?" "Once, sir." This generally means that the utensil has been emptied once, it having been used perhaps seven or eight times.

"Do you think the patient is much weaker than he was six weeks ago?" "Oh no, sir; you know it is very long since he has been up and dressed, and he can get across the room now." This means that the nurse has not observed that whereas six weeks ago he sat up and occupied himself in bed, he now lies still doing nothing; that, although he can "get across the room," he cannot stand for five seconds.

Another patient who is eating well, recovering steadily although slowly, from fever, but cannot walk or stand, is represented to the doctor as making no progress at all.

Want of truth the result of want of observation.[70]

It is a much more difficult thing to speak the truth than people commonly imagine. There is the want of observation *simple*, and the want of observation *compound*, compounded, that is, with the imaginative faculty. Both may equally intend to speak the truth. The information of the first is simply defective. That of the second is much more dangerous. The first gives, in answer to a question asked about a thing that has been before his eyes perhaps for years, information exceedingly imperfect, or says he does not know. He has never observed. And people simply think him stupid.

The second has observed just as little, but imagination immediately steps in, and he describes the whole thing from imagination merely, being perfectly convinced all the while that he has seen or heard it; or he will repeat a whole conversation, as if it were information which had been addressed to him; whereas it is merely what he has himself said to somebody else. This is the commonest of all. These people do not even observe that they have *not* observed nor remember that they have forgotten.

Courts of justice seem to think that anybody can speak "the whole truth and nothing but the truth," if he does but intend it. It requires many faculties combined of observation and memory to speak "the whole truth" and to say "nothing but the truth."

"I knows I fibs dreadful: but believe me, Miss,

I never finds out I have fibbed until they tells me so," was a remark actually made. It is also one of much more extended application than most people have the least idea of.

Concurrence of testimony, which is so often adduced as final proof, may prove nothing more, as is well known to those accustomed to deal with the unobservant imaginative, than that one person has told his story a great many times.

I have heard thirteen persons "concur" in declaring that a fourteenth, who had never left his bed, went to a distant chapel every morning at seven o'clock.

I have heard persons in perfect good faith declare, that a man came to dine every day at the house where they lived, who had never dined there once; that a person had never taken the sacrament, by whose side they had twice at least knelt at Communion; that but one meal a day came out of a hospital kitchen, which for six weeks they had seen provide from three to five and six meals a day. Such instances might be multiplied *ad infinitum* if necessary.

Questions as asked now (but too generally) of, or about patients, would obtain no information at all about them, even if the person asked of had every information to give. The question is generally a leading question: and it is singular that people never think what must be the answer to this question before they ask it; for instance, "Has he

Leading questions useless or misleading.

had a good night?" Now, one patient will think he has a bad night if he has not slept ten hours without waking. Another does not think he has a bad night if he has had intervals of dosing occasionally. The same answer has actually been given as regarded two patients—one who had been entirely sleepless for five times twenty-four hours, and died of it, and another who had not slept the sleep of a regular night, without waking. Why cannot the question be asked, How many hours' sleep has — had? and at what hours of the night? This is important, because on this depends what the remedy will be. If a patient sleeps two or three hours early in the night, and then does not sleep again at all, ten to one it is not a narcotic he wants,[71] but food or stimulus, or perhaps only warmth. If, on the other hand, he is restless and awake all night, and is drowsy in the morning, he probably wants sedatives, either quiet, coolness, or medicine, a lighter diet, or all four. Now the doctor should be told this, or how can he judge what to give? "I have never closed my eyes all night," an answer as frequently made when the speaker has had several hours' sleep as when he has had none, would then be less often said. Lies, intentional and unintentional, are much seldomer told in answer to precise than to leading questions. Another frequent error is to inquire, whether one cause remains, and not whether the effect which may be produced by a great many different causes, *not* inquired after, remains. As when it is asked, whether there was noise in the street last night; and if there were not, the patient is reported, without more ado, to have had a good night. Patients are completely taken aback by these kinds of leading questions, and give only the exact amount of information asked for, even when they know it to be completely misleading. The shyness of patients is seldom allowed for.

How few there are who, by five or six pointed questions, can elicit the whole case and get accurately to know and to be able to report *where* the patient is.

I knew a very clever physician, of large dispensary and hospital practice, who invariably began his examination of each patient with "Put your finger where you *be* bad." That man would never waste his time with collecting inaccurate information from nurse or patient. Leading questions always collect inaccurate information.

At a recent celebrated trial, the following leading question was put successively to nine distinguished medical men. "Can you attribute these symptoms to anything else but poison?" And out of the nine, eight answered "No!" without any qualification whatever. It appeared, upon cross-examination:—1. That none of them had ever seen a case of the kind of poisoning supposed. 2. That none of them had ever seen a case of the kind of disease to which the death, if not to poison,

Means of obtaining inaccurate information.

was attributable. 3. That none of them were even aware of the main fact of the disease and condition to which the death was attributable.

Surely nothing stronger can be adduced to prove what use leading questions are of, and what they lead to.

I had rather not say how many instances I have known, where, owing to this system of leading questions, the patient has died, and the attendants have been actually unaware of the principal feature of the case.

As to food patient takes or does not take.

It is useless to go through all the particulars, besides sleep, in which people have a peculiar talent for gleaning inaccurate information. As to food, for instance, I often think that most common question, How is your appetite? can only be put because the questioner believes the questioned has really nothing the matter with him, which is very often the case. But where there is, the remark holds good which has been made about sleep. The *same* answer will often be made as regards a patient who cannot take two ounces of solid food per diem, and a patient who does not enjoy five meals a day as much as usual.

Again, the question, How is your appetite? is often put when How is your digestion? is the question meant. No doubt the two things often depend on one another. But they are quite different. Many a patient can eat, if you can only "tempt his appetite." The fault lies in your not having got him the thing that he fancies. But many another patient does not care between grapes and turnips, —everything is equally distasteful to him. He would try to eat anything which would do him good; but everything "makes him worse." The fault here generally lies in the cooking. It is not his "appetite" which requires "tempting," it is his digestion which requires sparing. And good sick cookery will save the digestion half its work.

There may be four different causes, any one of which will produce the same result, viz., the patient slowly starving to death from want of nutrition.

1. Defect in cooking;
2. Defect in choice of diet;
3. Defect in choice of hours for taking diet;
4. Defect of appetite in patient.

Yet all these are generally comprehended in the one sweeping assertion that the patient has "no appetite."

Surely many lives might be saved by drawing a closer distinction; for the remedies are as diverse as the causes. The remedy for the first is, to cook better; for the second, to choose other articles of diet; for the third, to watch for the hours when the patient is in want of food; for the fourth, to show him what he likes, and sometimes unexpectedly. But no one of these remedies will do for any other of the defects not corresponding with it.

It cannot too often be repeated that patients are generally either too languid to observe these things, or too shy to speak about them; nor is it well that they should be made to observe them, it fixes their attention upon themselves.

Again, I say, what *is* the nurse or friend there for except to take note of these things, instead of the patient doing so?

More important to spare the patient thought than physical exertion.

It is commonly supposed that the nurse is there to spare the patient from making physical exertion for himself—I would rather say, that she ought to be there to spare him from taking thought for himself. And I am quite sure, that if the patient were spared all thought for himself and *not* spared all physical exertion, he would be the gainer. The reverse is generally the case in the private house. In the hospital it is the relief from all anxiety, afforded by the rules of a well-regulated institution, which has often such a beneficial effect upon the patient.

"Can I do anything for you?" says the thoughtless nurse—and the uncivil patient invariably answers "no"—the civil patient, "no, thank you." The fact is, that a real patient will rather go without almost anything than make the exertion of thinking *what* the nurse has left undone. And surely it is for her, not for him, to make this exertion. Such a question is, on her part, a mere piece of laziness, under the guise of being "obliging." She wishes to throw the trouble on the patient of nursing himself.

Again, the question is sometimes put, Is there diarrhoea? And the answer will be the same, whether it is just merging into cholera, whether it is a trifling degree brought on by some trifling indiscretion, which will cease the moment the cause is removed, or whether there is no diarrhoea at all, but simply relaxed bowels.

Means of obtaining inaccurate information as to diarrhoea.

It is useless to multiply instances of this kind. As long as observation is so little cultivated as it is now, I do believe that it is better for the physician *not* to see the friends of the patient at all. They will oftener mislead him than not. And as often by making the patient out worse as better than he really is.

In the case of infants, *everything* must depend upon the accurate observation of the nurse or mother who has to report. And how seldom is this condition of accuracy fulfilled!

It is the real test of a nurse whether she can nurse a sick infant. Of *it* she can never ask, "Can I do anything for you?"

A celebrated man,[72] though celebrated only for foolish things, has told us that one of his main objects in the education of his son, was to give him a ready habit of accurate observation, a certainty of perception, and that for this purpose one of his means was a month's course as follows:—he took the boy rapidly past a toy-shop; the father and son then described to each other as many of the objects as they could, which they had seen in passing the

Means of cultivating sound and ready observation.

windows, noting them down with pencil and paper, and returning afterwards to verify their own accuracy. The boy always succeeded best, *e.g.*, if the father described 30 objects, the boy did 40, and scarcely ever made a mistake.

How wise a piece of education this would be for much higher objects; and in our calling of nurses the thing itself is essential. For it may safely be said, not that the habit of ready and correct observation will by itself make us useful nurses, but that without it we shall be useless with all our devotion.

One nurse in charge of a set of wards not only carries in her head all the little varieties in the diets which each patient is allowed to fix for himself, but also exactly what each patient has taken during each day. Another nurse, in charge of one single patient, takes away his meals day after day all but untouched, and never knows it.

If you find it helps you to note down such things on a bit of paper, in pencil, by all means do so. Perhaps it more often lames than strengthens the memory and observation. But if you cannot get the habit of observation one way or other, you had better give up the being a nurse, for it is not your calling, however kind and anxious you may be.[73]

Surely you can learn at least to judge with the eye how much an oz. of solid food is, how much an oz. of liquid. You will find this helps your observation and memory very much, you will then say to yourself "A. took about an oz. of his meat to day;" "B. took three times in 24 hours about ¼ pint of beef tea;" instead of saying "B. has taken nothing all day," or "I gave A. his dinner as usual."

I have known several of our real old-fashioned hospital "sisters," who could, as accurately as a measuring glass, measure out all their patient's wine and medicine by the eye, and never be wrong. I do not recommend this,—one must be very sure of one's self to do it. I only mention it, because if a nurse can by practice measure medicine by the eye, surely she is no nurse who cannot measure by the eye about how much food (in oz.) her patient has taken. In hospitals those who cut up the diets give with quite sufficient accuracy, to each patient, his 12 oz. or his 6 oz. of meat without weighing. Yet a nurse will often have patients loathing all food and incapable of any will to get well, who just tumble over the contents of the plate or dip the spoon in the cup to deceive the nurse, and she will take it away without ever seeing that there is just the same quantity of food as when she brought it, and she will tell the doctor, too, that the patient has eaten all his diets as usual, when all she ought to have meant is that she has taken away his diets as usual.

Now what kind of a nurse is this?

Sound and ready observation essential in a nurse.

English
women have
great capacity
of but little
practice in
close observa-
tion.

It may be too broad an assertion, and it certainly sounds like a paradox. But I think that in no country are women to be found so deficient in ready and sound observation as in England, while peculiarly capable of being trained to it. The French or Irish woman is too quick of perception to be so sound an observer—the Teuton is too slow to be so ready an observer as the English woman might be. Yet English women lay themselves open to the charge so often made against them by men, viz., that they are not to be trusted in handicrafts to which their strength is quite equal, for want of a practiced and steady observation.[74] In countries, both Protestant and Roman Catholic, where women, both "secular" and "religious," (with average intelligence certainly not superior to that of, Englishwomen) are employed *e.g.*, in dispensing, men responsible for what these women do (not theorizing about man's and women's "missions"), have stated that they preferred the service of women to that of men, as being more exact, more careful, and incurring fewer mistakes of inadvertence.

Now certainly Englishwomen are peculiarly capable of attaining to this.

I remember when a child, hearing the story of an accident, related by some one who sent two nieces to fetch a "bottle of salvolatile from her room;" "Mary could not stir," she said, "Fanny ran and fetched a bottle that was not salvolatile, and that was not in my room."

Now this habit of inattention generally pursues a person through life. A woman is asked to fetch a large new bound red book, lying on the table by the window, and she fetches five small old boarded brown books lying on the shelf by the fire. And this, though she has "put that room to rights" every day for a month perhaps, and must have observed the books every day, lying in the same places, for a month, if she had any observation.

Habitual observation is the more necessary, when any sudden call arises. If "Fanny" had observed "the bottle of salvolatile" in "the aunt's room," every day she was there, she would more probably have found it when it was suddenly wanted.

There are two causes for these mistakes of inadvertence, 1. A want of ready attention; only part of the request is heard at all. 2. A want of the habit of observation.

To a nurse I would add, take care that you always put the same things in the same places; you don't know how suddenly you may be called on some day to find something, and may not be able to remember in your haste where you yourself had put it, if your memory is not in the habit of seeing the thing there always.

Some few of the instances in which nurses frequently fail in observation, may here be mentioned. There is a well-marked distinction between the excitable and what I will call the *accumulative* tem-

Difference of excitable and accumulative temperaments.

perament in patients. One will blaze up at once, under any shock or anxiety, and sleep very comfortably after it; another will seem quite calm and even torpid, under the same shock, and people say, "He hardly felt it at all," yet you will find him some time after slowly sinking. The same remark applies to the action of narcotics, of aperients, which, in the one, take effect directly, in the other not perhaps for twenty-four hours. A journey, a visit, an unwonted exertion, will affect the one immediately, but he recovers after it; the other bears it very well at the time, apparently, and dies or is prostrated for life by it. People often say how difficult the excitable temperament is to manage— I say how difficult is the *accumulative* temperament. With the first you have an out-break which you could anticipate, and it is all over. With the second you never know where you are— you never know when the consequences are over. And it requires your closest observation to know what *are* the consequences of what—for the consequent by no means follows immediately upon the antecedent—and coarse observation is utterly at fault.

Superstition the fruit of bad observation.

Almost all superstitions are owing to defective knowledge, to bad observation, to the *post hoc, ergo propter hoc;*[75] and bad observers are almost all superstitious. Farmers used to attribute disease among cattle to witchcraft; weddings have been attributed to seeing one magpie, deaths to seeing three;[76] and

I have heard the most highly educated now-a-days draw consequences for the sick closely resembling these.

Another remark: although there is unquestion- ably a physiognomy of disease as well as of health;[77] of all parts of the body, the face is perhaps the one which tells the least to the common observer or the casual visitor. Because, of all parts of the body, it is the one most exposed to other influences, besides health. And people never, or scarcely ever, observe enough to know how to distinguish between the effect of exposure, of robust health, of a tender skin, of a tendency to congestion, of suffusion, flushing, or many other things.[78] Again, the face is often the last to shew emaciation. I should say that the hand was a much surer test than the face, both as to flesh, colour, circulation, &c., &c. It is true that there are *some* diseases which are only betrayed at all by something in the face, *e.g.*, the eye or the tongue, as great irritability of brain by the appear- ance of the pupil of the eye. But we are talking of casual, not minute, observation. And few minute observers will hesitate to say that far more untruth than truth is conveyed by the oft repeated words, He *looks* well, or ill, or better or worse.

Wonderful is the way in which people will go upon the slightest observation, or often upon no observation at all, or upon some *saw* which the world's experience,[79] if it had any, would have pro- nounced utterly false long ago.

Physiognomy of disease little known.

I have known patients dying of sheer pain, exhaustion, and want of sleep, from one of the most lingering and painful diseases known, preserve, till within a few days of death, not only the healthy colour of the cheek, but the mottled appearance of a robust child. And scores of times have I heard these unfortunate creatures assailed with, "I am glad to see you looking so well." "I see no reason why you should not live till ninety years of age." "Why don't you take a little more exercise and amusement?" with all the other common-places with which we are so familiar.

There is, unquestionably, a physiognomy of disease. Let the nurse learn it.

The experienced nurse can always tell that a person has taken a narcotic the night before by the patchiness of the colour about the face, when the re-action of depression has set in; that very colour which the inexperienced will point to as a proof of health.

There is, again, a faintness, which does not betray itself by the colour at all, or in which the patient becomes brown instead of white. There is a faintness of another kind which, it is true, can always be seen by the paleness.

But the nurse seldom distinguishes. She will talk to the patient who is too faint to move, without the least scruple, unless he is pale and unless, luckily for him, the muscles of the throat are affected and he loses his voice.

Yet these two faintnesses are perfectly distinguishable, by the mere countenance of the patient.

Again, the nurse must distinguish between the idiosyncracies of patients. One likes to suffer out all his suffering alone, to be as little looked after as possible. Another likes to be perpetually made much of and pitied, and to have some one always by him. Both these peculiarities might be observed and indulged much more than they are. For quite as often does it happen that a busy attendance is forced upon the first patient, who wishes for nothing but to be "let alone," as that the second is left to think himself neglected.

Peculiarities of patients.

People have two ways of considering nursing. One is to consider it a troublesome and useless infliction (which it too often is), and to have as little of it as possible. The other is to consider it a "mystery." When a really good nurse is seen inducing a patient to do willingly what another nurse has entirely failed in, people look upon it as "genius," or as a kind of biological trick,[80] such as used to be practised some years ago in London.

Now, there is no "mystery" at all about it. Good nursing consists simply in observing the little things which are common to all sick, and those which are particular to each sick individual.

229

Some people have a curious power over animals. They can collect wild birds round them in a wood. This, once thought witchcraft, is now supposed to be some peculiar power, which we can't see into, like the calculating boy's.[81] It is nothing at all but the minute observation of the habits and instincts of birds.

So the "peculiar power" of one nurse, and the want of power of another over her patient, is nothing at all but minute observation in the former of what affects him, and want of observation in the latter.

In nothing is this more remarkable than in inducing patients to take food. A patient is sinking for want of it under one nurse; you put him under another, and he takes it directly. How is this? People say, oh! she has a command over her patients. It is no command. It is the way she feeds him, or the way she pillows his head, so that he can swallow comfortably. Opening the window will enable one patient to take his food; washing his face and hands another; merely passing a wet towel over the back of the neck, a third; a fourth, who is a depressed suicide, requires a little cheering to give him spirit to eat. The nurse amuses him with giving some variety to his ideas. I remember that, when very ill, the way in which one nurse put the spoon into my mouth enabled me to swallow, when I could not if I was fed by any one else.

It is just the observation of all these little things, no unintelligible "influence," which enables one woman to save life; it is the want of such observation which prevents another from finding the means to do so.

Even delirium, which seems to place the patient so out of the reach of all human relief, that he is shrieking and calling for you, and you cannot make him understand that you are there by him, is often increased by an awkward noise or touch, and yet the nurse who does so never perceives it.

Again, few things press so heavily on one suffering from long and incurable illness, as the necessity of recording in words from time to time, for the information of the nurse, who will not otherwise see, that he cannot do this or that, which he could do a month or a year ago. What is a nurse there for, if she cannot observe these things for herself? Yet I have known—and known too among those—and *chiefly* among those—whom money and position put in possession of everything which money and position could give—I have known, I say, more accidents, (fatal, slowly or rapidly,) arising from this want of observation among nurses than from almost anything else. Because a patient could get out of a warm bath alone a month ago—because a patient could walk as far as his bell a week ago, the nurse concludes that he can do so now. She has never observed

Nurse must observe for herself increase of patient's weakness, patient will not tell her.

the change; and the patient is lost from being left in a helpless state of exhaustion, till some one accidentally comes in. And this not from any unexpected apoplectic, paralytic, or fainting fit (though even these could be expected far more, at least, than they are now, if we did but *observe*). No, from the expected, or to be expected, inevitable, visible, calculable, uninterrupted increase of weakness, which none need fail to observe.

Again, a patient not usually confined to bed, is compelled by an attack of diarrhoea, vomiting, or other accident, to keep his bed for a few days; he gets up for the first time, and the nurse lets him go into another room, without coming in, a few minutes afterwards, to look after him. It never occurs to her that he is quite certain to be faint, or cold, or to want something. She says, as her excuse, Oh, he does not like to be fidgeted after. Yes, he said so some weeks ago; but he never said he did not like to be "fidgeted after," when he is in the state he is in now; and if he did, you ought to make some excuse to go in to him. More patients have been lost in this way than is at all generally known, viz., from relapses brought on by being left for an hour or two faint, or cold, or hungry, after getting up for the first time.

You do not know how small is the power of resistance in a weak patient—how he will succumb to habits of the nurse, which occasion him positive pain for the time and total prostration for the whole day, rather than remonstrate. A good nurse gets the patient into a good habit, such as washing and dressing at different times so as to spare his strength. A bad nurse succeeds, and the patient adopts her bad ways without a struggle. *Patients do what they are expected to do.* This is equally important to be remembered, for good as well as for bad.

Yet it appears that scarcely any improvement in the faculty of observing is being made. Vast has been the increase of knowledge in pathology— that science which teaches us the final change produced by disease on the human frame—scarce any in the art of observing the signs of the change while in progress. Or, rather, is it not to be feared that observation, as an essential part of medicine, has been declining?

Is the faculty of observing on the decline?

A high medical authority abroad (in a country where pathology is considered to be even farther advanced than in ours) says, Have you detected anything with the stethoscope? then it is already too late to do any good.

Which of us has not heard fifty times, from one or another, a nurse, or a friend of the sick, aye, and a medical friend too, the following remark:—"So A. is worse, or B is dead. I saw him the day before; I thought him so much better; there certainly was no appearance from which one could have expected so sudden (?) a change." I have never heard any one say, though one would think it the more natural thing,"There *must* have been *some* appearance, which I should have seen if I had but looked; let me try and remember what there was, that I may observe another time." No, this is not what people say. They boldly assert that there was nothing to observe, not that their observation was at fault.

Let people who have to observe sickness and death look back and try to register in their observation the appearances which have preceded relapse, attack, or death, and not assert that there were none, or that there were not the *right* ones.

Approach of death, paleness by no means an invariable effect, as we find in novels.

It falls to few ever to have had the opportunity of observing the different aspects which the human face puts on at the sudden approach of certain forms of death by violence; and as it is a knowledge of little use I only mention it here as being the most startling example of what I mean. In the nervous temperament the face becomes pale (this is the only *recognized* effect); in the sanguine temperament purple; in the bilious yellow, or every manner of colour in patches. Now, it is generally supposed that paleness is the one indication of almost any violent change in the human being, whether from terror, disease, or anything else. There can be no more false observation. Granted, it is the one recognized livery, as I have said—*de rigueur* in novels,[82] but nowhere else.

There are two habits of mind often equally misleading from correct conclusions:—(1.) a want of observation of conditions, and (2.) an inveterate habit of taking averages.

1. Men whose profession like that of medical men leads them to observe only, or chiefly, palpable and permanent organic changes are often just as wrong in their opinion of the result as those who do not observe at all. For instance, there is a cancer or a broken leg; the surgeon has only to look at it once to know; it will not be different if he sees it in the morning to what it would have been had he seen it in the evening. In whatever conditions the broken leg is, or is likely to be, there will still be the broken leg, until it is united. The same with many organic diseases. An experienced physician has but to feel the pulse once, and he knows that there is aneurism which will kill some time or other.

But with the great majority of cases, there is nothing of the kind; and the power of forming any correct opinion as to the result must entirely depend upon an enquiry into all the conditions in which the patient lives. In a complicated state of society in large towns, death, as every one of great experience knows, is far less often produced by any one organic disease, than by some illness, after many other diseases, producing just the sum of exhaustion necessary for death.

There is nothing so absurd, nothing so misleading as the verdict one so often hears: So-and-so has no organic disease,—there is no reason why he should not live to extreme old age; sometimes the clause is added, sometimes not: Provided he has quiet, good food, good air, &c., &c., &c.; the verdict is repeated by ignorant people *without* the latter clause; or there is no possibility of the conditions of the latter clause being obtained; and this, the *only* essential part of the whole, is made of no effect.

Observers look too much to what is palpable to their senses, not to what is implied by conditions.

I have known two cases, the one of a man who intentionally and repeatedly displaced a dislocation, and was kept and petted by all the surgeons, the other of one who was pronounced to have nothing the matter with him, there being no organic change perceptible, but who died within the week. In both these cases, it was the nurse who, by accurately pointing out what she had accurately observed, to the doctors, saved the one case from persevering in a fraud, the other from being discharged when actually in a dying state.

But one may even go further and say, that in diseases which have their origin in the feeble or irregular action of some function, and not in organic change, it is quite an accident if the doctor who sees the case only once a day, and generally at the same time, can form any but a negative idea of its real condition. In the middle of the day, when such a patient has been refreshed by light and air, by his tea, his beef tea, and his brandy, by hot bottles to his feet, by being washed and by clean linen, you can scarcely believe that he is the same person as he lay with a rapid fluttering pulse, with puffed eye-lids, with short breath, cold limbs, and unsteady hands, this morning. Now what is a nurse to do in such a case? Not cry, "Lord bless you, sir, why you'd have thought he were a dying all night." This may be true, but it is not the way to impress with the truth a doctor, more capable of forming a judgment from the facts, if he did but know them, than you are. What he wants is not your opinion, however respectfully given, but your facts. In all diseases it is important, but in diseases which do not run a distinct and fixed course, it is not only important, it is essential, that the facts the nurse alone can observe, should be accurately observed, and accurately reported to the doctor.

The nurse's attention should be directed to the Pulses. extreme variation there is not unfrequently in the pulse of such patients during the day. A very common case is this: Between 3 and 4 A.M. the pulse becomes quick, perhaps 130, and so thready it is not like a pulse at all, but like a string vibrating just underneath the skin. After this the patient gets no more sleep. About mid-day the pulse has come down to 80; and though feeble and compressible is a very respectable pulse. At night, if the patient has had a day of excitement, it is almost imperceptible. But, if the patient has had a good day, it is stronger and steadier and not quicker than at mid-day. This is a common history of a common pulse; and others, equally varying during the day, might be given. Now, in inflammation, which may almost always be detected by the pulse, in typhoid fever, which is accompanied by the low pulse that nothing will raise, there is no such great variation. And doctors and nurses become accustomed not to look for it. The doctor indeed cannot. But the variation is in itself an important feature.

Cases like the above often "go off rather suddenly," as it is called, from some trifling ailment of a few days, which just makes up the sum of exhaustion necessary to produce death. And everybody cries, Who would have thought it?— except the observing nurse, if there is one, who had always expected the exhaustion to come, from which there would be no rally, because she knew the patient had no capital in strength on which to draw, if he failed for a few days to make his barely daily income in sleep and nutrition.

Really good nurses are often distressed, because they cannot impress the doctor with the real danger of their patient; and quite provoked because the patient "will look," either "so much better" or "so much worse" than he really is "when the doctor is there." The distress is very legitimate, but it generally arises from the nurse not having the power of laying clearly and shortly before the doctor the facts from which she derives her opinion, or from the doctor being hasty and inexperienced, and not capable of eliciting them. A man who really cares for his patients, will soon learn to ask for and appreciate the information of a nurse, who is at once a careful observer and a clear reporter.

A nurse ought to be able to understand what the variations of the pulse imply, what its character indicates. It is not the absolute rate of the pulse which it signifies so much for you to know. At least, you ought to be able to form an accurate enough guess at its rate without counting. It is the character of the pulse which signifies. There is the "splashing" pulse, which implies aneurism. There is the pulse without an edge, which feels not like a ribbon, but a thread running along a space which it does not fill. There is the intermittent pulse of heart disease, the pulse of acute pleurisy, the pulse of peritonitis, the throbbing pulse which indicates acute inflammation or risk of haemorrhage. There is the rapid pulse of exhaustion in fever, which is the sign that the time has come for wine and stimulants. And upon the seizing of this time the patient's life constantly depends. The administration of the wine brings down the pulse. The doctor leaves orders that if re-action follows on depression, the wine is to be discontinued or the quantity diminished. This re-action is indicated by the pulse.

How can the nurse have any confidence in her

own work, how can she be the means of saving risk and suffering to her patient, if she is not made familiar with all these characters of pulse?

There is the low pulse which indicates the danger of gangrene or pyaemia. There is the pulse of apoplexy, which indicates the danger of bleeding,[83] sometimes practised even by unprofessional persons. There is the pulse of brain disease, the pulse of congestion, and many others. It is impossible to describe them on paper. They must be felt to be known. And it is a knowledge absolutely essential to a real nurse.

For this reason it is so necessary that her senses should be cultivated and acute. The same nurse who cannot distinguish by the ear the sound of her patient's bell will certainly not be able to distinguish by the touch the character of his pulse.[84] And she may commit frightful mistakes, which would make it better that she never should have had it put into her head to feel pulses at all.

To return to the observation of conditions.

To arrive at a sound judgment not only what the patient *is* but what he is likely to do must be taken into account.

I have heard a physician, deservedly eminent, assure the friends of a patient of his recovery. Why? Because he had now prescribed a course, every detail of which the patient had followed for years. And because he had forbidden a course which the patient could not by any possibility alter.

Undoubtedly a person of no scientific knowledge whatever but of observation and experience in these kinds of conditions, will be able to arrive at a much truer guess as to the probable duration of life of members of a family or inmates of a house, than the most scientific physician to whom the same persons are brought to have their pulse felt; no enquiry being made into their conditions.

In Life Insurance and such like societies, were they instead of having the persons examined by a medical man, to have the houses, conditions, ways of life, of these persons examined, at how much truer results would they arrive! W. Smith appears a fine hale man, but it might be known that the next cholera epidemic he runs a bad chance. Mr. and Mrs. J. are a strong healthy couple, but it might be known that they live in such a house, in such a part of London, so near the river that they will kill four-fifths of their children; which of the children will be the ones to survive might also be known.

2. Averages again seduce us away from minute observation. "Average mortalities" merely tell that so many per cent. die in this town, and so many in that, per annum. But whether A. or B. will be among these, the "average rate" of course does not tell. We know, say, that from 22 to 24 per 1,000 will die in London next year. But minute enquiries into conditions enable us to know that in such a district, nay, in such a street,—or even on one side of that street, in such a particular house, or even on one floor of that particular house, will be the excess of mortality; that is, the person

"Average rate of mortality" tells us only that so many per cent. will die. Observation must tell us *which* in the hundred they will be who will die.

will die who ought not to have died before old age.

Now, would it not very materially alter the opinion of whoever were endeavouring to form one, if he knew that from that floor of that house of that street the man came?

Much more precise might be our observations even than this and much more correct our conclusions.

It is well known that the same names may be seen constantly recurring on workhouse books for generations. That is, the persons were born and brought up, and will be born and brought up, generation after generation, in the conditions which make paupers. Death and disease are like the workhouse; they take from the same family, the same house, or in other words the same conditions. Why will we not observe what they are?

The close observer may safely predict that such a family, whether its members marry or not, will become extinct; that such another will degenerate morally and physically. But who learns the lesson? On the contrary, it may be well known that the children die in such a house at the rate of 8 out of 10; one would think that nothing more need be said; for how could Providence speak more distinctly?—yet nobody listens, the family goes on living there till it dies out, and then some other family takes it. Neither would they listen "if one rose from the dead."

In dwelling upon the vital importance of *sound* observation, it must never be lost sight of what observation is for. It is not for the sake of piling up miscellaneous information or curious facts, but for the sake of saving life and increasing health and comfort. The caution may seem useless, but it is quite surprising how many men (some women do it too), practically behave as if the scientific end were the only one in view, or as if the sick body were but a reservoir for stowing medicines into, and the surgical disease only a curious case the sufferer has made for the attendant's special information. This is really no exaggeration. You think, if you suspected your patient was being poisoned, say, by a copper kettle, you would instantly, as you ought, cut off all possible connection between him and the suspected source of injury, without regard to the fact that a curious mine of observation is thereby lost. But it is not everybody who does so, and it has actually been made a question of medical ethics, what should the medical man do if he suspected poisoning? The answer seems a very simple one,—insist on a confidential nurse being placed with the patient, or give up the case.

And remember, every nurse should be one who is to be depended upon, in other words, capable of being a "confidential" nurse. She does not know how soon she may find herself placed in such a situation; she must be no gossip, no vain talker;

What observation is for.

What a confidential nurse should be.

she should never answer questions about her sick except to those who have a right to ask them; she must, I need not say, be strictly sober and honest; but more than this, she must be a religious and devoted woman; she must have a respect for her own calling, because God's precious gift of life is often literally placed in her hands; she must be a sound, and close, and quick observer; and she must be a woman of delicate and decent feeling.[85]

Observation is for practical purposes.

To return to the question of what observation is for:—It would really seem as if some had considered it as its own end, as if detection, not cure, was their business; nay more, in a recent celebrated trial, three medical men, according to their own account, suspected poison, prescribed for dysentery, and left the patient to the poisoner. This is an extreme case. But in a small way, the same manner of acting falls under the cognizance of us all. How often the attendants of a case have admitted that they knew perfectly well that the patient could not get well in such an air, in such a room, or under such circumstances, yet have gone on dosing him with medicine, and making no effort to remove the poison from him, or him from the poison which they knew was killing him; nay, more, have sometimes not so much as mentioned their conviction in the right quarter—that is, to the only person who could act in the matter.

CONCLUSION.

———

THE whole of the preceding remarks apply even more to children and to puerperal women than to patients in general. They also apply to the nursing of surgical, quite as much as to that of medical cases. Indeed, if it be possible, cases of external injury require such care even more than sick.[86] In surgical wards, one duty of every nurse certainly is *prevention*. Fever, or hospital gangrene, or pyaemia, or purulent discharge of some kind may else supervene. Has she a case of compound fracture, of amputation, or of erysipelas, it may depend very much on how she looks upon the things enumerated in these notes, whether one or other of these hospital diseases attacks her patient or not. If she allows her ward to become filled with the peculiar close foetid smell, so apt to be produced among surgical cases, especially where there is great suppuration and discharge, she may see a vigorous patient in the prime of life gradually sink and die where, according to all human probability, he ought to have recovered. The surgical nurse must be ever on the watch, ever on her

Sanitary nursing as essential in surgical as in medical cases, but not to supersede surgical nursing.

guard, against want of cleanliness, foul air, want of light, and of warmth.

Nevertheless let no one think that because *sanitary* nursing is the subject of these notes, therefore, what may be called the handicraft of nursing is to be undervalued. A patient may be left to bleed to death in a sanitary palace.[87] Another who cannot move himself may die of bed-sores, because the nurse does not know how to change and clean him, while he has every requisite of air, light, and quiet. But nursing, as a handi-craft, has not been treated of here for three reasons: 1. that these notes do not pretend to be a manual for nursing, any more than for cooking for the sick; 2. that the writer, who has herself seen more of what may be called surgical nursing, *i.e.*, practical manual nursing, than, perhaps, any one in Europe, honestly believes that it is impossible to learn it from any book, and that it can only be thoroughly learnt in the wards of a hospital; and she also honestly believes that the perfection of surgical nursing may be seen practised by the old-fashioned "Sister" of a London hospital, as it can be seen nowhere else in Europe. 3. While thousands die of foul air, &c., who have this surgical nursing to perfection, the converse is comparatively rare.[88]

Children their greater susceptibility to the same things.

To revert to children. They are much more susceptible than grown people to all noxious influ-ences. They are affected by the same things, but much more quickly and seriously, viz., by want of fresh air, of proper warmth, want of cleanliness in house, clothes, bedding, or body, by startling noises, improper food, or want of punctuality, by dulness and by want of light, by too much or too little covering in bed, or when up,—by want of the spirit of management generally in those in charge of them. One can, therefore, only press the import-ance, as being yet greater in the case of children, greatest in the case of sick children, of attending to these things.

That which, however, above all, is known to injure children seriously is foul air, and most seriously at night. Keeping the rooms where they sleep tight shut up, is destruction to them. And, if the child's breathing be disordered by disease, a few hours only of such foul air may endanger its life, even where no inconvenience is felt[89] by grown-up persons in the same room.

The following passages, taken out of an excellent "Lecture on Sudden Death in Infancy and Childhood," just published, show the vital im-portance of careful nursing of children.[90] "In the great majority of instances, when death suddenly befalls the infant or young child, it is an *accident*; it is not a necessary, inevitable result of any disease from which it is suffering."

It may be here added, that it would be very desirable to know how often death is, with adults, "not a necessary, inevitable result of any disease."

Omit the word "sudden;" (for *sudden* death is comparatively rare in middle age;) and the sentence is almost equally true for all ages.

The following causes of "accidental" death in sick children are enumerated:—"Sudden noises, which startle—a rapid change of temperature, which chills the surface, though only for a moment —a rude awakening from sleep—or even an over-hasty, or an over-full meal"—"any sudden impression on the nervous system—any hasty alteration of posture—in short, any cause whatever by which the respiratory process may be disturbed."

It may again be added, that, with very weak adult patients, these causes are also (not often "suddenly fatal," it is true, but) very much oftener than is at all generally known, irreparable in their consequences.

Both for children and for adults, both for sick and for well (although more certainly in the case of sick children than in any others), I would here again repeat, the most frequent and most fatal cause of all is sleeping, for even a few hours, much more for weeks and months, in foul air, a condition which, more than any other condition, disturbs the respiratory process, and tends to produce "accidental" death in disease.

I need hardly here repeat the warning against any confusion of ideas between cold and fresh air. You may chill a patient fatally without giving him fresh air at all. And you can quite well, nay, much better, give him fresh air without chilling him. This is the test of a good nurse.

In cases of long recurring faintnesses from diseases, for instance, especially disease which affects the organs of breathing, fresh air to the lungs, warmth to the surface, and often (as soon as the patient can swallow) hot drink, these are the right remedies and the only ones. Yet, oftener than not, you see the nurse or mother just reversing this; shutting up every cranny through which fresh air can enter, and leaving the body cold, or perhaps throwing a greater weight of clothes upon it, when already it is generating too little heat.

"Breathing carefully, anxiously, as though respiration were a function which required all the attention for its purpose," is cited as a not unusual state in children, and as one calling for care in all the things enumerated above. That breathing becomes an almost voluntary act, even in grown up patients who are very weak, must often have been remarked.

"Disease having interfered with the perfect accomplishment of the respiratory function, some sudden demand for its complete exercise, issues in the sudden stand still of the whole machinery," is given as one process:—"Life goes out for want of nervous power to keep the vital functions in activity," is given as another, by which "accidental" death is not often brought to pass in infancy.

Also in middle age, both these processes may

be seen ending in death, although generally not suddenly. And I have seen, even in middle age, the "*sudden* stand-still" here mentioned, and from the same causes.

To sum up:—the answer to two of the commonest objections urged, one by women themselves, the other by men, against the desirableness of sanitary knowledge for women, *plus* a caution, comprises the whole argument for the art of nursing.

Reckless amateur physicking by women. Real knowledge of the laws of health alone can check this.

(1.) It is often said by men, that it is unwise to teach women anything about these laws of health, because they will take to physicking,—that there is a great deal too much of amateur physicking as it is, which is indeed true. One eminent physician told me that he had known more calomel given, both at a pinch and for a continuance, by mothers, governesses, and nurses, to children than he had ever heard of a physician prescribing in all his experience. Another says, that women's only idea in medicine is calomel and aperients. This is undeniably too often the case. There is nothing ever seen in any professional practice like the reckless physicking by amateur females. Many ladies, having once obtained a "blue pill" prescription from a physician,[91] will give and take it as a common aperient two or three times a week—with what effect may be supposed. The physician, being informed of it, substitutes for the prescription a comparatively harmless aperient pill. The lady complains that it "does not suit her half so well."[92]

If women will take or give physic, by far the safest plan is to send for "the doctor" every time. There are those who both give and take physic, who will not take pains to learn the names of the commonest medicines, and confound, *e.g.*, colocynth with colchicum.[93] This *is* playing with sharp-edged tools "with a vengeance."

There are also excellent women who will write to London to their physician that there is much sickness in their neighbourhood in the country, and ask for some prescription from him, which they "used to like" themselves, and then give it to all their friends and to all their poorer neighbours who will take it. Now, instead of giving medicine, of which you cannot possibly know the exact and proper application, nor all its consequences, would it not be better if you were to persuade and help your poorer neighbours to remove the dung-hill from before the door, to put in a window which opens, or an Arnott's ventilator,[94] or to cleanse and lime-wash their cottages? Of these things the benefits are sure. The benefits of the inexperienced administration of medicines are by no means so sure.

Homoeopathy has introduced one essential amelioration in the practice of physic by amateur females; for its rules are excellent, its physicking comparatively harmless—the "globule" is the one grain of folly which appears to be necessary to make any good thing acceptable.[95] Let then women, if they will give medicine, give homoeopathic medicine. It won't do any harm.

An almost universal error among women is the supposition that everybody *must* have the bowels opened once in every twenty-four hours, or must fly immediately to aperients. The reverse is the conclusion of experience.

This is a doctor's subject, and I will not enter more into it; but will simply repeat, do not go on taking or giving to your children your abominable "courses of aperients," without calling in the doctor.

It is very seldom indeed, that by choosing your diet, you cannot regulate your own bowels; and every woman may watch herself to know what kind of diet will do this; deficiency of meat produces constipation, quite as often as deficiency of vegetables; baker's bread much oftener than either. Home-made brown bread will oftener cure it than anything else.

A really experienced and observing nurse neither physics herself nor others. And to cultivate in things pertaining to health observation and experience in women who are mothers, governesses, or nurses, is just the way to do away with amateur physicking, and, if the doctors did but know it, to make the nurses obedient to them,—helps to them instead of hindrances. Such education in women would indeed diminish the doctor's work—but no one really believes that doctors wish that there should be more illness, in order to have more work.

(2.) It is often said by women, that they cannot know anything of the laws of health, or what to do to preserve their children's health, because they can know nothing of "Pathology," or cannot "dissect,"—a confusion of ideas which it is hard to attempt to disentangle. Pathology teaches the harm that disease has done. But it teaches nothing more. We know nothing of the principle of health, the positive of which pathology is the negative, except from observation and experience. And nothing but observation and experience will teach us the ways to maintain or to bring back the state of health. It is often thought that medicine is the curative process. It is no such thing; medicine is the surgery of functions, as surgery proper is that of limbs and organs. Neither can do anything but remove obstructions; neither can cure; nature alone cures. Surgery removes the bullet out of the limb, which is an obstruction to cure, but nature heals the wound. So it is with medicine; the function of an organ becomes obstructed; medicine, so far as we know, assists nature to remove the obstruction; but does nothing more. And what nursing has to do in either case, is to put the patient in the best condition for nature to act upon him. Generally, just the contrary is done. You think fresh air, and quiet

What pathology teaches. What observation alone teaches. What medicine does. What nature alone does.

and cleanliness extravagant, perhaps dangerous, luxuries, which should be given to the patient only when quite convenient, and medicine the *sine quâ non,* the panacea. If I have succeeded in any measure in dispelling this illusion, and in showing what true nursing is, and what it is not, my object will have been answered.

Now for the caution:—

What does *not* make a good nurse.

(3.) It seems a commonly received idea among men, and even among women themselves, that it requires nothing but a disappointment in love,[96] the want of an object, a general disgust or incapacity for other things, to turn a woman into a good nurse.

This reminds one of the parish where a stupid old man was set to be schoolmaster because he was "past keeping the pigs."

Apply the above receipt for making a good nurse to making a good servant. And the receipt will be found to fail.

Yet popular novelists of recent days have invented ladies disappointed in love or fresh out of the drawing-room turning into the war-hospitals to find their wounded lovers, and when found, forthwith abandoning their sick-ward for their lover, as might be expected. Yet in the estimation of the authors, these ladies were none the worse for that, but on the contrary were heroines of nursing.[97]

What cruel mistakes are sometimes made by

benevolent men and women in matters of business about which they can know nothing, and think they know a great deal.

The everyday management of a large ward, let alone of a hospital—the knowing what are the laws of life and death for men, and what the laws of health for wards—(and wards are healthy or unhealthy, mainly according to the knowledge or ignorance of the nurse)—are not these matters of sufficient importance and difficulty to require learning by experience and careful inquiry, just as much as any other art? They do not come by inspiration to the lady disappointed in love, nor to the poor workhouse drudge hard-up for a livelihood.

And terrible is the injury which has followed to the sick from such wild notions!

In this respect (and why is it so?), in Roman Catholic countries, both writers and workers are, in theory at least, far before ours. They would never think of such a beginning for a good working Superior or Sister of Charity. And many a Superior has refused to admit a *Postulant* who appeared to have no better "vocation" or reasons for offering herself than these.

It is true *we* make "no vows." But is a "vow" necessary to convince us that the true spirit for learning any art, most especially an act of charity, aright, is not a disgust to everything or something else? Do we really place the love of our kind (and of nursing, as one branch of it,) so low as this? What would the Mère Angélique of Port Royal,[98] what would our own Mrs. Fry have said to this?[99]

The two jargons of the day.

I would earnestly ask my sisters to keep clear of both the jargons now current everywhere (for they *are* equally jargons);[100] of the jargon, namely, about the "rights" of women, which urges women to do all that men do, including the medical and other professions, merely because men do it, and without regard to whether this *is* the best that women can do; and of the jargon which urges woman to do nothing that men do, merely because they are women, and should be "recalled to a sense of their duty as women," and because "this is women's work," and "that is men's," and "these are things which women should not do," which is all assertion and nothing more. Surely woman should bring the best she has, *whatever* that is, to the work of God's world, without attending to either of these cries. For what are they, both of them, the one *just* as much as the other, but listening to the "what people will say," to opinion, to the "voices from without?" And as a wise man has said, no one has ever done anything great or useful by listening to the voices from without.

You do not want the effect of your good things to be, "How wonderful for a *woman!*" nor would you be deterred from good things, by hearing it said, "Yes, but she ought not to have done this, because it is not suitable for a woman." But you want to do the thing that is good, whether it is "suitable for a woman" or not.

It does not make a thing good, that it is remarkable that a woman should have been able to do it. Neither does it make a thing bad, which would have been good had a man done it, that it has been done by a woman.

Oh, leave these jargons, and go your way straight to God's work, in simplicity and singleness of heart.

SUPPLEMENTARY CHAPTER.

What is a Nurse?

THIS book takes away all the poetry of nursing, it will be said, and makes it the most prosaic of human things. My dear sister, there is nothing in the world, except perhaps education, so much the reverse of prosaic—or which requires so much power of throwing yourself into others' feelings which you have never felt,[101]—and if you have none of this power, you had better let nursing alone.[102] The very alphabet of a nurse is to be able to interpret every change which comes over a patient's countenance, without causing him the exertion of saying what he feels.[103] What would many a nurse do otherwise than she does, if her patient were a valuable piece of furniture or a sick cow? I do not know. Yet a nurse must be something more than a lift or a broom. A patient is not merely a piece of furniture, to be kept clean and ranged against the wall, and saved from injury or breakage —though to judge from what many a nurse does and does not do you would say he was. But watch a good old-fashioned monthly nurse with the infant;[104] she is firmly convinced, not only that she understands everything it "says," and that no one else can understand it, but also that it understands everything she says, and understands no one else.

Now a nurse *ought* to understand in the same way every change of her patient's face, every change of his attitude, every change of his voice. And she ought to study them till she feels sure that no one else understands them so well. She may make mistakes, but she is *on the way* to being a good nurse. Whereas the nurse who never observes her patient's countenance at all, and never expects to see any variation, any more than if she had the charge of delicate china, is on the way to nothing at all. She never will be a nurse.

"He hates to be watched," is the excuse of every careless nurse. Very true. All sick people and all children "hate to be watched." But find a nurse who really knows and understands her children and her patients, and see whether these are aware that they have been "watched." It is not the staring at a patient which tells the really observant nurse the little things she ought to know. The best observer I know, a man whose labours among lunatics have earned for him the gratitude of Europe, appears to be quite absent. He leans back in his chair, with half-shut eyes, and, meanwhile, he sees everything, hears everything, observes everything: and you feel he knows you better than many who have lived with you twenty years. I believe it is this singular capacity of observation and of understanding what observed appearances imply, which gives him his singular influence over lunatics.

Appearance of watching not good nursing.

People often talk of a nurse who has been ten or fifteen years with the sick, as being an "experienced nurse." But it is observation only which makes experience; and a woman who does not observe might be fifty or sixty years with the sick and never be the wiser.

What is experience?

Nay more, experience sometimes tells in the opposite direction. "A man who practices the blunders of his predecessors,"[105] is often said to be "a practical man;" and she who perpetuates the "blunders of her predecessors" is often called an experienced nurse. The friends of a patient have been known to recommend the lodging in which he fell ill, just for the very reason which made him ill. A nurse has alleged as her reason for doing the things by which her predecessor ruined her own and her patient's health, that her predecessor "had always done them." People have taken a house because it had been emptied by death of all its occupants. These are they whom *no* experience will teach—viz., those who cannot see or understand the practical results of what they and others do. Now it is *no* reason that A did it for B to do it. It would be a reason if the results of A's doing it had been proved to be good.

What strikes one most with many women, who call themselves nurses, is that they have not learnt this A B C of a nurse's education. The A of a nurse ought to be to know what a sick human being is. The B to know how to behave to a sick human being. The C to know that her patient is a sick human being and not an animal.

A nurse must feel a calling for her occupation.

What is it to feel a *calling* for any thing? Is it not to do your work in it to satisfy your own high idea of what is the *right,* the *best,* and not because you will be "found out" if you don't do it? This is the "enthusiasm" which every one, from a shoemaker to a sculptor, must have, in order to follow his "calling" properly. Now the nurse has to do, not with shoes, or with chisel and marble, but with human beings; and if she, for her own satisfaction, does not look after her patients, no *telling* will make her capable of doing so.

A nurse who has such a "calling" will, for her own satisfaction and interest in her patient, inform herself as to the state of his pulse, which can be quite well done without disturbing him. She will have observed the state of the secretions, whether told to do so or not. Nay, the very appearance of them, a slight difference in colour, will betray to her observing eye that the utensil has not been emptied after each motion.

She will, in like manner, have observed the state of the skin, whether there is dryness or perspiration—the effect of the diet, of the medicines, the stimulants. And it is remarkable how often the doctor is deceived in private practice by not being told that the patient has just had his meal or his brandy. She will most carefully have watched any redness or soreness of the skin, always on her guard against bed sores. Any increasing emaciation will never come unknown to her.[106] She will be well acquainted with the different eruptions of fevers, measles, &c., and premonitory symptoms. She will know the shiver which betrays the formation of matter[107]—that which shows the unconscious patient's desire to pass water—that which precedes fever. She will observe the changes of animal heat in her patient, and whether periodical, and not consider him as a piece of inorganic matter, in keeping him warm or cool.

A nurse who has such a "calling" will look at all the medicine bottles delivered to her for her patients, smell each of them, and, if not satisfied, taste each. Nine hundred and ninety-nine times there will be no mistake, but the thousandth time there may be a serious mistake detected by her means. But if she does not do this for her own satisfaction, it is no use telling her, because you may be sure that she will use neither smell nor taste to any purpose. *A nurse with a calling.*

A nurse who has *not* such a "calling," will never be able to learn the sound of her patient's bell from that of others.[108] *A nurse without the nurse's calling.*

She will, when called to for hot brandy-and-water for her fainting patient, offer the weekly "Punch" (fact). Or she will wait to bring the cordial till she brings his tea (fact).

Under such a nurse, the patient never gets a hot drink. She pours out his tea, then she makes a journey to the larder for the butter, then she remembers that she has forgotten the toast, and has another journey to the kitchen fire to make the toast, then she fills a hot water bottle, and last of all she takes him his tea.

Such a nurse will never know whether her patient is awake or asleep. She will rouse him up to ask him "if he wants anything," and leave him uncared for when he *is* up.

She will make the room like an oven when he is feverish at night, and let out the fire when he is cold in the morning.

Such a nurse seems to have neither eyes, nor ears, nor hands.

She never touches any thing without a crash or an upset.

She does not shut the door, but pulls it after her, so that it always bursts open again.

She cannot rub in an embrocation without making a sore, which, in too many cases, never heals during the patient's life.

She catches up a cup and saucer in one hand, and pokes the fire with the other. Both of course come to "grief." Or she carries in a tray in one hand, and a coal scuttle in the other. Both of course tip out their contents. And she, in stooping to pick them up, knocks over the bedside table upon the patient with her head (fact).

Tables are made for things to stand upon—beds for patients to lie in.

But such a nurse puts down a heavy flower-pot upon the bed, or a large book or bolster which has rolled upon the floor.

Yet these things are not done by drinking Mrs. Gamps, but by respectable women, receiving their guinea a-week in private families.[109]

A man's definition of a nurse.

Yet no *man*, not even a doctor, ever gives any other definition of what a nurse should be than this—"devoted and obedient."[110]

This definition would do just as well for a porter. It might even do for a horse. It would not do for a policeman. Consider how many women there are who have nothing to devote—neither intelligence, nor eyes, nor ears, nor hands. They will sit up all night by the patient, it is true; but their attendance is worth nothing to him, nor their observations to the doctor.

Cases have been known where the patient was cold before the nurse had observed he was dead—and yet she was not asleep—many cases where she supposed him comfortably sleeping, and he was insensible—very many where she never knew he was dying, unless he told her so himself.

But let no woman suppose that obedience to the doctor is not absolutely necessary. Only, neither doctor nor nurse lay sufficient stress upon *intelligent* obedience, upon the fact that obedience *alone* is a very poor thing.

I have known an obedient nurse, told not to disturb a very sick patient as usual at ten o'clock with some customary service which she used to perform for him then, actually leave him in the dark all night, alleging this order as her reason for not carrying in his night-light as usual.

Everybody has known the window left open in heavy fog or rain, or shut when the patient was fainting, by such obedient nurses.

There seems to be no medium for them between a furnace of a fire and no fire at all; and one is actually obliged in this variable climate to divide the year into two parts, and tell them—"Now no fire," "Now fire;" as if they were volunteer riflemen. You cannot trust them to make a *small* fire, although in England it is a question whether, except when the air without is hotter than the air within, patients are not always the better of some fire, if only to promote ventilation. But no; such nurses make it impossible.

Again, ladies generally give the definition of a good nurse as "sober, honest, and chaste."[111] But would this not do for any other description of female service? Do you ask no more than this even from your cook or your housekeeper?

A lady's definition of a nurse.

When you reflect how little, in England, women's powers of observation are exercised, how the prevailing impression is that almost any woman will do for a nurse, provided she is thus "sober" and "kind"—it seems most important that clinical instruction, so to speak, should be given to every nurse where alone it can be given,—in a hospital.

The elements of a nurse's duty.

The merest element of this is to call upon a nurse to observe the state of the pulse,—the effect of the diet,— of sleep, whether it has been disturbed,—whether there have been startings up in bed—a common mark of fatal disease; whether it has been a heavy, dull sleep, with stertorous breathing; whether there has been twitching of the bed-clothes,—to observe the state of the expectoration, the rusty expectoration of pneumonia, the frothy expectoration of pleurisy, the viscid mucous expectoration of bronchitis, the blood-streaked, dense, heavy expectoration which often occurs in consumption,—the nature of the cough itself by which the expectoration is expelled,—to observe the state of the secretions (yet nine-tenths of all nurses know nothing about these), whether the motions are costive or relaxed, and what is their colour, or whether there are alternations every few days of diarrhoea, and of no action of the bowels at all; whether the urine is high-coloured or pale, excessive or scanty, muddy or clear, or whether it is high-coloured when the bowels do not act and pale when there is diarrhoea; whether there is ever blood in the motions, —in children, whether there are worms. All these things most nurses do not appear to consider it their business to observe.

The condition of the breathing and the position in which the patient breathes most easily, is another thing essential for the nurse to observe. In heart-complaints life is often extinguished by the patient "accidentally" falling into a position in which he cannot breathe—and life preserved by an "accidental" change of position. Now, what a thing it is to have to say of a nurse that it was not through her means, but through an "accident" that her patient was able to breathe.

Another essential duty of the nurse is, to observe the action of medicine;—as, for instance, that of quinine. The sore throat, the deafness, the tight feeling in the head, are well known effects of quinine. But the loss of memory it often occasions, is seldom known except to a very observant nurse. Indeed, she has often not memory enough herself to remember that the patient has forgotten.

A good nurse scarcely ever asks a patient a question—neither as to what he feels nor as to what he wants. But she does not take for granted, either to herself or to others, that she knows what he feels and wants, without the most careful observation and testing of her own observations.

But why, for instance, should a nurse ask a private patient every day, "Please, sir, shall I bring your coffee?" or "your broth?" or whatever it is,—when she has every day brought it to him at that hour. One would think she did it for the sake of making the patient speak. Now, what the patient most wants is never to be called upon to speak about such things.

No sick man (in the *educated* classes) ever wishes for anything, in respect to his nurse, but that she should be as much out of the room as possible—a sufficient proof of what nursing *is now*: which, like other practical things, *is* always the consequence of what it is supposed it *ought to be*. A patient says, when his friends express uneasiness lest he should not be able to summon his nurse, "The last thing I should do, if I were worse, would be any thing to bring my nurse into the room, at least if I had my senses."

"Afraid of my nurse."

Such is nursing now. Amongst educated people, there

is not one-half the fear of dying alone that there is of the nurse coming into the room.

Observations which might be made by the sick bed.

There are a great many observations, of much importance, both physiologically and practically, which might be made by nurses, if they were educated to observation, and, indeed, can only be made by nurses or those who are always with the sick.

I indicate them with the greatest diffidence, because of the little that is known upon them, and of my having no experience but my own to speak from.

Such are—

The different idea of time formed by the patient with the quick pulse and the patient with the slow pulse.

Dugald Stewart and other metaphysicians have speculated as to how we form our idea of time.[112]

Without entering into any speculation, my experience is, that to the quick pulse the Arabian fables of a man putting his head underwater, and the seconds appearing to him years, are all but realized.

A nurse's unpunctuality of ten minutes inflicts upon such a patient the idea of hours.

By the low, slow pulse, on the other hand, the lapse of time is almost unheeded.

Again, the physical difference of death-beds by different diseases, is little observed. Patients who die of consumption very frequently die in a state of seraphic joy and peace; the countenance almost expresses rapture. Patients who die of cholera, peritonitis, &c., on the contrary, often die in a state approaching despair. The countenance expresses horror.

In dysentery, diarrhoea, or fever, the patient often dies in a state of indifference.

Again, in some cases, even of consumption and peritonitis, there are alternations almost of ecstacy and of despondency. In the lives of the "Saints," and in religious biographies we often find such death-beds described truly enough. But then the patient and friends make unwise exertions to bring back the state of rapture, quite unaware that it may be only a physical state. And if it does not return, both may perhaps consider that its absence is a token of a state of "reprobation," or "backsliding."[113]

Friends, in all these cases, are apt to judge most unfairly of the spiritual state of the sick from the physical manifestations.

Again, the question of temperaments is almost entirely unstudied in England for any practical purpose, except by medical men. And some patients are thought to suffer much less, some much more, than they really do. I have known a Celt rouse the whole hospital because his toes were cold. While, if an Anglo-Saxon said his back was cold, he was generally within 24 hours of death. An Anglo-Saxon man feels twice as much pain as he says; an Anglo-Saxon woman three times as much. You may generally believe half of what a Celtic man says he feels; and one-tenth of what a Celtic woman says.

Again, there are cases of disease of many classes and orders, which generate nervous power, without any balance of vital or digestive power, which is excessively misleading. The opposite case ceases to be able to produce brain power when the vital powers are exhausted. It falls asleep and eats. And its life is saved. But the first goes on able to think long after its powers of sleeping and eating are at an end, and neither patient himself nor others have any idea how ill he is. He dies simply because the powers of life go out.

These are two instances only of many varieties.

Again, there is a kind or stage of delirium which is often mistaken for dreaming, and *vice versâ*. Dreams almost always refer to times long ago. So does the low gentle delirium before death. I have known great criminals talk of their mother's garden (like innocent children), just before death. And it has been supposed to be a sign of "grace."

Delirium and the visions produced by opium, generally refer to present things. The patient distorts what has very lately passed or just passed (or what is actually passing) around him, to his own imaginations.

I was once taken to see a great actress in Lady Macbeth. To me it appeared the mere transference upon the stage of a death-bed, such as I had often witnessed. So, just before death, have I seen a patient get out of bed, and feebly re-enact some scene of long ago, exactly as if walking in sleep.[114]

There are many other physical observations, by which metaphysical questions might probably be solved. But it requires the world's accurate experience to gather data for them.

I only indicate a few.

CONVALESCENCE.

Hints for the sick will not do for convalescene.

Many, indeed most, of the hints given for sickness will not do for convalescence; for instance, the *patient's* fancies about diet are often valuable indications to follow —the *convalescent's* often the reverse.

Every nurse should make it a point to ascertain what are the signs of approaching convalescence. In all diseases these signs are more or less the same, but they are, of course, modified by the seat of the disease, as well as by its nature.

Difference of sickness and convalescence.

During disease, the system is engaged in throwing off dead or poisonous matters—during convalescence, in repairing waste. As soon as the vital powers have been freed there is a spring, as it were, towards health, operating irregularly, sometimes in the direction of one set of organs, sometimes of another. This is most remarkable in surgical injury, where there is fracture in more than one place. The patient distinctly feels like a set of little carpenters at work with little hammers, first at one fracture, then at another, never at both at once. Remark that a surgical patient *may*, and ought to be, in perfect health, during recovery from an accident—it is the fault of something else than the injury if he is not.

When the diseased action has terminated, and convalescence has fairly set in, the patient very often has longings, especially for articles of food, which, if incautiously indulged, may lead to violent re-action, or even to relapse. The digestive functions are beginning to recover their power,—the most prominent symptom of which is increased appetite for food exceeding in quantity or quality (or both) what the stomach can digest. The utmost caution is necessary on the part of the nurse to prevent mischief from this cause. The medical attendant is, of course, the best judge of the food and regimen required; but during convalescence he is not there day by day, very often not above once or twice a week; and the nurse, at one of the most important periods of her patient's life, is left almost to herself—she has to be doctor and nurse too. It, therefore, very much depends upon her knowledge and experience whether the convalescence is to be slowly and steadily advanced, or whether it may not receive some rude check, throwing the patient back for weeks.

It has happened that a single well-meant but ill-directed indulgence has ended in death.

In dieting convalescents, as a rule it is safer to keep *within* the patient's appetite than to satisfy it, and especially to go beyond it. Indeed, to satisfy the appetite of a convalescent is to go beyond what is required for nourishment, for the appetite is ahead of the power of digesting material to supply the waste occasioned by disease.

Margin notes:
Surgical patients should not be ill.

Restraint necessary in convalescence.

Convalescent appetites.

The nurse has often to deal not only with the patient's appetite, but with the officiousness of his friends. Some unwholesome, perhaps poisonous, delicacy is one of the first offerings generally made by them. The nurse should be on the watch against this—she ought to remember that her responsibility only ends when her services have been discontinued, and that she is really the person to see that the patient is dieted in strict conformity with the doctor's orders.

On the other hand, it may be that the main difficulty in the recovery is the patient's *want* of appetite, most likely to occur where he has no change of air. In such cases the nurse must exercise the same care in regard to diet and the times at which it is to be given, as is indicated for sickness at Chap. VI.

There are other indulgences besides those of the stomach which require to be kept under check. Some patients are apt to over-exert themselves in various ways, to incur unnecessary exposure and fatigue, perhaps to be followed by sitting in a draught. Friends often carry on long and exhausting conversations, or prolonged readings, at one time, which are followed by a loss of vital power to the patient, requiring some time for its recovery. Errors in too much or too little clothing have also to be guarded against; but as a rule convalescents require warm clothing.

In all these things, a convalescent is, so to speak, like a child; neither mind nor body has recovered its proper tone, and, for a certain time differing in different diseases, the nurse has to guide him by her own experience. She has this great advantage, that she has watched the whole progress of the case, from the point of danger up to that of recovery, and by keeping the whole chain in view she will be able to find the right course.

It is not meant that she is to be like Sancho Panza's physician, and order every thing to be removed from table;[115] she is there as before to exercise common sense and discretion. She must study her convalescent just as faithfully as she has studied her patient.

The activity and craving of the imagination, is like that of the stomach, extraordinary in some convalescents, especially in convalescents from fever. They have often an excessive craving for novels, not character novels, but melodramatic and incident novels. And if they cannot obtain such, they will, with singular lucidity of memory and vigour of fancy, go over novels in their head which they have not read for twenty years. And they often state that never in their lives did they know what the pleasures of fancy were before. It is well not to let this go too far, as the terrors of some ghost story or appalling crime will have the same vividness in their imagination, and, creeping in unawares, become uncontrollable even to the degree of preventing sleep.

Convalescent imaginations.

Change, a change of air, is of the very first importance as soon as the disease has "taken a turn." Everybody must have remarked how a person recovering remains sometimes for weeks without making any progress, yet with apparently nothing the matter with him. The change from a ground-floor to an upstairs ward will sometimes hasten a patient's recovery. The mere move to what *he* considers the "convalescent" ward will give him a fillip. Change is essential. He must go to another place, or even only to another room. Then he immediately begins to "pick up." This is every-day experience. But with the poor, "change of air" is next to impossible. And people, without large experience, and who have never had a severe illness themselves to enlighten them, have little idea how large a class there is (and for how long a time) who require an intermediate place between hospital and a convalescent Institution where there is *no* nursing. A place with the most careful nursing and every hospital comfort, *together with country air,* would save many lives

Change of air essential.

from being spent in the Union Workhouse, many from requiring poor-law relief at all, many from giving birth to unhealthy families, and many premature deaths.

Convalescent institutions.

There are those to whom this subject appears unimportant; such people say, when a sick man is convalescing, he is doing well, and there is an end of it. They never consider that convalescence has its degrees and its course the same as disease. And that you may have a very long convalescence instead of a short one, or perhaps no convalescence at all, by simply entertaining the habit of thought that "there is an end of it."

Convalescents require nursing as well as country air.

Such people do not see "why convalescents are to be *nursed* at all." And yet persons who have taken the pains to watch are perfectly well aware that many cases would be irretrievably lost but for careful nursing. Some would become permanent invalids; others burdens to themselves and their friends for the rest of their days. There may be return to *life;* but return to health and usefulness depends upon the *after*-nursing in almost all cases. Careful nursing has done in a few weeks what uncareful medical observation has declared it impossible to do in less than two years. Long convalescence ending in relapse or death is by no means unfrequent among the poor, many of whom leave hospital to make way for more necessitous cases long before they are able to return to their customary employment.

Follow these people to their homes, and what do you find? A straightened household, overtaxed to the utmost by a long illness of its head or support, receiving back, perhaps from expected death, its head (not to be a *support* but) to be a farther call upon its exhausted resources for nursing, clothing, and above all for suitable food and comforts. There can be no doubt that these defective convalescences, gone through in bad air and in the absence of almost every requisite, eventually go to swell the Registrar's Death List.

The question naturally arises, whether in contributing to a "County Hospital," one has done one's whole duty in this matter. Healthy people don't thrive very wcell if they sleep among sick people. Is it rational to imagine that convalescents can do so either? Would it not appear a main point in regard to all hospitals in populous districts for each to have its convalescent branch at a convenient distance in the open country into which recovering cases should be drafted from the hospital wards as speedily as possible?

My own conviction is that, next to removing hospitals entirely out of towns, there is nothing which would add so much to the efficiency of these institutions, or, at the same time, be so great a blessing to the sick poor as henceforth to look on convalescence as a state as much requiring its special conditions and management as sickness; and to provide for it accordingly.

I rejoice to think that steps are being made in this direction both in London and Manchester.

CHILDREN IN LONDON.

It may be imagined that all these remarks apply only to the nursing of sick, whereas, in reality, there is another class, for whom they are equally important—and those are children—not sick, but "delicate," chiefly children of the richer classes, who, in spite of every care and no little expense, become a source of incessant anxiety to their parents, from excessive or from ignorant nursing.

To save not only the sick but "delicate" children— "delicate," owing to excessive nursing —chiefly in the class who can afford too much of every thing artificial.

Many children who, during their stay in the country, are blooming in full vigour, are, during their town life, in an incredibly short time, transformed into delicate hot-house plants, for whose lives parents tremble after an hour's exposure to fresh air and cold. This is the result

Not "London air" but London life does it.

of their being transplanted into an artificial overtrained and over-nursed hot-house life, without having fresh air, or free exercise *ad libitum*,[116] with altered diet, altered habits, coercion and restriction meeting them at every turn; and all this in badly constructed, badly ventilated, badly warmed houses, in a large town. All the good that has been built up during six months in the country, in a healthful life, is generally lost in one month of town life.

Good gained in the country lost.

The popular belief is, that London air does it all; that children cannot thrive in it; and that all that is to be done is to keep them there for as short a time as possible.

But we forget the effect of the "air of London houses" and of London habits.

As to healthiness of site, there is a great difference between Hampstead, Camberwell, and Belgravia. The most densely populated and most filthy parts of a town are not the best neighbours to windward. The most elevated and exposed positions are generally the healthiest; the lowest to leeward of nuisances, under the shelter of the more elevated parts, generally the unhealthiest.

The low western districts, under the lee of London nuisances, are the recipients of foul air from the less healthy districts of London, whenever the wind comes from that direction; and yet people like to live there, because it is the "West End."

Difficult to poison a house in the country, in London very little will do it.

A house in the country isolated in healthy and pure air defies almost any amount of ignorance to make it unhealthy (and often one sees no little),[117] but in the atmosphere of London very little indeed will do it.

Houses generally are not built to be ventilated. There is no way for the foul air to go out, and there is no way for fresh air to get in. The best popular test, because affecting everybody's senses, is the length of time which most houses retain the smell of dinner; some houses are seldom without it in the garrets. The only place whence

Constant "smell of dinner" test.

the air of many a house is drawn is the basement and the kitchen.

The air both of basement and kitchen should be so pure as never to be offensive. Nothing offensive has any right to be there. Keep the air inside your house as pure as the air outside, by all means; a proper use of windows will enable you to do this, but never think of ventilation as a substitute for cleanliness.

But to return to children, how do they live in these houses? In the country they spend at least half their time in the open air; but in town, 99 hours out of 100 are spent in the house, and when they do go out, they go like dogs in leashes. This does away with all the healthy influence of play, of muscular exercise; there is not a run nor a laugh, nor a warm and red and healthy-looking face, and in many cases the delicate ones are packed up in a carriage to take the imaginary airing like a dose of medicine.

Children in town go out (when they do) like dogs in leashes, or in a carriage.

Then that traditionary dread on the part of nurses of a "north-easter,"[118] which in their minds comprises about three-fourths of the compass. This dread is certainly justified when children have had a year's training as hot-house plants, which makes them like invalids after ten years' residence in the tropics, and which actually succeeds in producing that educational monstrosity, rheumatic phthisicky invalids, of fifteen.[119]

All this artificial fear not necessary, though it soon creates some foundation for itself.

An amount of schooling which would be a fair allowance for twelve months is often condensed into a period of six or four months in London, on account of the greater facilities for tuition; at all events the "pupils" sit in the school-room, they sit in the drawing-room, they sleep in their bedroom or nursery, one closer than the other, one warmer than the other (sometimes they *sleep in warmed rooms,* the most injurious error in the régime of all young people), they do everything by order, everything according to rule, they become pale, lifeless shadows, in which there

Well-instructed lifeless victims.

is no health, or strength, or spirit; nerves, muscles, and mind are all equally wanting in healthful exercise.[120]

Three injuries to children.

I would add three other things, which exercise a terrible influence on the health of this class of children:—

1. I have seen people of large fortune exile their children (without the least scruple) to a north nursery (*qy.* nursery of scrofula),[121] which never had one breath of sun-purified air; and these the most affectionate and anxious of parents.

2. The habit of having children "in to dessert." It is often said that this is the only time when a busy father can see his children. But, if there is "company," surely his seeing them then is not much good; and, if there is not, why must he see them over sweetmeats and wine?

3. I wonder whether many housekeepers' experience is the same as mine—viz., that in London houses "renewing" papers and furniture means putting a fresh paper a-top of a dirty one, and tacking a fresh chintz a-top of a dirty one,—aye, to *three* and FOUR deep!! No wonder some London houses are always musty, if cleanliness has no more conscience than this! This clearly affects all the inmates; children only suffer in a greater degree.

Appetite-test; in country—in town.

The effects on the body are sometimes best tested by the state of appetite. Children who in the country have excellent appetites for animal, vegetable, and farinaceous food, for meat, milk, fruit, home-made bread, during their hothouse existence come down to bread and butter, tea, pastry, with an occasional orange. Is it a wonder that the stock should deteriorate under such "forcing?"

Tea not to be given to children as to sick.

Don't treat your children like sick—don't dose them with tea; especially nervous and irritable children, who gain a little transient relief from it at the inevitable cost of their power of nutrition. Why not let them eat meat and drink half a glass of light beer, or milk? If they can't, rely upon it somebody is to blame, not the child nor the child's natural appetite.

Give them fresh, light, sunny, and open schoolrooms, Summary. cool bedrooms, plenty of out-of-door exercise, facing even cold and wind and weather in sufficiently warm clothes and with sufficient exercise, plenty of amusement and play (free and according to the children's own schemes, not by order), more liberty and nature and less schooling and cramming and forcing and training; with more attention to food; less attention to physic—and you will find it possible to keep children in better health, even in the "air of London."

NOTE UPON SOME ERRORS IN NOVELS.

Novels do much to spread and stereotype popular errors and ignorances, forming, as they do now, so large a proportion of the reading of women of all classes. A few of the most common errors in novels are these:—

1. The joys of convalescence.—People must have had very different constitutions when they could rush back to life in the way recounted in fiction. In these days, for people of middle age, in the large towns of highly civilized communities, recovery (?) from severe illness is seldom recovery at all—is often delayed by relapse,—and is never anything but a struggle, slow and by no means "joyful." The assisting and encouraging, instead of overwhelming, convalescence is one of the most difficult and important duties of the nurse. Taking for granted that the patient is in a state of enjoyment, or even ease, is folly. Often, when he has no engrossing interest or affection, he is regretting the being called back to life which has then no zest for him. Or when these instantly re-seize their hold

on him, he is making a painful effort to fulfil duties for which he feels himself totally unequal.

2. The loves of cousins are a favourite topic. The authors never think how they are assisting to thwart the plans of God for the human race.

3. Sick-beds and death-beds are painted with colours and descriptions which not only the novelist never could have seen, but which no one ever did see. There is perhaps but one novel-writer who is an exception to this.

In England, of all human experience, sickness and death have met with the least faithful observation. The materials of course are there, but the careful study is altogether wanting. The "death-bed" of almost every one of our novels is as mere a piece of stage-effect as is the singing-death of a PRIMA DONNA in an opera. One would think death did not exist in reality. Shakespeare is the only author who has ever touched the subject with truth, and his truth is only on the side of art.

4. In novels, lives are saved by "*strong* jelly!" (what does *strong* jelly mean?) and by other things equally absurd.

5. The heroine always braves "contagion;" and then dies of it with her whole family or charge. More shame for her if they do!

Now, it is a question whether disease and death should be made matters of fiction at all. But if authors choose to write about such grave interests, surely it is not too much to ask that they will at least take the trouble to observe before they describe. Why should they encourage serious and even fatal mistakes? Why should they not inform themselves, for instance, as to what "infection" is, and make their heroine prevent it for others and herself, not partake in it, if such is to be the scene of her labours?

The true definition of infection is, that it is a means of spreading disease, which, when it exists, proves neglect or ignorance on the part of somebody, doctor, nurse, or relative; or that the place where it occurs is not fit for habitation, either by sick or by well.

METHOD OF POLISHING FLOORS.

The object of this proceeding is only to obtain a good surface polish, in order to obviate the necessity of scrubbing. In all wood floors, except those of oak, a complete saturation, either with bees-wax or with *laque,* or with any indestructible material which may be thought better, so as to render the grain of the wood impervious, is the only thing perfectly safe for hospitals.[122]

Let the floors if not of oak be stained of that colour, but not too dark. No water should ever touch the boards after they are stained.

Bees-wax should be carefully prepared by scraping it into a vessel, and covering it with spirits of turpentine; it should stand *covered over* until the wax is melted. It takes some hours to melt.

If the wax is dirty (as is often the case) melt it in the oven and then pour it carefully into another vessel leaving all sediment behind.

The wax should be only just soft enough to admit of its being well rubbed in, and off the boards.

Keep the softened wax always clean after it is made. If accidentally the polish becomes soiled, melt it again, and pour off the sediment as before. In applying it proceed as follows:—

1. Sweep the floor and wipe it clean from dust.

2. Spread the wax on the floor with discretion, *using very little.*

3. Take a soft thick cloth and rub it in well.

4. Take a second thick soft cloth and rub any superfluous wax off thoroughly.

5. If you use a polishing brush do so after this second cloth.

6. Then take a *soft duster* and polish, rubbing *briskly*. This process should be repeated twice a week.

N.B.—Be very careful to have your cloths *large* enough so that you may never have to rub twice with the same *dirty* piece, but always *fold* the cloth afresh as you go on.

Wash all the cloths after once using them. Do not wash the brush; put some turpentine into a plate, and rub the brush in it; pick out the little bits from it with a fork or stick. It should not require cleaning very often, if only used after the second cloth.

Floors if properly done, ought never to require beeswaxing more than twice a week. The high polish which the boards acquire repels dust and dirt.

A clean soft floor brush, and a clean soft cloth passed over once a day ought to remove all trace of dust.

This process does not require any additional labour or any more allowance of time than oft-repeated scouring. The boards once in good condition require no more labour than is expended in the ordinary ways by which rooms and wards are cleaned; with the additional benefit of being more healthy, and of saving patients exposure to damp exhalation from wet boards.

Before this plan was adopted floors of certain hospitals, owing to the constant passing and re-passing, had to be scrubbed every day. The stained boards have stood the test of seven years' experience, and they have been kept in order by women and girls at the same amount of time which they before bestowed upon the scrubbing system.

Note Upon Employment of Women.

People have written of late years immensely upon the non-"market" for "female labour," the want of "demand," or of "field," for the "industrial" employment of "women." My experience is, that the "demand" is many times greater than the *supply,* that the market for "female labour" is large, but the *labourers* are few. I limit myself to my own personal experience and particular field, and of course to paid labour. I do not avail myself of information collected as to other employments, such as that of teachers, both in families and in national schools, in which experience is the same as mine is in nursing. As to nursing, then, I have had, during the last three years, several hundreds of applications to recommend qualified matrons or superintendents of institutions—qualified missionary or parish nurses (*i.e.,* to nurse in a parish with a salary, derived not from Boards of Guardians but from proprietors in the parish)—qualified sick nurses for private families, for hospitals, and workhouses. Now, in all this the lack was of qualified nurses to fill the places, not of places for the nurses, had they existed, to fill. At a rough guess, I should say that about one-third of these applicants offered ample remuneration; another third fixed no rate, but were willing to enter into any agreement suitable to the qualifications of the nurse; and the remaining third, (principally workhouses and provincial hospitals), offered a sum which could not have obtained the qualifications they required in any case.

I can only re-echo, as to nurses, what *Fraser* says as to "national school teachers," that "the demand" "at this moment far exceeds the supply of qualified persons."[123]

If all the crowd of female writers who have enlarged on the employment of women, on women's just right to a field, and to adequate pay for their labour, were each to train (or to put into the way of training), ten women to supply the demand which is *already* open, we can hardly hesitate as to what the superiority of the result would be.

I am permitted to say by a friend who has (instead of writing about) tried it upon her own premises, in the matter of *female printers,* that the experiment has fully succeeded, that the women earn good and even high wages (from 15s. to 25s. per week), that they do not work long hours, but have time over for domestic employment, and still the enterprise pays itself.

NOTE AS TO THE NUMBER OF WOMEN EMPLOYED AS NURSES IN GREAT BRITAIN.[124]

25,466 were returned, at the census of 1851, as nurses by profession, 39,139 nurses in domestic service,*[12] and 2,822 midwives.[125] The numbers of different ages are shown in Table A, and in Table B their distribution over Great Britain.

To increase the efficiency of this class, and to make as many of them as possible the disciples of the true doctrines of health, would be a great national work.

For there the material exists, and will be used for nursing, whether the real "conclusion of the matter" be to nurse or to poison the sick. A man, who stands perhaps at the head of our medical profession, once said to me, "I send a nurse into a private family to nurse my Patient, but I know that the result is only to do him harm."

* A curious fact will be shown by Table A, viz., that 18,122 out of 39,139, or nearly one-half of all the nurses, in domestic service, are between 5 and 20 years of age; "while of public or professional nurses, about the same *proportion* are over sixty years of age."

Now a nurse means any person in charge of the personal health of another. And, in the preceding notes, the term *nurse* is used indiscriminately for amateur and professional nurses. For, besides nurses of the sick and nurses of children, the numbers of whom are here given, there are friends or relations who take temporary charge of a sick person, there are mothers of families. It appears as if these unprofessional nurses were just as much in want of knowledge of the laws of health as professional ones.

Then there are the school-mistresses of all national and other schools throughout the kingdom. How many of children's epidemics originate in these! Then the proportion of girls in these schools, who become mothers or members among the 64,600 nurses recorded above, or schoolmistresses in their turn. If the laws of health, as far as regards fresh air, cleanliness, light, &c., were taught to these, would this not prevent some children being killed, some evil being perpetuated? On women we must depend, first and last, for personal and household hygiene—for preventing the family from degenerating in as far as these things are concerned. Would not the true way of infusing the art of preserving its own health into the human race be to teach the female part of it in schools and hospitals, both by practical teaching and by simple experiments, in as far as these illustrate what may be called the theory of it?

GREAT BRITAIN.

TABLE A.—AGES.

Nurses.	All Ages.	Under 5 Years.	5—	10—	15—	20—	25—	30—	35—	40—	45—	50—	55—	60—	65—	70—	75—	80—	65 and Upwards
Nurse (not Domestic Servant).....	25,466	...	...	...	...	624	817	1,118	1,359	2,223	2,748	3,982	3,456	3,825	2,542	1,568	746	311	147
Nurse (Domestic Servant).....	39,139	...	508	7,259	10,355	6,537	4,174	2,495	1,681	1,468	1,206	1,196	833	712	369	204	101	25	16

TABLE B.—AGED 20 YEARS OF AGE, AND UPWARDS.

	Great Britain and Islands in the British Seas.	England and Wales.	Scotland.	Islands in the British Seas.	1st. Division. London.	2nd Division. South Eastern.	3rd Division. South Midland.	4th Division. Eastern Counties.	5th Division. South Western Counties.	6th Division. West Midland Counties.	7th Division. North Midland Counties.	8th Division. North Western Counties.	9th Division. Yorkshire.	10th Division. Northern Counties.	11th Division. Monmouth and Wales.
Nurse (not Domestic Servant).....	25,466	23,751	1,543	172	7,807	2,878	2,286	2,408	3,055	1,225	1,003	970	1,074	402	343
Nurse (Domestic Servant).....	21,017	18,945	1,922	150	5,061	2,514	1,252	959	1,737	2,283	957	2,135	1,023	410	614

Editor's Notes

1. Thomas Babington Macaulay, Baron Macaulay (25 October 1800–27 December 1859), historian, politician, and writer.
2. The bitterness of the east wind is reflected in the proverb, "When the wind is in the east, it is neither good for man nor beast" (*Oxford Dictionary of English Proverbs*, edited by F. P. Wilson, 3rd edition [Oxford, 1970], p. 893).
3. Robert Angus Smith (1817–1884), in a lecture before the Royal Institution in 1859, described the method by which he compared the relative amounts of organic impurities of the air in different locations (*Dictionary of National Biography*).
4. In 1861 this is called "a restorative process."
5. "Flannel" means "flannel underclothing."
6. In 1861, "for the housemaid to do this, or for the charwoman to do that," is changed to "for anybody else to do what their patients want."
7. In 1861 these last two sentences are generalized to "These are common everywhere. And yet people are surprised that their children, brought up in 'country air,' suffer from children's diseases."
8. Changes made in 1861 are discussed in the Introduction, above, p. 28.
9. The changes to this passage in 1861 are discussed in the Introduction, above, p. 39. A pound cake is one in which the main ingredients each weigh about a pound. In her famous Victorian *Book of Household Management*, Mrs. Beeton gives this recipe for "two nice-sized cakes": "1 lb. of butter, 1 ¼ lb. of flour, 1 lb. of pounded loaf sugar, 1 lb. of currants, 9 eggs, 2 oz. of candied peel, ½ oz. of citron, ½ oz. of sweet almonds; when liked, a little pounded mace" (Mrs. Isabella Beeton, *The Book of Household Management*, Entirely New Edition [Five Hundred and Fifty-eighth Thousand] [London, 1892], number 2514).
10. The changes to this passage are discussed in the Introduction, above, p. 23. Elizabeth Gaskell comments on the habits of the idle rich in Chapter xviii of *Mary Barton*:

    > Mrs. Carson was . . . indulging in the luxury of a headache. . . . "Wind in the head," the servants called it. But it was the natural consequence of the state of mental and bodily idleness in which she was placed. Without education enough to value the resources of wealth and leisure, she was so circumstanced as to command both. It would have done her more good than all the ether and sal-volatile she was daily in the habit of swallowing, if she might have taken the work of one of her own housemaids for a week . . . and gone out into the fresh morning air, without all the paraphernalia . . . in which she was equipped before setting out for an "airing," in the closely shut-up carriage.

11. *Quod erat demonstrandum* is a Latin phrase, here meaning "the thing which had to be proven." Nightingale sarcastically suggests that the army deliberately recruits only those who have been turned down by life insurance companies as bad risks on grounds of poor health.
12. This is to prevent the sudden noise from hooves and carriage wheels passing by.

13. Nightingale included a separate "Note on Contagion and Infection" in *Subsidiary Notes as to the Introduction of Female Nursing into Military Hospitals in Peace and in War* (1858), pp. 128–132:

> '"Contagion" . . . means the communication of disease from person to person by contact. . . . Infection acts through the air. . . . Epidemics . . . teach, not that "current contagions" are "inevitable" but that, unless nature's laws be studied and obeyed, she will infallibly step in and vindicate them, sooner or later.'

"Current" here means "running" or "quickly spreading."

In "Sanitary Condition of Hospitals and Hospital Construction," one of the two papers read on her behalf at the Liverpool meeting of the National Association for the Promotion of Social Science, in October, 1858 (p. v), and published in *Notes on Hospitals* (1858), Nightingale gives more detail about the source of her ideas. There she writes (p. 6) that "The history of the doctrine of 'Contagion' is given by Dr. Adams in his very learned translation of the works of Paulus Ægineta, Vol. I, p. 284—(Sydenham Society). . . . Aretaeus appears to be the first medical author who believed in contagion. Galen seems to have held the doctrine of infection'; but the word was understood to have first been used by Virgil with reference 'to contagious diseases among cattle'" (*Eclogues,* I and *Georgics,* III, 464). See also, C. E. Rosenberg, "Florence Nightingale on Contagion: The Hospital as a Moral Universe," in C. Rosenberg, ed., *Healing and History* (New York, 1979), pp. 116–135; and V. Nutton, "The Seeds of Disease: An Explanation of Contagion and Infection from the Greeks to the Renaissance," *Medical History* xxvii (1983), 1–34.

14. The spelling is changed to "whooping-cough" in 1868.

15. Nightingale contributed letters to *The Builder*, edited by the spirited reformer George Godwin. Although she has been accredited with the authorship of the "three papers from *The Builder*" published in *Notes on Hospitals* (1859), pp. 89–108, Anthony King, "Hospital Planning: Revised Thoughts on the Origin of the Pavilion Principle in England," *Medical History* x (1966), 360–373, correctly attributes them to John Roberton, though "edited, and perhaps added to, by Godwin" (p. 371). Nightingale was clearly influenced by the articles in *The Builder*, many of which during 1857 to 1859 were devoted to the subject of hospital ventilation. See below, in Chapter IX.—Light, and also Ruth Richardson, "George Godwin of *The Builder*: Indefatigable Journalist and Instigator of a Fine Victorian Visual Resource," *Visual Resources* vi, (1989), 121–140.

16. *Caeteris paribus* means "other things being equal."

17. In so far as Nightingale scrupulously corrected the 1861 text, I have adopted "her nurse's presence" over "his nurse's presence," the reading in the second version. In the first version of *Notes on Nursing* (1860), only the earliest copies published read "his nurse's presence," which was then altered to "her nurse's presence." The second version was evidently set in type from one of these early copies. Whilst the third version of 1861 was itself set in type from the second, Nightingale was careful to change the pronoun to "her."

18. A *sine qua non* is an essential without which something could not exist.

19. This remarkably sarcastic description of the women's rights press is minimized in 1861 to "It is . . . when there so much talk about 'woman's mission.'"

20. Cook, *Life of Florence Nightingale*, i. 454, indicates Nightingale's source for this quotation in the painter C. R. Leslie's *Autobiographical Recollections*, edited by Tom Taylor (1860), i. 169, where he cites William Lamb, second Viscount Melbourne (1779–1848).

21. In 1861 this sentence begins, "All likings and aversions of the sick towards different persons will."

22. Crinoline, a stiff composite cloth of horse-hair and linen or cotton, was introduced about 1830. One popular use was for full, self-supporting skirts, or for petticoats. By 1851 the word came to represent the distended petticoat itself. (See the quotations in the *Oxford English Dictionary*.)

23. "Fancy" means "imaginary" here.

24. "Calculate" means "arrange" here.

25. In 1861, "deprecate" becomes "remonstrate against."

26. In 1868, the passage "*You* will . . . traceable," reads: "*You* will not suffer by knowing what you have done—the poor patient will, although *he* may not know either. It will not be directly traceable to its real cause."

27. "Fancy patients" means "patients who imagine their illnesses."

28. In 1861 the wording of "hypochondriacs . . . nurse" becomes "would-be invalids. To distinguish between real and fancied disease is an important thing for a nurse to be able to do."

29. Throughout both *The Iliad* and *The Odyssey* Homer describes the debates of the gods as they decide to influence the fate of mortals. What Homer provides a reader with in poetry, in order to add an extra dimension of insight, is an unacceptable complication in real life, especially to the sick.

30. "Houdin" is J. E. Robert-Houdin (1805–1871), the famous Parisian magician, who in 1859 published his autobiography, *Confidences d'un Prestidigitateur*. A translation was published in London in the same year. Nightingale refers to him once more in her manuscript annotation on "a celebrated man" under "Means of cultivating sound and ready observation," in Chapter XIII.—Observation of the Sick.

31. In 1868, "opium" is changed to "opiate."

32. Compare the wording of Nightingale's letter of June 8, 1859, to Aitken, cited in the Introduction, above, p. 13.

33. "Home, sweet home" is from the opera *Clari* (first performed May 8, 1823) by Sir Henry Rowley Bishop (1786–1855).

34. This air, which translates as "Seated at the foot of a willow," is from Rossini's opera *Otello* (1816), an adaptation of Shakespeare's *Othello*.

35. "The superior . . . often been" becomes in 1861, "Persons suffering severe paroxysms of pain are much more cheerful than persons suffering from nervous weakness. This has often been."

36. In May 1855 Nightingale suffered an attack of Crimean fever. Cook (i. 258) records that the "hut in which she lay was immediately behind those of the wounded soldiers. The attack of fever was sharp, and she was, as she afterwards admitted to her friends, 'very near to death.'"

37. In 1861, "these painful . . . he wants" becomes "these painful ideas are far better dismissed by amusing the invalid, or by showing him something pretty, than by arguing with him."

38. In 1861 "more of the *entente cordiale*" becomes "more of making common cause."

39. Nightingale realized the potential to misinterpret here, and changed the wording in 1861 to "The breaking of it always brings on more or less dislike to taking food."

40. In 1861, "brought in to" was misprinted as "brought into," and emended in 1868 to "brought to." The words "in a state perfectly perceptible," and the following euphemism "peccant article," become in 1861 the more direct "in a state loathsome" and "bad article."

41. Dr. Robert Christison (1797–1882) was Professor of Medical Jurisprudence (1822–32), and then of Materia Medica and Therapeutics (1832–1877), in the University of Edinburgh. A baronetcy was conferred upon him in 1871. In his "Notes and Observations on Medical Practice," in the *Monthly Journal of Medicine* xx (1855), 1–9, part 2, "On Preserved Meat-juice," he describes the advantages over beef-tea of the newly produced concentrated extract of meat. Nightingale quotes directly from pp. 8–9, with slight adaptations.

    In preparing her *Notes on Matters Affecting the Health, Efficiency, and Hospital Administration of the British Army* (1858), Nightingale consulted Christison "on dietetics" (Cook, *Life*, i. 352). Sue Goldie, *A Calendar of the Letters of Florence Nightingale* (Oxford, 1977), fiche 5. D4. 439 (n. 2), notes Christison's contribution to the volume, Appendix XIV, pp. viii-x, and xi-xvii.

42. Nightingale contradicts herself in the opening of Chapter IX.—Light, where she claims that "second only to their need of fresh air is their need of light."

43. I have broken this very long paragraph twice: here, where the topic shifts to sleeplessness, and again where it addresses patients' tastes.

44. The *Oxford English Dictionary* cites this passage under *diluent,* "A substance which increases the proportion of water in the blood and other bodily fluids."

45. In 1861, "It is . . . service" reads, "It is often recommended to persons about to go through great fatigue, either from the kind of work."

46. Christison, in "Notes and Observations on Medical Practice," in the *Monthly Journal of Medicine* xx (1855), p. 9, cites the study by Dr. Julius Lehmann, "Ueber den Kaffee als Getränk in chemis-physiologischer Hinsicht" (A Consideration of Coffee as a Drink in Chemical-physiology), *Annalen der Chemie und Pharmacie* lxxxvii (Neue Reihe, Band xi) (1853), 205–215. Lehmann observes the difference in two subjects on fixed diets of the volume of urine, and the weight in grams of its phosphate, sodium chloride, and urea content, first without and then with coffee. Less weight of phosphate, sodium chloride, and urea are excreted in urine when coffee is drunk (Christison says, "will reduce the daily waste by a fourth part"). Although Lehmann does "weigh the man" in the initial description of his subjects, Nightingale's expression, "find the fact from his weight," is

ambiguous enough to be misconstrued. As the only weight mentioned by Christison is "an ounce of roasted coffee," Nightingale may here be paraphrasing some intermediary source.

47. This is tea made from the leaf of the blackthorn.

48. In 1861, "saturated with organic matter" reads "both from his own perspiration."

49. In 1861, "an adult" is changed to "a grown up man."

50. This passage is cited in the *Oxford English Dictionary*, which notes that it describes a form of air-bed. In 1861 this sentence is reduced to "The best bedding, either for sick or well, is an *iron* bedstead, (no vallance, of course), and hair mattress."

51. In 1861, "two or three feet" becomes "three or four feet."

52. In 1861 the two preceding sentences are reduced to "Not a few cases of scrofula among children proceed from the habit of sleeping with the head under the bed clothes, and so breathing air already breathed, and full of perspiration from the skin. The same with sick."

53. In 1861, "temperature . . . atmosphere" becomes "wind or by damp."

54. A Witney blanket is one made from the heavy, loose woollen material with a nap made at Witney in Oxfordshire.

55. Introducing a discussion of "Deficiency of Light" in *Notes on Hospitals* (1859), p. 11, Nightingale notes that "The effect of light on health and disease has been ably discussed in an article on light in the August number, 1858, of the "North British Review." Its importance has been long recognized in the medical profession, as may be learned from the writings of Sir Andrew Wylie, Dr. Milne Edwards, and Mr. Ward." John Roberton, in "Hospital Construction—Wards," reprinted from *The Builder* (1858) in Nightingale's *Notes on Hospitals* (1859), pp. 99–100, writes on

> the injurious effects of absence of light on peculiar classes of disease. But the only experimental evidence we have hitherto obtained is that given by Sir James Wylie in regard to certain hospitals and barracks at St. Petersburg. In some of these hospitals there were rooms without direct light; and the sick and wounded treated in these dark chambers yielded only a fourth part of the recoveries when compared with patients treated in the light rooms. Nearly twice the number of invalids, it was also found, were received from the dark side of the barracks as from the light side. Dr. Edwards, who has paid particular attention to the effect of light upon health, has given equally strong testimony to its preventive and curative efficacy.

See p. 182, and note 1.

The review articles in *The North British Review* are unsigned, but the article to which Nightingale alludes, "Researches on Light—Sanatory—Scientific and Aesthetical," lvii (August, 1858), 177–210, is attributed in W. E. Houghton, ed., *The Wellesley Index to Victorian Periodicals* (Toronto, 1966-), i. 682, to the expert David Brewster. She could hardly have missed this item, as the very next article, "Our Army In India," heads its reviews, *Report of the Commissioners on the Regulations Affecting the Sanatory Condition of the Army*, 1858, and the *Appendix thereto. Answers To Questions Addressed to Miss Nightingale by the Commissioners.*

56. Here Nightingale gives light as next in importance to fresh air, but in the chapter "What Food?" (above, p. 167) she has already staked a claim for food in this hierarchy.

57. In 1861, "there is cretinism" is paraphrased as "there idiots grow;" "there is the degeneracy and weakliness" as "there are the weakly."

58. The phrase "into the sun" is changed in 1868 to "to live in the sun."

59. By "private patients," Nightingale means "patients nursed in their homes" rather than those in hospitals; compare the change from "private sick" to "sick at home" in the chapter "Personal Cleanliness," p. 196 and p. 373.

60. "Blacks" are particles of soot.

61. In 1861 this sentence is altered to "This is called 'putting the room to rights.'"

62. For "Berlin *lackered* floor," 1861 has "old-fashioned polished oak floor." In *Notes on Hospitals* (1859), p. 15, Nightingale describes the floors used in the hospitals of Berlin: "oiling and *lackering, i.e.,* saturating the floor with linseed-oil, and then rubbing it over with a peculiar *laque* varnish, and polishing it so as to resemble French polish." Both this and the French *parquet*, finished by "filling up the grain of the wood (which ought to be oak) with bees-wax and turpentine," "render the floor non-absorbent," though the "Prussian floor requires re-preparing every three years."

   See also the section, "Method of Polishing Floors" in the "Supplementary Chapter," above, p. 279.

63. See below, "Health of Houses," p. 318.

64. "Their name is Legion," means "they are innumerable." The expression originates in Mark v. 9, the reply of the unclean spirit to Jesus, "My name is Legion: for we are many." The exact words used here occur in Charles Dickens's *Dombey and Son* (1848), near the end of chapter 54, when that most beautiful of wronged women, Edith, the second Mrs. Dombey, turns her invective against her husband's assistant and her seducer, Carker. When he demands, "What devil possesses you?," she launches into him: " 'Their name is Legion,' she replied, uprearing her proud form as if she would have crushed him, 'you and your master have raised them in a fruitful house, and they shall tear you both. False to him, false to his innocent child. . . .' " This child is Florence Dombey, the sensitive and caring heroine of the work. Edith Dombey's anger may well be echoed in the mood exhibited by Nightingale's frustrated patient.

65. This may be a quotation from a nineteenth-century adaptation of Shakespeare's *As You Like It*, alluding to the character receiving an overwhelming amount of attention.

66. From 1859 onwards, Nightingale's health remained so precarious that she often believed herself near death. She lived in this state until August 13, 1910.

67. I have removed an asterisk after "patient," made redundant with the incorporation of "Absurd statistical . . . sick" into the text.

68. In 1861 this is reduced to "says nothing but 'Oh!' and 'Ah!' ".

69. A similar idea about being able to imagine oneself in the shoes of a sick person is expressed in the opening of "What Is A Nurse?," above, p. 258.

70. See below, the "Appendix on Method of Training Nurses," paragraph six, p. 410.
71. In 1861, "narcotic" is altered to "sleeping dose."
72. Nightingale notes, on p. 63 of the copy of the first version of *Notes on Nursing* inscribed to "Selena Bracebridge[,] from the Authoress," that this is "Houdin the conjuror." The copy is in the Florence Nightingale Museum. She previously referred to Robert-Houdin in the chapter on "Noise," above, p. 141, at note 30. There is only one other annotation in the Bracebridge copy, the identification of the novel *Sword and Gown* referred to in the Introduction, above, p. 21.

    The ensuing paragraph is a close adaptation of a passage in J. E. Robert-Houdin, *Memoirs*, translated by Lascelles Wraxall (London, 1859), ii. 6.
73. Compare the wording, "and if you have none of this power, you had better let nursing alone," in the second sentence of "What Is A Nurse?," above, p. 258, at note 102.
74. The spelling "practiced," where "practised" is now used, was current during the nineteenth century.
75. This describes a faulty argument that derives its conclusion not from first premises, but rather from an assumption: "this is the situation, therefore, because this is the situation."
76. The nearest version of the proverb in *The Oxford Dictionary of English Proverbs*, 3rd ed., revised by F. P. Wilson (Oxford, 1970), p. 596, is from Devonshire, "One [magpie] for sorrow, two for mirth, three for a wedding, and four for death." Nightingale records a variation.
77. The "physiognomy" of a disease consists of those observable aspects of it that indicate its character.
78. I have added a comma after "skin," bringing the punctuation into accord with the first version. Here in the second version the word "skin" falls at the end of a line, a position in which it is not unusual to find that the following punctuation is missing.
79. A "saw" is not here just a proverbial saying, but rather one which embraces some untenable belief about disease.
80. Nightingale's expression "biological trick" is her colloquialism for the practice of "electro-biology," "animal-magnetism," or "mesmerism," all now equated with hypnotism.
81. The reference is to a child prodigy in arithmetic.
82. That is, "obligatory in novels."
83. Apoplexy is the surge of effusion of blood, during which occurrence, blood-letting or "bleeding" may be dangerous.
84. The willingness to "learn the sound of her patient's bell" is stressed in "What Is A Nurse?," p. 261 (at note 108).
85. This paragraph, without its heading, is tacked on at the end of "What Is A Nurse?" in 1861.
86. In the first sentence, Nightingale in 1861 simplifies "puerperal women" to "women in childbed," and in this third sentence "cases of external injury" becomes simply "accidents."
87. See the Introduction, above, p. 10.
88. "Who have . . . perfection" means "who are given perfect care as far as the ideals of surgical nursing go."

89. The word in this text is "left." However, as no suitable meaning exists for the combination "convenience is left," I take this to be a typesetting error and adopt "felt" from the first version.

90. This reference is included in the first version of *Notes on Nursing*, composed during 1859. Nightingale quotes from and paraphrases the lecture by Charles West, M.D., Physician to the Hospital for Sick Children, "On Sudden Death in Infancy and Childhood," "Delivered at the Hospital for Sick Children, Nov. 12 1859," and published in *The Medical Times and Gazette* xl (New Ser. xix) (1859), 521–524, in the individual part issued on November 26, 1859.

91. A blue pill is "a mercurial pill of anti-bilious operation" (*Oxford English Dictionary*).

92. In this passage, "Many ladies . . . complains," is substantially changed in 1861, where it reads:

> "Many women, having once obtained a 'bottle' from a druggist, or a pill from a quack, will give and take it for anything and everything. . . . The doctor, being informed of it, substitutes for it some proper medicine. The woman complains."

93. Colocynth is a purgative drug; colchicum was used in treating gout and rheumatism.

94. See below, in the chapter "Health of Houses," p. 320.

95. Nightingale places the word globule between inverted commas to point out its special usage as the term for a pill used in homoeopathy.

96. In 1861, "a disappointment in love" becomes "a loving heart."

97. In the Florence Nightingale Museum copy of *Notes on Nursing* inscribed "Selena Bracebridge[,] from the Authoress," Nightingale's annotation reads "*Sword and Gown*." This novel by George Alfred Lawrence is discussed in the Introduction, above, p. 21. The heroine, Cecil Tresilyan, is perhaps the inspiration behind Nightingale's description of nurses "turning into the war-hospitals to find their wounded lovers, and when found, forthwith abandoning their sick-ward for their lover." Royston Keene, left for dead by the enemy, is sent to Scutari where he regains consciousness under the care of Cecil, for whom he has an unfulfilled passion:

> His right hand still grasped hers, firmly; and her delicate cheek was pillowed on his shoulder; the fingers of his other hand played gently with a long, glossy chestnut tress that had escaped from the prison of the close cap she wore. So they remained, for a long time—no sound passing between them, beyond half-formed whispers of endearment; no one came in to molest them: there was work enough and to spare, that night, for all in Scutari. The thought of interruption never crossed Cecil's mind for an instant. Always careless and defiant of conventionality, or the world's opinion, she was tenfold more reckless now. . . . [Keene, sensing death approaching, sends her away.] She leant down, without speaking, and their lips met in a long, passionate kiss. . . . [He dies before she returns in the morning.]
>
> When Cecil Tresilyan saw that same sight the next morning, she did not scream or faint. Neither then nor afterwards, did she prove herself unworthy of her haughty lover, by demonstrating or parading her sorrows. . . . It is

needless to give all the details of the hospital service that occupied her till the conclusion of the war set her free. . . . (pp. 306–308).

98. On April 28, 1861, Nightingale wrote to her "Dear Papa," "I cannot give up my belief that the Mere Angelique was one of the most efficient because most practical religious deliverers the world has had" (British Library MS. Add. 45790, fols. 207b-208). Jacqueline Marie Angélique Arnauld (1591–1661) became abbess of Port Royal, a convent of Cistercian nuns near Versailles, in 1602. She became a firm adherent of the Jansenist movement, which stressed the benevolence of God's grace and opposed the powerful Jesuits.

99. Elizabeth Fry (1780–1845), a philanthropist and prison reformer, in 1840 founded the English Protestant Sisters of Charity (G. Bowman, *The Lamp and the Book* [London, 1967], p. 22).

100. Nightingale expands on this reference to jargon in a letter of September 12, 1860 to John Stuart Mill:

> I refer to an American world, consisting of female M.D.s, etc., and led by a Dr. Eliz[th] Blackwell,—and though the latter is a dear and intimate and valued friend of mine, I re-assert that her world talks a "jargon" and a very mischievous one—that their female M.D.s have taken up the worst part of a male M.D.-ship of 30 years ago and that, while medical education is what it is—a subject upon which I may talk with some "connaissance de cause",—instead of wishing to see more Doctors made by women joining what there are, I wish to see as few Doctors, either male or female, as possible. For, mark you, the women have made no improvement: they have only tried to be "men," and they have only succeeded in being third rate men.

(British Library MS. Add. 45787, fols. 10–11. Another copy in the Boston University Library, N62: Box 2, Folder 4, is transcribed in M. Vicinus and B. Nergaard, *Ever Yours, Florence Nightingale* [London, 1989], pp. 209–210).

Elizabeth Blackwell (1821–1910) was the first woman to graduate M.D. in America (1849), and the first woman doctor on the English Medical Register. Born British, she grew up and was educated in America. In 1857 she established a hospital in New York staffed only by women, and shortly after took up residence in England. In February 1859 she wrote from London to her sister, Dr. Emily Blackwell, that on a visit to Malvern she had discussions with Nightingale "in relation to a school for nurses which she wishes to establish" (E. Blackwell, *Pioneer Work in Opening the Medical Profession to Women, And Autobiographical Sketches* (London, 1895; reprinted London, [1914]), p. 175). On Blackwell's relationship with Nightingale from 1851 onwards, see Z. Cope, *Florence Nightingale and the Doctors* (London, 1958), pp. 144–7.

101. This passage is discussed in the Introduction, above, p. 26. A parallel idea is expressed in "Chattering Hopes and Advices," above, p. 207.

102. Compare the wording in "Observation of the Sick," above, p. 222, at note 73.

103. This passage is discussed in the Introduction, above, p. 27.

104. In the quaint terms of the *Oxford English Dictionary*, a monthly nurse is "a sick-nurse who attends a woman lying in during the first month after

her accouchement." The illustration given is drawn from the following passage in Charles Dickens's *Martin Chuzzlewit*, chapter xix:

> Mr. Pecksniff had been to the undertaker, and was now upon his way to another officer in the train of mourning: a female functionary, a nurse, and watcher, and performer of nameless offices about the persons of the dead: whom he had recommended. Her name . . . was Gamp. . . .
>
> This lady lodged at a bird-fancier's, next door but one to the celebrated mutton-pie shop, and directly opposite to the original cats'-meat warehouse. . . . Mrs. Gamp being, in her highest walk of art, a monthly-nurse, or, as her sign-board boldly had it, "Midwife".

105. This sentence begins "A farmer "who . . . " in 1861.
106. In 1861, this reads, "Any loss of flesh will never take place unknown to her."
107. In 1861, "the formation of matter" reads "that matter is forming."
108. The ability to distinguish "the sound of her patient's bell" is stressed in "Observation of the Sick," above, p. 261.
109. The 1861 version is discussed in the Introduction, above, p. 20.
110. In 1861 this becomes "Yet we are often told that a nurse needs only to be 'devoted and obedient.'"
111. This passage is discussed in the Introduction, above, p. 19.
112. Dugald Stewart (1753–1828) was an eminent Scottish philosopher, ten volumes of whose *Collected Works* were published in Edinburgh between 1854 and 1858.
113. Nightingale comments on the falsity of moral interpretation placed upon a person's demeanour at death—if he looks ill at ease, he is said either to have been rejected by God, or he is falling away from Christian faith.
114. In Shakespeare's *Macbeth* (V.i.22 onwards) Lady Macbeth walks in her sleep reenacting the murder of Duncan (II.ii).
115. In chapters 6 and 7 of Cervantes' novel *Don Quixote*, the hero of that name goes mad and terrorizes the countryside by living out a fantasy that he is a medieval knight. The curate and the barber (physician) undertake to burn Don Quixote's library of chivalric romances, wall up the room, and tell him that a magician has made the lot disappear. This actually occurs immediately before he recruits his simple neighbour Sancho Panza as his squire.
116. "Ad libitum" means "at pleasure" or "as they will."
117. The parenthesis means, "and often one sees a great deal of ignorance."
118. In London, a wind from the north-east can be exceptionally cold. The harshness of the east wind in proverbial; see above, p. 69.
119. "Rheumatic phthisicky" means suffering from catarrh and asthma, but could also imply consumption.
120. This accumulation of sentences is mentioned in relation to other aspects of Nightingale's prose style in the Introduction, above, p. 24.
121. By "*qy.*" she indicates the interrogative, "Is this not for certain a nursery which induces scrofula?"
122. This introductory paragraph is printed between square brackets in the original text.

123. The first article that Nightingale herself published in *Fraser's Magazine* was the controversial "A Note on Pauperism" (March, 1869); see Cook, *Life of Florence Nightingale*, ii. 164. This journal is referred to above, in the Introduction, p. 21.

124. Nightingale has taken this title, the first two paragraphs and the asterisked note, and Tables A and B directly from her *Subsidiary Notes as to the Introduction of Female Nursing into Military Hospitals in Peace and in War* (1858), section 3, pp. 20–21.

125. In *Subsidiary Notes* this number was 2,882.

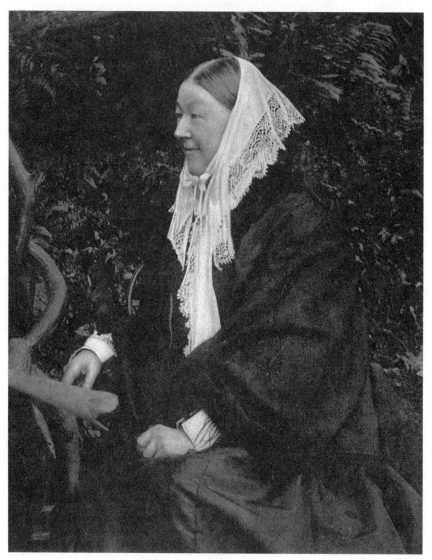

Florence Nightingale ca. 1890.

Part
Three

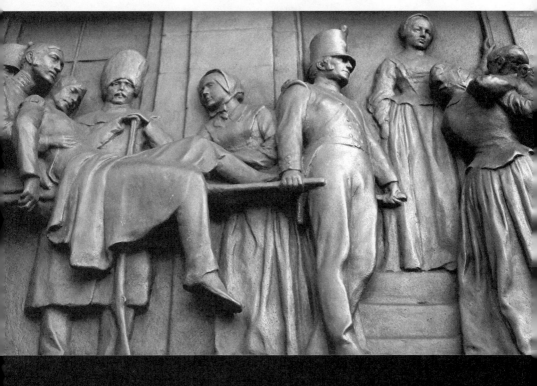

Notes on Nursing
for

The Labouring Classes

1868 EDITION

NOTES ON NURSING

FOR

THE LABOURING CLASSES.

BY

FLORENCE NIGHTINGALE.

NEW EDITION

LONDON:

HARRISON, 59, PALL MALL,

Bookseller to the Queen and H.R.H. the Prince of Wales.

1868.

This Edition has been made for the use of the Labouring Classes, with some abridgment, with considerable additions, and with a supplementary Chapter on Children.

September, 1867.   F. N.

PREFACE.

THE following notes are by no means intended as a rule of thought by which nurses can teach themselves to nurse, still less as a manual to teach nurses to nurse. They are meant simply to give hints for thought to women who have personal charge of the health of others. Every woman, or at least almost every woman, in England has, at one time or another of her life, charge of the personal health of somebody, whether child or invalid, — in other words, every woman is a nurse. Every day sanitary knowledge, or the knowledge of nursing, or in other words, of how to put the constitution in such a state as that it will have no disease, or that it can recover from disease, takes a higher place. It is recognized as the knowledge which every one ought to have — distinct from medical knowledge, which only a profession can have.

If then, every woman must, at some time or other of her life, become a nurse, *i.e.*, have charge of somebody's health, how immense and how valuable would be the produce of her united experience if every woman would think how to nurse.

I do not pretend to teach her how, I ask her to teach herself, and for this purpose I venture to give her some hints.

CONTENTS.

		PAGE
I.	VENTILATION AND WARMING	8
II.	HEALTH OF HOUSES	20
III.	PETTY MANAGEMENT	34
IV.	NOISE	39
V.	VARIETY	50
VI.	TAKING FOOD	53
VII.	WHAT FOOD	58
VIII.	BED AND BEDDING	63
IX.	LIGHT	67
X.	CLEANLINESS OF ROOMS AND WALLS	69
XI.	PERSONAL CLEANLINESS	74
XII.	CHATTERING HOPES AND ADVICES	77
XIII.	OBSERVATION OF THE SICK	84
XIV.	CONVALESCENCE	95
XV	WHAT IS A NURSE?	97
XVI.	"MINDING BABY"	103
	CONCLUSION	108
	APPENDIX	112

NOTES ON NURSING:

WHAT IT IS AND WHAT IT IS NOT.

IN watching disease, both in private houses and in public hospitals, the thing which strikes the experienced observer most forcibly is this, that the symptoms or the sufferings generally considered to be unavoidable and peculiar to the disease are very often not symptoms of the disease at all, but of something quite different—of the want of fresh air, or of light, or of warmth, or of quiet, or of cleanliness, or of punctuality and care in the administration of diet, of each or of all of these. And this quite as much in private houses and cottages as in hospitals.

The process of repairing the body which Nature has instituted, and which we call disease, has been hindered by some want of knowledge or attention, in one or in all of these things, and pain, suffering, or interruption of the whole process sets in.

If a patient is cold, if a patient is feverish, if a patient is faint, if he is sick after taking food, if he has a bed-sore, it is generally the fault not of the disease, but of the nursing.

I use the word nursing for want of a better. It has been limited to signify little more than the administration of medicines and the application of poultices. It ought to signify the proper use of fresh air, light, warmth, cleanliness, quiet, and the proper choosing and giving of diet—all at the least expense of vital power to the patient.

It has been said and written scores of times, that every woman makes a good nurse. I believe, on the contrary, that the very elements of nursing are all but unknown.

By this I do not mean that the nurse is always to blame. Bad construction of rooms and houses, and other bad arrangements often make it impossible to nurse. But the art of nursing ought to include such arrangements as alone make what I understand by nursing possible.

If we are asked, Is such or such a disease a restorative process? Can such an illness be unaccompanied with suffering? Will any care prevent such a patient from suffering this or that?—I humbly say, I do not know. But when you have done away with all that pain and suffering, which in patients are the symptoms not of their disease, but of the absence of one or all of the above-mentioned essentials to the success of Nature's restorative processes, we shall then know what are the symptoms of and the sufferings inseparable from the disease.

Another and the commonest exclamation which will be instantly made is—Would you do nothing, then, in cholera, fever, &c.?— so deep-rooted and universal is the conviction that to give medicine is to be doing something, or rather everything; to give air, warmth, cleanliness, &c, is to do nothing. The reply is, that in these and many other similar diseases the exact value of particular remedies and modes of treatment is by no means ascertained, while there is universal experience as to the extreme importance of careful nursing in determining the issue of the disease.

II. The very elements of what constitutes good nursing are as little understood for the well as for the sick. The same laws of health or of nursing, for they are in reality the same, obtain among the well as among the sick. The breaking of them produces only a less violent consequence among the former than among the latter,—and this sometimes, not always.

It is constantly objected,—"But how can I obtain this medical knowledge? I am not a doctor. I must leave this to doctors."

Oh, mothers of families! You who say this, do you know that one in every seven infants in this civilized land of England perishes before it is one year old? That, in London, two in every five die before they are five years old? And, in the other great cities of England, nearly one out of two?

Upon this fact the most wonderful deductions have been strung. For a long time an announcement something like the following has been going the round of the papers:—"More than 25,000 children die every year in London under 10 years of age; therefore we want a Children's Hospital." Last spring there was a paper issued, and divers other means taken to this effect:— "There is a great want of knowledge about health in women: therefore we want a Women's Hospital." Now, both the above facts are too sadly true. But what is the consequence? The causes of the enormous child mortality are perfectly well known; they are chiefly want of cleanliness, want of ventilation, careless dieting and clothing, want of white-washing; in one word, want of *household* care of health. The remedies are just as well known; and among them is certainly not the establishment of a Child's Hospital. This may be a want; just as there may be a want of hospital room for adults. But the Registrar-General would certainly never think of giving us, as a cause for the high rate of child mortality in (say) Liverpool, that there was not sufficient hospital room for children; nor would he urge upon us, as a remedy, to found a hospital for them.*

Again, women, and the best women, are wofully deficient in knowledge about health; although it is to women that we must look, first and last, for its application, as far as *household* care of health is concerned. But who would ever think of citing the institution of a Women's Hospital as the way to cure this want?

"The life duration of babies is the most delicate test" of sanitary conditions. Granted that nearly half the whole population of English cities dies before it is five years old, is all this premature suffering and death necessary? Or did Nature intend mothers to be always accompanied by doctors? Or is it better to learn any thing rather than to learn the laws which are to preserve your offspring?

At present neither mothers of families of any class, nor schoolmistresses of any class, nor nurses of children, nor nurses of hospitals, are taught anything about those laws which God has assigned to the relations of our bodies with the world in which He has put them. In other words, the laws which make these bodies, into which He has put our minds, healthy or unhealthy organs of those minds, are all but unlearnt. Not but that these laws—the laws of life—are in a certain measure understood, but not even mothers think it worth their while to study them—to study how to give their children healthy existences. They call it medical or physiological knowledge, fit only for doctors.

Again, we are constantly told,—"But the circumstances which govern our children's healths are beyond our control. What can we do with winds? There is the east wind. Most people can tell before they get up in the morning whether the wind is in the east."

To this one can answer with more certainty than to the former objections. Who is it who knows when the wind is in the east? Not the Highland drover, certainly, exposed to the east wind, but the "young lady" who is worn out with the want of exposure to fresh air, to sunlight, &c. Put the latter under as

---

* This very year, 1868, a health report on Manchester has appeared, which is virtually to this effect:—Let the town breed as much infectious disease as it likes; put the cases into big infirmaries; this is the way to cure Manchester, to build hospitals to cure people after they have been killed.

healthy circumstances as the former, and she too will not know when the wind is in the east.

I.—VENTILATION AND WARMING.

THE very first rule of nursing, the first and the last thing upon which a nurse's attention must be fixed, the first essential to the patient, without which all the rest you can do for him is as nothing, with which I had almost said you may leave all the rest alone, is this: TO KEEP THE AIR HE BREATHES AS PURE AS THE EXTERNAL AIR, WITHOUT CHILLING HIM. Yet what is so little attended to? Even where it is thought of at all, there are the most extraordinary misconceptions about it. Even in admitting air into the patient's room or ward, few people ever think where that air comes from. It may come from a passage, always unaired, always full of the fumes of gas, dinner, of various kinds of mustiness: from an underground kitchen, sink, wash-house, water-closet, dung-heap, or even, as I myself have had sorrowful experience, from open sewers loaded with filth; and with this the patient's room or ward is aired, as it is called—poisoned, it should rather be said. Always air from the air without, and that, too, through those windows, through which the air comes freshest. From a closed court, especially if the wind do not blow that way, air may come as stagnant as from any inside passage.

Again, a thing I have often seen in the sleeping rooms of private houses and cottages. The fire-place is carefully fastened up with a board; the windows are rarely or never opened; perhaps they are not made to open, or they open only at the bottom; perhaps some kind of stores are kept in the room; no breath of fresh air can by possibility enter into that room. The air is as stagnant, musty, and corrupt as it can by possibility be made. It is quite ripe to breed small-pox, scarlet fever, diptheria, or anything else you please.

Yet people, or worse still, children will sleep in that room without any previous airing. And the door will be left open all day in order to make the adjoining sitting-room or "houseplace" as foul as possible too, for ten to one the window of the sitting-room is kept closed.

The common idea as to rooms is that they may safely be left with window and chimney-board both closed—sealed up if possible—to keep out the dust, it is sometimes said; and that no harm will happen when inmates are put in. The question is often asked—But when ought the windows to be opened? The answer is—When ought they to be shut?

A short time ago a man walked into a back kitchen in Queen's-square, and cut the throat of a poor consumptive creature sitting by the fire. The murderer did not deny the act, but simply said, "It's all right." Of course he was mad.

But in our case, the extraordinary thing is that the victim says, "It's all right," and that we are not mad. Yet, although we "nose" the murderers in the musty, unaired, unsunned room, the scarlet fever which is behind the door, or the fever and hospital gangrene which are stalking among the crowded beds of a hospital ward, we say, "It's all right."

With a proper supply of windows, and a proper supply of fuel in open fire-places, fresh air is comparatively easy to secure when your patient or patients are in bed. Never be afraid of open windows then. People don't catch cold in bed. This is a popular fallacy. With proper bed-clothes and hot bottles, if necessary, you can always keep a patient warm in bed, and well ventilate him at the same time.

But a careless nurse, be her rank and education what it may, will stop up every cranny, and keep a hot-house heat when her patient is in bed,—and, if he is able to get up, leave him comparatively unprotected. The time when people take cold (and there are many ways of taking cold, besides a cold in the nose) is when they first get up after the two-fold exhaustion of dressing and of having had the skin relaxed by many hours, perhaps days, in bed, and thereby rendered more incapable of re-action. Then the same temperature which refreshes the patient in bed may destroy the patient just risen. And common sense will point out that, while purity of air is essential, a temperature must be secured which shall not chill the patient. Otherwise the best that can be expected will be a feverish re-action.

To have the air within as pure as the air without, it is not necessary, as often appears to be thought, to make it as cold.

In the afternoon again, without care, the patient whose vital powers have then risen, often finds the room as close and oppressive as he found it cold in the morning. Yet the nurse will be terrified if a window is opened.

It is very desirable that the windows in a sick room should be such as that the patient shall, if he can move about, be able to open and shut them easily himself.* In fact, the sick room is very seldom kept aired if this is not the case—so very few people have any perception of what is a healthy atmosphere for the sick. The sick man often says, "This room, where I spend twenty-two hours out of the twenty-four, is fresher than the other where I only spend two. Because here I can manage the windows myself." And it is true.

In a little book on nursing, published a short time ago, we are told, that "with proper care it is very seldom that the windows cannot be opened for a few minutes twice in the day to admit fresh air from without." I should think not; nor twice in the hour either. It only shows how little the subject has been considered.

Of all methods of keeping patients warm the very worst certainly is to depend for heat on the breath and bodies of the sick. I have known many a nurse keep her invalid's windows always closed, thus exposing the invalid to all the dangers of an infected atmosphere, because she was afraid that, by admitting fresh air, the temperature would be too much lowered. This is a destructive fallacy.

To attempt to keep a room warm at the expense of making the sick repeatedly breathe their own hot, damp, putrid atmosphere is a certain way to delay recovery or to destroy life.

Do you ever go into the bed-rooms of any persons of any class, whether they contain one, two, or twenty people, whether they hold sick or well, at night, or before the windows are opened in the morning, and ever find the air anything but unwholesomely close and foul? And why should it be so? And of how much importance is it that it should not be so? During sleep, the human body, even when in health, is far more injured by the influence of foul air than when awake. Why can't you keep the air all night, then, as pure as the air without in the rooms you sleep in? But for this, you must have sufficient outlet for the impure air you make yourself to go out; sufficient inlet for the pure air from without to come in. You must have open chimneys, open windows, or ventilators; no close curtains round your beds; no shutters or curtains to your windows, none of the con-

---

* NOTE.—Delirious fever cases, where there is any danger of the patient jumping out of window, are of course, exceptions. It is absolutely necessary that such cases should be kept cool and well-aired. I would undertake, with four gimlets, to save all risk of accidents, by merely preventing the sashes, both upper and lower, from being opened more than a few inches.

trivances by which you undermine your own health or destroy the chances of recovery of your sick.

Open the window above, not below. If your windows do not open above, the sooner they are made to do so the better. An inch or two will be enough for two people in a moderately-sized bed-room in winter. In a children's nursery or bed-room more will be required, according to the number. The worst place to admit air, either into a sick room or hospital ward, is at or near the level of the floor. I like casement windows better than sash windows, for this reason, that you *cannot* open a casement or French window as I see all women doing—an inch and a half of the lower sash—just on purpose *not* to air the room and to give you the rheumatism by the draught. Air admitted in this situation cools the floor and the lower strata of air; and if the patient is able to step out of bed, the cold air may give him a dangerous chill. During mild weather and summer time your windows may be wide open. In this, as in other things, common sense must be used. Ventilation of a bed-room or a sick room does not mean throwing the window up to the top, or drawing it down as far as it will come; still less does it mean opening the windows at intervals and keeping them shut between times, thereby subjecting the patient to the risk of frequent and violent alternations of temperature. It means simply keeping the air fresh.

The true criterion of ventilation is to step out of the sitting-room, bed-room, or sick room, in the morning, into the open air. If, on returning to it, you feel the least sensation of closeness, the ventilation has not been enough, and that room has been unfit for either sick or well to sleep in.

It is very odd how much more regard gardeners have for their plants than women have for their children or patients. If you were a gardener, you would know that, if you admitted air into your green-houses, as almost all women do into their rooms, viz., by a chink at the bottom of the window, the plants opposite that chink would die from the cutting air, and the plants above the chink would die for *want* of air. The air throughout a room is never changed by a draught in the lower part of the room. But it is changed by an open window in the upper part.

I have observed fifty times the death of poor unfortunate plants transferred to rooms aired after this fashion by the care of stupid women. What must it then be for their children or patients?

It is a curious fact, which you may any day observe for yourself, that the air admitted from a chink at the top of your window will circulate throughout the room—will keep it perfectly fresh without a draught, while, with a much wider chink near the bottom, it will be both close and draughty.

Do give yourself the trouble to open the window from the top. It is nothing but laziness which prevents your doing so. Add to this you can generally make a bad chimney smoke by the chink below—rarely by the chink above.

Again, you may any day observe for yourself how smells *drift*. If there is a corner in your room where there is no window, or where you never open the window, especially if it be at the end of a narrow room, any smell from any mess or dirt, from any-thing doing on the fire, will be stronger there than at the spot, or at any other spot in the room. Nay, it will even remain there long after the dirt is removed, and the smell gone from the spot. Yet such a corner as this is the one generally chosen for a sick bed to stand in. You can easily satisfy yourself by actual experi-ment of what I say. It is true even with regard to the scent of flowers. It is this which makes it so dangerous to leave the bed-room door open into a passage. You are quite sure to have the smell of any smoking, of any gas or candle, of any water-closet or sink, drifting into the place you sleep in, or worse where your sick person lies.

Of all places, public or private schools, where a number of children or young persons sleep in the same dormitory, require some test of freshness to be constantly applied. If it be hazardous for two children to sleep together in an unventilated bed-room, it is more than doubly so to have four, and much more than trebly so to have six under the same circumstances. People rarely remember this; yet, if parents were as solicitous about the air of school bed-rooms as they are about the food the children are to eat, and the kind of education they are to receive, at school, depend upon it due attention would be bestowed on this vitally important matter, and they would cease to have their children sent home either ill, or because scarlet fever or some other "cur-rent contagion" had broken out in the school.* There are schools where attention is paid to these things, and where "children's epidemics" are unknown.

* NOTE.—Nineteen cases out of every twenty of Scarlatina, in one London parish, were traced to the state of the public schools. In order to prevent such "schools from being the hot-beds of epidemic disease," there should be more space for each child, "proper ventilation," &c., &c.

How much sickness, death, and misery are produced by the present state of many factories, warehouses, workshops, and work-rooms! The places where poor dressmakers, tailors, letter-press printers, and other similar trades have to work for their living, are generally in a worse condition than any other portion of our worst towns. Many of these places of work were never constructed for such an object. They are badly adapted garrets, sitting-rooms, or bed-rooms, generally of an inferior class of house. No attention is paid to cubic space or ventilation. The poor workers are crowded on the floor to a greater extent than occurs with any other kind of over-crowding. In many cases 100 cubic feet would be considered by employers an extravagant extent of space for a worker. The constant breathing of foul air, saturated with moisture, and the action of such air upon the skin, makes the inmates peculiarly liable to cold, which is a sign indeed of the danger of chest disease to which they are exposed. In such places and under such circumstances of constrained posture, want of exercise, hurried and insufficient meals, long exhausting labour, and foul air—is it wonderful that a great majority of them die early of chest diseases? Intemperance is a common evil of these workshops. The men can only complete their work under the influence of stimulants, which help to undermine their health and destroy their morals, while hurrying them to premature graves. Employers rarely consider these things. Healthy work-rooms are no part of the bond into which they enter with their work-people. They pay their money, which they reckon their part of the bargain. And for this wage the workman or work-woman has to give work, health, and life.

Do men and women who employ fashionable tailors and milliners ever think of these things?

And yet the master is no gainer. His goods are spoiled by foul air and gas fumes, his own health and that of his family suffers, and his work is not so well done as it would be were his people in health. It is now admitted to be cheaper for all manufacturing purposes to have pure soft water than hard water. And the time will come when it will be found cheaper to supply shops, warehouses, and work-rooms with pure air than with foul air.

But the work-people themselves are not always without blame. In badly constructed work-places, where ventilation is at all times difficult, and where the workers have in consequence become very sensitive to cold, instead of using their common sense, they will frequently paste up every chink and crevice through which fresh air can reach them. This is especially the case with sedentary trades, such as tailors and dressmakers, and many perish from consumption in consequence. Indeed it has been said that "a decline" is the general disease of which they die. Have we not also heard of the Sheffield grinders refusing to make use of simple contrivances to protect their health, and dying early in consequence? Work-people should remember that health is their only capital, and they should come to an understanding among themselves to secure pure air in their places of work, which is one of the prime agents of health. This *would* be worth a "Trades' Union," almost worth a "strike."

The senses of nurses, mothers, workmen and workwomen, become so dulled to foul air that they are perfectly unconscious of what an atmosphere they have let their children, patients, or charges sleep in, or in which they themselves work. It is a bad habit which requires to be got rid of by education and fore-thought.

Oh! the crowded national school! in it how many children's epidemics have their origin! Ought not parents to say, "I will not send my child to that school. I will not trust my son or my daughter in that tailor's or milliner's workshop." And the dormitories of our great boarding schools! Scarlet fever would be no more ascribed to contagion but to its right cause, if parents would but use their common sense.

We should hear no longer of "mysterious dispensations," nor of "plague and pestilence" being "in God's hands," when, so far as we know, He has put them into our own.

For the sick, *warming* is a necessary part of ventilation.

A careful nurse will keep a constant watch over her sick, especially weak cases, to guard against the loss of vital heat by the patient himself. In certain diseased states much less heat is produced than in health; and there is a constant tendency to the decline and death of the vital powers by the call made upon them to sustain the heat of the body. Cases where this occurs should be watched with the greatest care from hour to hour, I had almost said from minute to minute. The feet and legs should be examined by the hand from time to time, and whenever a tendency to chilling is discovered, hot bottles, hot bricks, or warm flannels, with some warm drink, should be made use of until warmth is restored. The fire should be, if necessary, replenished.

Patients are frequently lost in the latter stages of disease from want of attention to such simple precautions. The nurse may be trusting to the patient's diet, or to his medicine, or to the occasional dose of stimulant which she is directed to give him, while the patient is all the while sinking from want of a little external warmth. Such cases happen at all times, even during the height of summer. This fatal chill is most apt to occur towards early morning, at the period of the lowest temperature of the twenty-four hours, and at the time when the effect of the preceding day's diets is exhausted.

Generally speaking, you may expect that weak patients will suffer cold much more in the morning than in the evening. The vital powers are much lower. If they are feverish at night, with burning hands and feet, they are almost sure to be chilly and shivering in the morning. But nurses are very fond of heating the foot-warmer at night, and of neglecting it in the morning, when they are busy. I should reverse the matter.

What can nurses be thinking of who put a bottle of boiling water to the patient's feet, hoping that it will keep warm all the twenty-four hours? Of course, every time he touches it, it wakes him. It sends the blood to the head. It makes his feet tender. And then the nurse leaves it in the bed after it has become quite cold. A hot bottle should never be hotter than it can be comfortably touched with the naked hand. It should not be expected to keep warm longer than eight hours. Tin foot-warmers are too hot and too cold. Stone bottles are the best, or India-rubber; but careless nurses make sad havoc with the latter, by putting in water too hot, or by letting the screw get out of order, and the patient be deluged in his bed.

All these things require common sense and care. Yet perhaps in no one single thing is so little common sense shown, in all ranks, as in nursing.

The art of nursing, as now practised, seems to be expressly constituted to unmake what God had made disease to be, viz., a restorative process.

The extraordinary confusion between cold and ventilation, in the minds of even well-educated people, illustrates this. To make a room cold is by no means necessarily to ventilate it. Nor is it at all necessary, in order to ventilate a room, to chill it. Yet, if a nurse finds a room close, she will let out the fire, thereby making it closer, or she will open the door into a cold room, without a fire, or an open window in it, by way of improving the ventilation. The safest atmosphere of all for a patient is a good fire and an open window, excepting in extremes of temperature. (Yet no nurse can ever be made to understand this.) To ventilate a small room without draughts of course requires more care than to ventilate a large one.

But it is often observed that nurses who make the greatest outcry against open windows are those who take the least pains to prevent dangerous draughts. The door of the patients' room *must* sometimes stand open to allow of persons passing in and out, or heavy things being carried in and out. The careful nurse will keep the door shut while she shuts the windows, and then, and not before, set the door open, so that a patient may not be left sitting up in bed, perhaps in a profuse perspiration, directly in the draught between the open door and window. Neither, of course, should a patient, while being washed or in any way exposed, remain in the draught of an open window or door.

It is truly provoking to see stupid women bring into disrepute the life-spring of the patient, viz., fresh air, by their stupidity. Chest and throat attacks may undoubtedly be brought on by the nurse letting her sick run about without slippers, flannel or dress-ing gowns, in a room where she has left the wintry wind blowing in upon them, without taking any precaution if they should leave their beds. Certain beds are sometimes pointed out, in a kind of helpless way, as being predestined to bronchitis, because of the "draught from the door." Why should there be a draught from the door? If there be, why should the draught fall on a patient? Is there no such thing as a screen to be had; or if the bed space be in a draught which cannot be prevented, why not remove the bed? But a careless woman will come into the sick room and leave the door open till she goes out again, for no reason that any-body can discover but her own blindness. And she will leave the window open over her patient who is washing or sitting up in a night-dress, and then say, "He has taken cold from the open window." He has taken cold from your own thoughtlessness. Neither leaving doors open nor drawing down windows over your patients when the surface is exposed is ventilation. It is simply carelessness.

Another extraordinary fallacy is the dread of night air. What air can we breathe at night but night air? The choice is between pure night air from without, and foul night air from within. Most people prefer the latter. An unaccountable choice. What will they say, if it is proved to be true that fully one-half of all the disease we suffer from is occasioned by people sleeping with their windows shut! A window open at the top most nights in the year can never hurt any one. In great towns night air is often the best and purest air to be had in the twenty-four hours. I could better understand shutting the windows during the day in towns than during the night, for the sake of the sick. The absence of smoke, the quiet, all tend to making night the best time for airing patients. The air in London is never so good as after ten o'clock at night.

The only time when it can be unsafe to open the window at night is when the air is more foul without than within. This may be the case in close back courts, with open privies and middensteads in them (nuisances which ought not to be permitted to exist in towns), or at hours when there is a sudden fall of temperature.

Always air your room, then, from the outside air, if possible. Windows are made to open; doors are made to shut—a truth which seems extremely difficult of apprehension. I have seen a careful nurse airing her patient's room through the door near to which were two gaslights (each of which consumes as much air as eleven men), a kitchen, a close passage, the atmosphere in which consisted of gas, paint, foul air, never changed, full of effluvia, including a current of sewer air from an ill-placed sink, ascending in a continual stream by a well-staircase, and discharging themselves constantly into the patient's room. The window of the said room, if opened, was all that was desirable to air it. Every room must be aired from without—every passage from without—but the fewer passages there are, the better.

If we are to preserve the air within as pure as the air without, it is needless to say that the chimney must not smoke. Almost all smoky chimneys can be cured—from the bottom, not from the top. Often it is only necessary to have an inlet for air to supply the fire, which is feeding itself, for want of this, from its own chimney. On the other hand, almost all chimneys can be made to smoke by a careless nurse, who lets the fire get low, and then overwhelms it with coal; not, as we verily believe, in order to spare herself trouble (for very rare is unkindness to the sick), but from not thinking what she is about.

In laying down the principle that the first object of the nurse must be to keep the air breathed by her patient as pure as the air without, it must not be forgotten that everything in the room which can give off effluvia, besides the patient, evaporates itself into his air. And it follows, that there ought to be nothing in the room, excepting him, which *can* give off effluvia* or moisture. Out of all damp towels, &c., which become dry in the room, the damp, of course, goes into the patient's air. Yet this "of course" seems as little thought of as if it were an obsolete fiction. How very seldom you see a nurse who acknowledges by her practice that nothing at all ought to be aired in the patient's room, that nothing at all ought to be cooked at the patient's fire! Indeed, the arrangements often make this rule impossible to observe.

If the nurse be a very careful one, she will, when the patient leaves his bed, but not his room, open the sheets wide, and throw the bedclothes back, in order to air his bed. And she will spread the wet towels or flannels carefully out upon a horse, in order to dry them. Now either these bedclothes and towels are not dried and aired, or they dry and air themselves into the patient's air. And whether the damp and effluvia do him most harm in his air or in his bed, I leave to you to determine, for I cannot.

Even in health people cannot repeatedly breathe air in which they live with impunity, on account of its becoming charged with unwholesome matter from the lungs and skin. In disease, where everything given off from the body is highly noxious and dangerous, not only must there be plenty of ventilation to carry off the effluvia, but everything which the patient passes must be instantly removed away, as being more noxious than even the emanations from himself.

Of the fatal effects of the effluvia from the excretions it would seem unnecessary to speak, were they not so constantly neglected. Concealing the utensil behind the vallance to the bed seems all the precaution which is thought necessary for safety in private nursing. Did you but think for one moment of the atmosphere under that bed, the saturation of the under side of the mattress with the warm evaporations, you would be startled and frightened too!

The use of any chamber utensil *without a lid* should be utterly

---

* NOTE.—"Effluvia" is a very fine word, and might he replaced by the word "smell." But smells only shew where effluvia are, and are not the effluvia themselves; and it is most dangerous to remove smells without removing the offensive thing itself, for God put the smell there to shew us the danger.

abolished, whether among sick or well. You can easily convince yourself of the necessity of this absolute rule, by taking one with a lid and examining the under side of that lid. It will be found always covered, whenever the utensil is not empty, by condensed offensive moisture. Where does that go when there is no lid?

But never, never should the possession of this indispensable lid confirm you in the abominable practice of letting the chamber utensil remain in a patient's room unemptied, except once in the twenty-four hours, *i. e.*, when the bed is made. Yes, impossible as it may appear, I have known the best and most attentive nurses guilty of this; aye, and have known, too, a patient afflicted with severe diarrhoea for ten days, and the nurse, a very good one, not know of it, because the chamber utensil (one with a lid) was emptied only once in the twenty-four hours. As well might you have a sewer under the room, or think that in a water-closet the plug need be pulled up but once a day. Also take care that your *lid*, as well as your utensil, be always thoroughly rinsed.

If a nurse declines to do these kinds of things for her patient, "because it is not her business," I should say that nursing was not her calling. I have seen surgical "sisters," women whose hands were worth to them two or three guineas a-week, down upon their knees scouring a room or hut, because they thought it otherwise not fit for their patients to go into. I am far from wishing nurses to scour. It is a waste of power. But I do say that these women had the true nurse-calling—the good of their sick first, and second only the consideration what it was their "place" to do—and that women who wait for anybody else to do what their patients want, when their patients are suffering, have not the *making* of a nurse in them.

Earthenware, or if there is any wood, highly polished and varnished wood, are the only materials fit for patients' utensils. The very lid of the old abominable close-stool is enough to breed a pestilence. It becomes saturated with offensive matter, which scouring is only wanted to bring out. I prefer an earthenware lid as being always cleaner. But there are various good new-fashioned arrangements.

A slop-pail should never be brought into a sick room. It should be a rule invariable, rather more important in the private house than elsewhere, that the utensil should be carried directly to the water-closet, emptied there, rinsed there, and brought back. There should always be water and a cock in every water-closet for rinsing. But even if there is not, you must carry water there to rinse with. I have actually seen, in the sick room, the utensils emptied into the foot-pan, and put back, unrinsed under the bed. I can hardly say which is most abominable, whether to do this or to rinse the utensil in the sick room. In the best hospitals it is now a rule that no slop-pail shall ever be brought into the wards, but that the utensils shall be carried direct to be emptied and rinsed at the proper place. I would it were so in every house!

Let no one ever depend upon fumigations, "disinfectants," and the like, for purifying the air. The offensive thing, not its smell, must be removed. I wish all disinfecting fluids invented made an "abominable smell" that they forced you to open the windows and to admit fresh air. That would be a useful invention.

II.—HEALTH OF HOUSES

THERE are five essential points in securing the health of houses: —

1. Pure air.
2. Pure water.

3. Efficient drainage.
4. Cleanliness.

5. Light.

Without these no house can be healthy. And it will be unhealthy just in proportion as they are not.

1. To have pure air, your house must be so built as that the outer air shall find its way with ease to every corner of it. House builders hardly ever consider this. The object in building a house is to obtain the largest interest for the money, not to save doctor's bills to the tenants. But, if tenants should ever become so wise as to refuse to occupy unhealthily built houses, builders would speedily be brought to their senses. As it is, they build what pays best. And there are always people foolish enough to take the houses they build. And if in the course of time the families die off, as is so often the case, nobody ever thinks of blaming any but Providence for the result. Ill-informed people help to keep up the delusion, by laying the blame on "current contagions." Bad houses do for the healthy what bad hospitals do for the sick. Once insure that the air in a house is stagnant, and sickness is certain to follow.

No one thinks how much disease might be prevented even in the country, by simply attending to providing the cottages with fresh air.

I know whole districts in the south of England where, even when the windows are sashed, the sashes are never made to open at the top.

I know whole districts in the north of England where, even in quite new cottages, the bedroom windows are not made to open at all, excepting a single pane, generally placed low down in the window. Now, if this open pane were in the upper row of the upper sash, it would be all very well. Very tolerable ventilation is procured by this means. But if it is in the lower row, it is all very bad. It does nothing but produce a draught setting inwards, actually driving the foul air upon the inmates, and not letting it out at all.

Only satisfy yourself of all these things by experiment for yourself.

What happens in a cottage? The rooms are always small and generally crowded. One or two rooms have to serve for all household purposes. And the air in them, especially at night, is stagnant and foul. Almost always there are closets or corners without either light or air, which make the whole house musty. And the house has itself hardly ever sufficient light.

Now, it is quite impossible to lay down a general rule without knowing the particular case.

It is for the father of the family to decide.

Sometimes an additional pane of glass, made to open and shut, and put into the wall where it is wanted, will make a cottage sweet which always was musty.

Sometimes a sky-light, made to open, will make an attic wholesome which never was habitable before.

Every careful woman will spread out the bedding daily to the light and air.

No window is safe, as has often here been said, which does not open at top, or where at least a pane in the upper row of the upper sash does not open.

In small crowded rooms, I again repeat, the foul air is all above the chimney-breast, and is therefore quite ready to be breathed by the people sitting in the room or in bed. This air requires to be let off; and the simplest way of doing it is one of these, viz.:—

1. An Arnott's ventilator in the chimney close to the ceiling.

2. An air-brick in the wall at the ceiling.

3. A pane of perforated glass in a passage or stair-window.

The large old fire-place, under which three or four people can sit—still to be seen in cottages of the south of England and in old manor-houses—is an immense benefit to the air of the room. Pity it has disappeared in all new buildings![1]

But never stop up your chimney. Of whatever size it is, it is a good ventilator.

And during almost every night of the year, pull your window an inch down *at the top*. Remember, AT THE TOP.

To clergymen, district-visitors, and landlords may be said, Help the people to carry out these improvements. They are often more willing to do so than you are to help. You will thus do infinitely more good than by supporting hospitals and dispensaries for them when they are ill of foul air. Why not prevent the illness which comes of foul air?

The main objection of working-people to fresh air is the cold. Warm the air introduced into cottage-rooms by passing it through some fire-clay contrivance behind the grate and heated by the fire, —the air to be admitted to the heating cavity direct from the outside, and entering the room above the chimney-piece. You can economise half the fuel by some of the new cottage-grates.

2. Pure water is more general in houses than it used to be; thanks to the exertions of a few. Within the last few years, a large part of London was in the daily habit of using water polluted by the drainage of its sewers and water-closets. This has happily been remedied. But, in many parts of the country, well-water of a very impure kind is used for domestic purposes. And when epidemic disease shows itself, persons using such water are almost sure to suffer. Never use water that is not perfectly colourless and without taste or smell. And never keep water in an open tub or pail in a sitting-room or bed-room. Water absorbs foul air, and becomes foul and unwholesome in consequence, and it damps the air in the room, making it also unwholesome.

The following way of purifying village wells is a good one. When well-water is impure, this generally arises from foul water filtering in through the dirty ground near the well's mouth. To cure this, the earth should be dug away all round the well's mouth to a distance of six feet from the brickwork, and to a depth of six or seven feet below the surface. The cavity is then to be filled up with clean sand and rammed hard down. This stops the entrance of foul water into the well.

3. It would be curious to ascertain by inspection, how many houses said to be drained are really well-drained. Many people would say, surely all or most of them. But many people have no idea in what good drainage consists. They think that a sewer in the street, and a pipe leading to it from the house is good drainage. All the while the sewer may be nothing but a place from which sickness and ill health are being poured into the house. No house with any untrapped, unventilated drain-pipe communicating immediately with an unventilated sewer, whether it be from water-closet, sink, or gully-grate, can ever be healthy. An untrapped sink may at any time spread fevers and other diseases among the inmates of a palace.

Country cottages suffer from bad drainage quite as much as, if not more than, town houses. The best that can be said about their floors is that they are on the level of the ground, instead of being a foot *or more* above it, as they ought to be, with the air playing freely below the boards. Most frequently, however, the floors are not boarded, but are merely made of earth or of porous brick, which absorbs a large quantity of moisture, and keeps damp cold air always about the feet. Perhaps most frequently of all, the floor has been worn away several inches below the level of the ground, and of course after every wet day the floor is wet and sloppy. One would think this bad enough, but it is not the worst. Sometimes a dung-hill, or a pig-sty is kept so close to the door that the foul water from it, after rain, may be seen flowing over the house floor.

It frequently happens when cottages are built on hill-sides that the cottage wall is built against the damp earth, instead of being separated from it, and the water from the hill keeps both walls and floors constantly damp. There are whole villages in which one or more, or even all of these defects exist, and the natural result is fever, scarlet fever, measles, rheumatism, &c.

People are astonished that they are not healthy in the country, as if living in the country would save them from attending to any of the laws of health more than living in a town.

Now then, here is a whole field for activity—for saving human life and health. Is there nobody in the parish who would take such matters up, and go from house to house to examine into them? A little common sense, a little labour, which in nine cases out of ten could be found by the people themselves, a few shillings of expense at the outside, and no costly machinery of any kind, would put the whole thing to rights, and save health, life, and poor-rates.

Did you ever observe on looking over an extensive landscape after sunset that there were certain groups of houses over which the first fog settled sooner than over others? The fog is nature's way of showing that the houses and their neighbourhood are saturated with moisture from the neglects above specified. These fogs also point out where the fever or cholera will come.

To remedy this state of things, the ground requires to be drained or trenched, the earth cut away, the floors raised above the level of the ground, and dung-hills and pig-sties removed as far as possible from the houses. These things can always be placed in such a way as that the natural drainage removes all that is offensive about them, at least away from the house.

Another not uncommon cause of sickness among village people is a puddle of foul water or an offensive ditch. The former can always be filled up with earth, or drained away by a little spade labour. As regards the latter, there is nothing in which more good could be done than by laying a drain-pipe in the bottom of the ditch and filling the earth in over it to a sufficient distance on either side the houses.

People often put up with nuisances from dunghills and pig-sties, on account of the value of the matter itself. Value there is certainly. But the question is whether the nuisance is necessary; and whether, in preventing nuisance, money would not be saved?

"All foul smell indicates disease, and loss of money," says Mr. Chadwick.[2] Never live in a house which smells. Either don't take it, or examine where the smell comes from, and put a stop to it; but never think of living in it until there is no smell. A house which smells is a hot-bed of disease.

But though such smells always indicate danger, says the same authority, it does not always follow that there is no danger when there is no smell. The danger is often greater, when the smell which gives warning is gone. Therefore remove the thing itself and not only the smell.

One of the most common causes of disease in towns is having privies and cesspools, ashpits or *middensteads* close to the houses. There are great and rich cities and towns which justly pride themselves on their drainage, their water-supply, their paving, and surface cleansing, and yet have more death in their dwellings than many towns where no such works have been carried out. In all these cases, the domestic filth of the population is allowed to accumulate among the houses, in close courts, polluting the soil underneath and the air within the houses to such a degree, that, in spite of the draining, water-supply, and paving, excellent as these may be, the people suffer from exactly double the sickness and death which ought to fall to their lot. There is no way of putting a stop to this terrible loss of life, except by putting an end to these privies and cesspits, and bringing in drainage and water-closets, as has been done in many of the very worst districts of London, and throughout the whole of the dwelling-houses of improved towns.

An attempt is often made to shield these neglects under the plea that "so much has been done already." But the ready reply is "these things ought you to have done, and not to have left the others undone."

As regards country cottages, if a safe outlet for the sewage can be obtained, cottages can be very cheaply drained. The pipes required will cost about a shilling per lineal yard, and a soil-pan can be put up for ten shillings additional more or less.

The worst class of nuisances are certainly those I have referred to in which the local authorities, who ought to be the uncompromising protectors of the health of the poor, attempt to palliate their own deficiencies. But there is another class in which people injure each other by committing nuisance or keeping their premises in a filthy condition. In the present state of the law this can be avoided by bringing reasonable complaint before the authorities who will see the law enforced. It often happens, however, that the poor are too ill-informed or too apathetic to take any such step, and it is at this point that they can often be most efficiently assisted by the clergyman or district visitor, in whom a knowledge of the law, as it bears on the health of the parishioners, would often be the means of saving sickness as well as "parish rates." Unhealthy houses, those whoso inmates suffer most from sickness and mortality, are well known to parish doctors, officers of health, and to other medical practitioners. The simple question, "Show us the houses which yield the largest amount of fever or other epidemic disease?" addressed to any of these officers will enable the finger to be laid at once on the plague spots of the parish, and show where the poor require help, or advice, or both, in having their houses drained, cleansed, lime-washed, or venti-lated.

Among the more common causes of ill-health in cottages is overcrowding. There is perhaps only a single room for a whole family, and not more than 150 or 200 cubic feet for each inmate. Nothing can make such a room healthy. Ventilation would im-prove it, but still it would be unhealthy. The only way to meet this overcrowded state of cottages is by adding rooms, or by building more cottages on a better model.

The ordinary oblong sink is an abomination. That great surface of stone, which is always left wet, is always exhaling into the air. I have known whole houses and hospitals smell of the sink. I have met just as strong a stream of sewer air coming up the back staircase of a grand London house from the sink, as I have ever met at Scutari; and I have seen the rooms in that house all ventilated by the open doors, and the passages all *un*ventilated by the closed windows, in order that as much of the sewer air as possible might be conducted into and retained in the bed-rooms. It is wonderful!

Another great evil in house construction is carrying drains underneath the house. Such drains are never safe. All house drains should begin and end outside the walls. Many people will readily say, how important are these things. But how few are there who trace disease in their households to such causes! Is it not a fact that, when scarlet fever, measles, or small-pox appear among the children, the very first thought which occurs is, "where" the children can have "caught" the disease? And the parents immediately run over in their minds all the families with whom they may have been. They never think of looking at home for the source of the mischief. If a neighbour's child is seized with small-pox, the first question which occurs is, whether it had been vaccinated. No one would undervalue vaccination; but it becomes of doubtful benefit when it leads people to look abroad for the source of evils which exist at home.[3]

4. Without cleanliness, within and without your house, ventila-tion is comparatively useless. In certain foul districts poor people used to object to open their windows and doors because of the foul smells that came in. Rich people like to have their stables and dunghill near their houses. But does it ever occur to them that with many arrangements of this kind it would be safer to keep the windows shut than open? You cannot have

the air of the house pure with dung heaps under the windows. These are common everywhere. And yet people are surprised that their children, brought up in "country air," suffer from children's diseases. If they studied nature's laws in the matter of children's health, they would not be so surprised.

There are other ways of having filth inside a house besides having dirt in heaps. Old papered walls of years' standing, dirty carpets, dirty walls and ceilings, uncleaned furniture, pollute the air just as much as if there were a dung heap in the basement. People are so unaccustomed to consider how to make a home healthy, that they either never think of it at all, and take every disease as a matter of course, to be "resigned to" when it comes "as from the hand of Providence;" or if they ever entertain the idea of preserving the health of their household as a duty, they are very apt to commit all kinds of "negligences and ignorances" in performing it.

Even in the poorest houses, washing the walls and ceilings with quick-lime wash twice a year, would prevent more disease than you wot of.

5. A dark house is always an unhealthy house, always an ill-aired house, always a dirty house. Want of light stops growth, and promotes scrofula, rickets, &c., &c., among the children.

People lose their health in a dark house, and if they get ill they cannot get well again in it. More will be said about this farther on.

Three out of many "negligences and ignorances" in managing the health of houses generally, I will here mention as specimens —1. That the mistress of any building, large or small, does not think it necessary to visit every hole and corner of it every day. How can she expect others to be more careful to maintain her house in a healthy condition than she who is in charge of it? — 2. That it is not considered essential to air, to sun, and to clean every room, whether inhabited or not; which is simply laying the ground ready for all kinds of diseases. —3. That the window is considered enough to air a room. Have you never observed that any room without a fire-place is always close? And, if you have a fire-place, would you cram it up not only with a chimney-board, but perhaps with a great wisp of brown paper, in the throat of the chimney—to prevent the soot from coming down, you say? If your chimney is foul, sweep it; but don't expect that you can ever air a room with only one opening; don't suppose that to shut up a room is the way to keep it clean. It is the best way to foul the room and all that is in it.

But again, to look to all these things yourself (and here I speak to school-mistresses, mothers of large families, and matrons), does not mean to do them yourself. "I always open the windows," the head in charge often says. If you do it, it is by so much the better, certainly, than if it were not done at all. But can you not insure that it is done when not done by yourself? Can you insure that it is not undone when your back is turned? This is what being "in charge" means. And a very important meaning it is, too. The former only implies that just what you can do with your own hands is done—the latter, that what ought to be done is always done.

And now, you think these things trifles, or at least exaggerated. But what you "think" or what I "think" matters little. Let us see what God thinks of them. God always justifies His ways. While we are "thinking," He has been teaching. I have known cases of sickness quite as severe in private houses as in any of the worst towns, and from the same cause, viz., foul air. Yet nobody learnt the lesson. Nobody learnt *anything* at all from it. They went on *thinking*—thinking that the sufferer had scratched his thumb, or that it was singular that everybody should have "whitlows," or that something was "much about this year; there is always sickness in our house." This is a favourite mode of thought—leading *not* to inquire what is the uniform cause of these general "whitlows," but to stifle all inquiry. In what sense is "sickness" being "always there," a justification of its being "there" at all?

What was the cause of sickness being in that nice private house? It was, that the sewer air from an ill-placed sink was carefully conducted into all the rooms by sedulously opening all the doors, and closing all the passage windows. It was that the slops were emptied into the foot pans;—it was that the utensils were never properly rinsed;—it was that the chamber crockery was rinsed with dirty water;—it was that the beds were never properly shaken, aired, picked to pieces, or changed. It was that the carpets and curtains were always musty;—it was that the furniture was always dusty;—it was that the papered walls were saturated with dirt;—it was that the floors were never cleaned; —it was that the empty rooms were never sunned, or cleaned, or aired;—it was that the cupboards were always reservoirs of foul air;—it was that the windows were always tight shut up at night;—it was that no window was ever regularly opened, even in the day, or that the right window was not opened. A person gasping for air might open a window for himself. But the people were not taught to open the windows, to shut the doors; or they opened the windows upon a dank well between high walls, not upon the airier court; or they opened the room doors into the unaired passages, by way of airing the rooms. Now all this is not fancy, but fact. In that house there have been in one summer six cases of serious illness: all the *immediate* products of foul air. When, in temperate climates, a house is more un-healthy in summer than in winter, it is a certain sign of some-thing wrong. Yet nobody learns the lesson. Yes, God always justifies His ways. He is teaching while you are not learning. This poor body loses his finger, that one loses his life. And all from the most easily preventible causes.

God lays down certain physical laws. Upon His carrying out such laws depends our responsibility (that much abused word); for how could we have any responsibility for actions, the results of which we could not foresee?—which would be the case if the carrying out of his laws were *not* certain. Yet we seem to be continually expecting that He will work a miracle—*i.e.*, break His own laws expressly to relieve us of responsibility.

"With God's Blessing he will recover" is a common form of parlance. But "with God's blessing" also, it is, if he does *not* recover; and "with God's blessing" that he fell ill; and "with God's blessing" that he dies, if he does die. In other words, *all* these things happen by God's laws, which *are* His blessings, that is, which are all to contribute to teach us the way to our best happiness. Cholera is just as much His "blessing" as the exempt-tion from it. It is to teach us how to obey His laws. "With God's blessing he will recover," is a common form of speech with people who, all the while, are neglecting the means on which God has made health or recovery to depend.

I must say a word about servants' bed-rooms. From the way they are built, but oftener from the way they are kept, and from no intelligent inspection whatever being exercised over them, they are almost invariably dens of foul air, and the "servants' health" suffers in an "unaccountable"(?) way, even in the country. For I am by no means speaking only of London houses where too often servants are put to live under the ground and over the roof. But in the country I have known three maids, who slept in the same room, ill of scarlet fever. "How catching it is!" was of course the remark. One look at the room, one smell of the room was quite enough. It was no longer "unaccountable." The room was not a small one; it was up stairs, and it had two large windows—but nearly every one of the neglects enumerated above was there.

Servants might do much to prevent illness in their miserably neglected bed-rooms by attending to cleanliness, by leaving the chimney open, and especially by opening the window an inch or two at the top through the night. The window ought, of course, to be wide open all day, when the weather will allow of it.

The houses of the grandmothers and great-grandmothers of this generation, at least the country houses, with front door and back door always standing open, winter and summer, and a thorough draught always blowing through—with all the scrubbing, and cleaning, and polishing, and scouring which used to go on,—the grandmothers, and still more the great-grandmothers, always out of doors, and never with a bonnet on except to go to church,—these things, when contrasted with our present "civilized" habits, entirely account for the fact so often seen of a great-grandmother, who was a tower of physical strength, descending into a grandmother, perhaps a little less strong, but still sound as a bell and healthy to the core, into a mother languid and confined to her house, and lastly, into a daughter sickly and confined to her bed. For, remember, even with a general decrease of mortality you may often find a race thus degenerating and still oftener a family. You may see poor little feeble washed-out rags, children of a noble stock, suffering morally and physically, throughout their useless, degenerate lives, and yet people who are going to marry and to bring more such into the world, will consult nothing but their own convenience as to where they are to live, or how they are to live.

That consumption is induced by the foul air of houses, *i.e.*, by air fouled by human bodies, more than by all other causes put together, is now certain. It is often said, even by doctors, as throwing doubt upon this fact, that "young ladies," who do not, it is supposed, live in a "vitiated atmosphere," yet die of consumption. But do these people know the up-stair habits of this class?—I do, or did. And of all classes there are two, viz., "young ladies," and soldiers, who are the most exposed to the influences which produce consumption. Both sleep, and partly live, in foul air. A "young lady," advised to open her window and her curtains at night, has been known to say that "it would spoil her complexion." From this close, foul air both the "young lady," and the soldier go out at night in all weathers,—the one to "parties," the other to sentry duty; both enter into more foul air,—the one in crowded ball-rooms, the other in guard-rooms; both go home in damp night air after the skin and lungs have been oppressed by over-crowding and want of ventilation, and both suffer from chest diseases, especially from consumption.

Insufficient and unwholesome food is an auxiliary in some people to the work of consumption.

The object of spoiling her digestion is still further forwarded by many a woman by the practice of taking continual and powerful aperients; or, if the process of exhaustion is far advanced, by taking opium, gin, or some cordial. It is little known how far this practice prevails.

Could we devise a course more likely first to ruin the general health and sow the seeds, and then act as a forcing-house, of consumption?

Again, people often point to the frequency of consumption in some families to prove its "hereditary nature." Therefore it is "inevitable." It is, indeed, extremely likely that if one or two deaths occur from consumption in a family there will be many more; for the whole family has been so mismanaged, that it is very unlikely that it should not attack other members in succession, just as children's epidemics do. But because seventeen persons, who eat poisoned sugar-plums at Bradford, several out of the same family, all die, is it a reason for supposing their poisoning "hereditary," "contagious," or the result of a "family predisposition"?

Once more; it is indeed to be feared that weakness of digestion, or bad health, *is* becoming "hereditary" in many women, which also "predisposes" to consumption, and which, more than anything else, tends to the degeneracy of a family or race. Weakness of digestion depends upon habits; primarily and directly upon want of fresh air; secondarily and indirectly upon idleness or unhealthy work, or excitement, unwholesome food, abuse of stimulants and aperients, and other exhausting habits.

It has been often stated that intermarriage, marrying cousins is a fruitful source of family weakness and want of health; but is it considered that other habits descending from parents to offspring, such, for instance, as intemperance, breathing foul air, living in gloomy unhealthy localities and the like, also tend to want of health?

In healthy "registration" districts, the mortality is low, and the annual proportion of births is also low, but in unhealthy districts the mortality rises, while at the same time the proportion of births increases, showing that in such districts the circuit of life is shortened.

Now as to these children ushered into existence in the midst of such excessive mortality!

Has not every one had the opportunity of comparing the full healthy development of a child born in a healthy country district with the thin, ill-fed, undeveloped or ill-developed frame of the child born in an unhealthy town? And is not the conclusion irresistible that the unhealthy town child belongs to a lower family type than the healthy country child? A process of physical deterioration has been going on notwithstanding the increase of births; and of these two classes of children about a third of the country children die before they reach the age of five years, while of the town children a half die before that period, and a large proportion of those who survive their fifth year are puny, sickly people, whose early deaths go to swell the local mortality.

These are momentous facts, if people would only ponder them, and act on the lessons they are teaching.

With regard to the health of houses where there is a sick person, it often happens that the sick room is made a ventilating shaft for the rest of the house; for while the house is kept as close, unaired, and dirty as usual, the window of the sick room is kept a little open always, and the door occasionally. Now, there are certain sacrifices which a house with one sick person in it does make to that sick person. Why can't it keep itself thoroughly clean and unusually well-aired, out of regard to the sick person?

We must not forget what, in ordinary language, is called "Infection;"—a thing of which people are generally so afraid that they frequently follow the very practice in regard to it which they ought to avoid. Nothing used to be considered so infectious or contagious as small-pox; and people, not very long ago, used to cover up patients with heavy bed-clothes, while they kept up large fires, and shut the windows. Small-pox, of course, under this management, was very "infectious." People are somewhat wiser now in their management of this disease. They have ventured to cover the patients lightly and to keep the windows open; and we hear much less of the "infection" of small-pox than we used to do. But do people in our days act with more wisdom on the subject of "infection" in fevers—scarlet fever, measles, &c. — than their forefathers did with small-pox? Does not the popular idea of "infection" involve that people should take greater care of themselves than of the patient? That, for instance, it is safer not to be too much with the patient, not to attend too much to his wants?

True nursing knows nothing of infection, except to prevent it. Cleanliness and fresh air from open windows, with unremitting attention to the patient, are the only defence a true nurse either asks or needs.

Wise and humane management of the patient is the best safeguard against infection.

Is it not living in a continual mistake to look upon diseases, as we do now, as separate things, which must exist, like cats and dogs? instead of looking upon them as conditions, like a dirty and a clean condition, and just as much under our own control; or rather as the reactions of a kindly nature, against the conditions in which we have placed ourselves.

I was brought up, both by scientific men and ignorant women, distinctly to believe that small-pox, for instance, was a thing of which there was once a first specimen in the world, which went on propagating itself, in a perpetual chain of descent, just as much as that there was a first dog (or a first pair of dogs), and that small-pox would not begin itself any more than a new dog would begin without there having been a parent dog.

Since then I have seen with my eyes and smelt with my nose small-pox growing up in first specimens, either in close rooms or in overcrowded wards, where it could not by any possibility have been "caught," but must have begun.

Nay, more, I have seen diseases begin, grow up, and pass into one another. Now, dogs do not pass into cats.

I have seen, for instance, with a little overcrowding, continued fever grow up; and with a little more, typhoid fever; and with a little more, typhus, and all in the same ward or hut.

Would it not be far better, truer, and more practical if we looked upon disease in this light?

There are not a few popular opinions, in regard to which it is useful at times to ask a question or two. For example, it is commonly thought that children must have what are commonly called "children's epidemics," "current contagions," &c.; in other words, that they are born to have measles, whooping-cough, perhaps even scarlet fever, just as they are born to cut their teeth, if they live.

Now, do tell us, why must a child have measles?

Oh, because, you say, we cannot keep it from infection—other children have measles—and it must take them—and it is safer that it should.

But why must other children have measles? And if they have, why must yours have them too?

If you believed in, and observed the laws for preserving the health of houses which inculcate cleanliness, fresh air, whitewashing, and other means, and which, by the way, *are laws*, as implicitly as you believe in the popular opinion, for it is nothing more than an opinion, that your child must have children's epidemics, don't you think that, upon the whole, your child would be more likely to escape altogether?

III.— PETTY MANAGEMENT.

ALL the results of good nursing may be spoiled or utterly negatived by one defect, viz., in petty management, or, in other words, by not knowing how to manage, that what you do when you are there shall be done when you are not *there*. The most devoted friend or nurse cannot be always there. Nor is it desirable that she should. And she may give up her health, all her other duties, and yet, for want of a little management, be not one-half so efficient as another who is not one-half so devoted, but who has this art of multiplying herself—that is to say, the patient of the first will not really be so well cared for as the patient of the second.

It is as impossible in a book to teach a person in charge of sick how to *manage*, as it is to teach her how to nurse. Circumstances must vary with each different case. But it *is* possible to press upon her to think for herself:—Now, what does happen during my absence? I am obliged to be away on Tuesday. But fresh air, or punctuality, is not less important to my patient on Tuesday than it was on Monday. Or: At 10 p.m. I am never with my patient; but quiet is of no less consequence to him at 10 than it was at 5 minutes to 10.

Curious as it may seem, this very obvious consideration occurs comparatively to few; or, if it does occur, it is only to cause the devoted friend or nurse to be absent fewer hours or fewer minutes from her patient—not to arrange so as that no minute and no hour shall be for her patient without the essentials of her nursing.

A very few instances will be sufficient, not as precepts, but as illustrations.

A stranger will burst in by mistake to the patient's sick-room, after he has fallen into his first doze, giving him a shock, the effects of which are irremediable, though he himself laughs at the cause, and probably never even mentions it. The nurse, who is, and is quite right to be, at her supper, has not provided that the stranger shall not lose his way and go into the wrong room.

The patient's room may always have the window open. But the passage outside the patient's room may never have one open. Because it is not understood that the charge of the sick-room extends to the charge of the passage. And thus, as often happens, the nurse makes it her business to turn the patient's room into a ventilating shaft for the foul air of the whole house.

An empty room, a newly painted room, an uncleaned closet or cupboard, may often become a reservoir of foul air for the whole house, because the person in charge never thinks of arranging that these places shall be always aired, always cleaned; she merely opens the window herself "when she goes in."

An excellent paper, the *Builder*, mentions the lingering of the smell of paint for a month about a house as a proof of want of ventilation. Certainly—and, where there are windows to open, and these are never opened to get rid of the smell of paint, it is a proof of want of management in using the means of ventilation. Of course the smell will then remain for months. Why should it go?

An agitating letter or message may be delivered, or an important letter or message *not* delivered; a visitor whom it was of consequence to see, may be refused, or one whom it was of still more consequence *not* to see, may be admitted—because the person in charge has never asked herself this question:—What is done when I am not there?

Why should you let your patient ever be surprised, except by thieves? I do not know. In England, people do not come down the chimney, or through the window, unless they are thieves. They come in by the door, and somebody must open the door to them.

At all events, one may safely say, a nurse cannot be with the patient, open the door, eat her meals, take a message, all at one and the same time. Nevertheless the person in charge never seems to look the impossibility in the face.

Add to this that the *attempting* this impossibility does more to increase the poor patient's hurry and nervousness than anything else.

It is never thought that the patient remembers these things if you do not. He has not only to think whether the visit or letter may arrive, but whether you will be in the way at the particular day and hour when it may arrive. So that your *partial* measures for "being in the way" yourself, only increase the necessity for his thought. Whereas, if you could but arrange that the thing should always be done whether you are there or not, he need never think at all about it.

For the above reasons, whatever a patient *can* do for himself, it is better, *i.e.*, less anxiety, for him to do for himself, unless the person in charge has the spirit of management.

Always tell a patient, and tell him beforehand, when you are going out, and when you will be back, whether it is for a day, an hour, or ten minutes. You fancy perhaps that it is better for him if he does not find out your going at all, better for him if you do not make yourself "of too much importance" to him; or else you cannot bear to give him the pain or the anxiety of the temporary separation.

No such thing. You *ought* to go, we will suppose. Health or duty requires it. Then say so to the patient openly. If you go without his knowing it, and he finds it out, he never will feel secure again that the things which depend upon you will be done when you are away; and in nine cases out of ten he will be right. If you go out without telling him when you will be back, he can take no measures nor precautions as to the things which concern you both, or which you do for him.

If you look into the reports of trials or accidents, and especially of suicides, or into the medical history of fatal cases, it is almost incredible how often the whole thing turns upon something which has happened because "he," or still oftener "she," "was not there." But it is still more incredible how often, how almost always this is accepted as a sufficient reason, a justification; why, the very fact of the thing having happened is the proof of its not being a justification. The person in charge was quite right not to be "*there,*" he was called away for quite sufficient reason, or he was away for a daily recurring and unavoidable cause: yet no provision was made to supply his absence. The fault was, not in his "being away" but, in there being no management to supplement his "being away." When the sun is under a total eclipse, or during his nightly absence, we light candles. But it would seem as if it did not occur to us that we must also supplement the person in charge of sick or of children, whether under an occasional eclipse, or during a regular absence.

In institutions where many lives would be lost, and the effect of such want of management would be terrible and patent, there is less of it than in the private house.*

But in both, the institution and the private house, let whoever is in charge keep this simple question in her head (*not*, how can I always do this right thing myself? but), how can I provide for this right thing to be always done?

Then, when anything wrong has actually happened in consequence of her absence, which absence we will suppose to have been quite right, let her question still be (*not*, how can I provide against any of such absences? which is neither possible nor desirable, but), how can I provide against anything wrong arising out of my absence?

Many people seem to think that the world stands still while they are away, or at dinner, or ill. If the sick have an accident during that time, is it their fault, not yours? I once heard an official justly told, "Patients, Sir, will not stop dying, while we are in church."

It is the invariable sign of a bad nurse and manager when her excuse that such a person was neglected, or such a thing was left undone, is that she was "out of the way." What does that signify? The thing that signifies is, that the neglect should not happen.

*Note.—The simple precaution of removing cords by which a patient can hang himself, razors by which he can cut his throat, out of his way, when inclined to do such things, is much neglected, especially in private nursing. Many inquests upon suicides shew this, and the friends are invariably absolved by the verdict!!

How few men, or even women, understand, either in great or in little things, what it is the being "in charge"—I mean, know how to carry out a "charge." From the most colossal calamities, down to the most trifling accidents, results are often traced (or rather not traced) to such want of someone "in charge" or of his knowing how to be "in charge." A short time ago the bursting of a funnel-casing on board the finest and strongest ship that ever was built, on her trial trip, destroyed several lives, and put several hundreds in jeopardy—not from any undetected flaw in her new and untried works—but from a tap being closed which ought not to have been closed—from what every child knows would make its mother's tea-kettle burst. And this simply because no one seemed to know what it is to be "in charge," or *who* was in charge. Nay more, the jury at the inquest actually altogether ignored the same, and apparently considered the tap "in charge," for they gave as a verdict "accidental death."

This is the meaning of the word, on a large scale. On a much smaller scale, it happened, a short time ago, that an insane person burnt herself slowly and intentionally to death, while in her doctor's charge, and almost in her nurse's presence. Yet neither was considered "at all to blame." The very fact of the accident happening proves its own case. There is nothing more to be said. Either they did not know their business, or they did not know how to perform it.

To be "in charge" is certainly not only to carry out the proper measures yourself but to see that every one else does so too; to see that no one either wilfully or ignorantly thwarts or prevents such measures. This is the meaning which must be attached to the word by (above all) those "in charge" of sick and of children, whether of numbers or of individuals; and indeed I think it is with the latter that it is least understood.

As the jury seems to have thought the tap was in charge of the ship's safety, so mistresses now seem to think the house is in charge of itself. They neither know how to give orders, nor how to teach children or servants to obey orders—*i.e.*, to obey intelligently, which is the real meaning of all discipline.

Elder children are often the most efficient assistants a mother or school-mistress can have in carrying out her "charge." At the best public schools this is so well understood that the highest boys often keep order better than the master himself, who taught them how. It is less well understood in families, where many a burnt child would have been saved if the mother had understood how to put the elder boy or girl in charge when she was out washing. But I have seen in a careful family the elder child of even five years old exercising this charge over a little one of two, and much better than a grown-up woman sometimes.

Again, people who are in charge often seem to have a pride in feeling that they will be "missed," that no one can understand or carry on their arrangements, their system, books, accounts, &c., but themselves. It seems to me that the pride is rather in carrying on a system, in keeping stores, closets, books, accounts, &c., so that anybody can understand and carry them on—so that, in case of absence or illness, one can deliver everything up to others and know that all will go on as usual, and one shall never be missed.

IV.— NOISE.

UNNECESSARY noise, or noise that creates an expectation in the mind, is that which hurts a patient. It is rarely the loudness of the noise, the effect upon the organ of the ear itself, which appears to affect the sick. How well a patient will generally bear, *e.g.*, the putting up of a scaffolding close to the house, when he cannot bear the talking, still less the whispering, especially if it be of a familiar voice, outside his door.

There are certain patients, no doubt, especially where there is slight concussion or other disturbance of the brain, who are affected by mere noise. But intermittent noise, or sudden and sharp noise, in these as in all other cases, affects far more than continuous noise—noise with jar far more than noise without. Of one thing you may be certain, that anything which wakes a patient suddenly out of his sleep will invariably put him into a state of greater excitement, do him more serious, aye, and lasting mischief, than any continuous noise, however loud.

Never to allow a patient to be waked, intentionally or accidentally, is a *sine qua non* of all good nursing. If he is roused out of his first sleep, he is almost certain to have no more sleep. It is a curious but quite intelligible fact that, if a patient is waked after a few hours' instead of a few minutes' sleep, he is much more likely to sleep again. Because pain, like irritability of brain, perpetuates and intensifies itself. If you have gained a respite of either in sleep, you have gained more than the mere respite.

Both the probability of recurrence and of the same intensity will be diminished, whereas both will be terribly increased by want of sleep. This is the reason why sleep is so all-important. This is the reason why a patient, waked in the early part of his sleep loses, not only his sleep, but his power to sleep. A healthy person who allows himself to sleep during the day will lose his sleep at night. But it is exactly the reverse with the sick generally; the more they sleep the better will they be able to sleep.

A good nurse can apply hot bottles to the feet, or give the nourishment ordered, hour by hour, without disturbing, but rather composing the patient. I have seen one of the (would-be) careful nurses neglect to warm the legs of a patient, invariably cold in the early morning, because "she did not like to disturb him." Such an excuse stamps a woman at once as incapable of her trust.

I have often been surprised at the thoughtlessness (resulting in cruelty, quite unintentional), of friend or of doctor who will hold a long conversation just in the room or passage adjoining to the room of the patient, who is either every moment expecting them to come in, or who has just seen them, and knows they are talking about him. If he is an amiable patient, he will try to occupy his attention elsewhere and not to listen—and this makes matters worse—for the strain upon his attention and the effort he makes are so great that it is well if he is not worse for hours after. If it is a whispered conversation in the same room, then it is absolutely cruel; for it is impossible that the patient's attention should not be involuntarily strained to hear. Walking on tip-toe, doing anything in the room very slowly, are injurious, for exactly the same reasons. A firm, light, quick step, a steady quick hand are what you want; not the slow, lingering, shuffling foot, the timid, uncertain touch. Slowness is not gentleness, though it is often mistaken for such; quickness, lightness, and gentleness are quite compatible. Again, if friends and doctors did but watch, as nurses can and should watch, the features sharpening, the eyes growing almost wild, of fever patients who are listening for the persons to come in, whose voices they hear at the door, these would never run the risk again of creating such expectation, or irritation of mind. Such unnecessary noise has undoubtedly induced or aggravated delirium in many cases. I have known such. In one case death ensued. It is but fair to say that this death was attributed to fright. It was the result of a

long whispered conversation, within sight of the patient, about
an impending operation; but any one who has known the cheerful coolness, with which the certainty of an operation will be
accepted by any patient, capable of bearing an operation at all,
if it is properly communicated to him, will hesitate to believe
that it was mere fear which produced, as was averred, the fatal
result in this instance. It was rather the uncertainty, the
strained expectation as to what was to be decided upon.

I need hardly say, that the other common course, namely, for a
doctor or friend to leave the patient and communicate his opinion
on the result of his visit to the friends just outside the patient's
door, or inside the adjoining room, after the visit, but within
hearing or knowledge of the patient is, if possible, worst of all.

Affectation, like whispering or walking on tip-toe, is peculiarly
painful to the sick. An affectedly quiet voice, an affectedly
sympathising voice, like an undertaker's at a funeral, sets all
their nerves on edge. Advice, such as what I have been giving,
does more harm than good, if it only makes people *affect* composure and quiet, when with the sick. Better almost make your
natural noise.

It is, I think, alarming, peculiarly at this time, when there is
so much talk about "woman's mission," to see that the dress of
women is daily more and more unfitting them for any "mission,"
any usefulness at all. It is unfitted for all domestic purposes. A
man is now a more handy and far less objectionable being in a
sick room than a woman. Compelled by her dress, every woman
now either shuffles or waddles—only a man can cross the floor of
a sick room without shaking it! What is become of woman's
light step?—the firm, light, quick step we have been asking for?

Unnecessary noise, then, is the most cruel absence of care
which can be inflicted either on sick or well. For, in all these
remarks, the sick are only mentioned as suffering in a greater
proportion than the well from precisely the same causes.

Unnecessary (although slight) noise injures a sick person much
more than necessary noise (of a much greater amount).

All likings and aversions of the sick towards different persons
will be found to resolve themselves very much, if not entirely,
into presence or absence of care in these things.

A nurse who rustles (I am speaking of nurses professional and
unprofessional) is the horror of a patient, though perhaps he does
not know why.

The fidget of silk and of crinoline, the crackling of starched petticoats, the rattling of keys, the creaking of stays and of shoes, will do a patient more harm than all the medicines in the world will do him good.

The "noiseless step" of woman means nothing at this day. Her skirts (and well if they do not throw down some piece of furniture) will at least brush against every article in the room as she moves.

Fortunate it is if her skirts do not catch fire—and if the nurse does not give herself up a sacrifice together with her patient, to be burnt in her own petticoats. In two years, 1863–4, no fewer than 630 females, of all ages, were burnt to death by their clothes catching fire. If the crinoline age begins after 10, and continues onwards, then 277 lives are known to have been sacrificed by fire during two years only to this absurd and hideous custom. But the Registrar-General tells us that a far greater number of deaths by fire take place among women, where the manner is not stated. Thus, in 1864 alone, the deaths by fire, without the deaths by scalding, among girls and women above the age of 10, were no less than 395. And if to these we add those who are not killed outright, but crippled for life, the account to be laid at the door of women's clothes is cruel indeed! But if people will be stupid, let them take measures to protect themselves from their own stupidity—measures which every chemist knows, such as putting alum into starch, which prevents starched articles of dress from blazing up.

I wish, too, that people who wear crinoline could see the indecency of their own dress as other people see it. A respectable elderly woman stooping forward, in crinoline, exposes quite as much of her own person to the patient lying in the room as any dancer does on the stage. But no one will ever tell her this unpleasant truth.

Again, one nurse cannot open the door without making everything rattle. Or she opens the door unnecessarily often, for want of remembering all the articles that might be brought in at once.

I have seen an expression of real terror pass across a patient's face, whenever a nurse came into the room who stumbled over the fire irons, &c.

I have seen patients, scarcely able to crawl, get out of bed before such a nurse came in and put out of her way everything she could throw down,—shut the window, sure that she would leave the door open—hide everything they were likely to want, (not because they had no right to have it, but because she would inadvertently put it out of their reach).

A good nurse will always make sure that no door or window in her patient's room shall rattle or creak; that no blind or curtain shall, by any change of wind through the open window, be made to flap—especially will she be careful of all this before she leaves her patients for the night. If you wait till your patients tell you, or remind you of these things, where is the use of their having a nurse? There are more shy than exacting patients in all classes; and many a patient passes a bad night, time after time, rather than remind his nurse every night of all the things she has forgotten.

If there are blinds to your windows, always take care to have them well up, when they are not being used. A little piece slipping down, and flapping with every draught, will distract a patient.

All hurry or bustle is peculiarly painful to the sick. And when a patient has compulsory occupations to engage him, instead of having simply to amuse himself, it becomes doubly injurious. The friend who remains standing and fidgeting about while a patient is talking business to him, or the friend who sits and proses, the one from an idea of not letting the patient talk, the other from an idea of amusing him,—each is equally inconsiderate. Always sit down when a sick person is talking business to you, show no signs of hurry, give complete attention and full consideration if your advice is wanted, and go away the moment the subject is ended.

Always sit within the patient's view, so that when you speak to him he has not painfully to turn his head round in order to look at you. Everybody involuntarily looks at the person speaking. If you make this act a wearisome one on the part of the patient you are doing him harm. So also if by continuing to stand you make him continuously raise his eyes to see you. Be as motionless as possible, and never gesticulate in speaking to the sick.

Never make a patient repeat a message or request, especially if it be some time after. Occupied patients are often accused of doing too much of their own business. They are instinctively right. How often you hear the person, charged with the request of giving the message or writing the letter, say half an hour afterwards to the patient, "Did you appoint 12 o'clock?" or, "What did you say was the address?" or ask perhaps some much more agitating question—thus causing the patient the effort of memory, or worse still, of decision, all over again. It is really less exertion to him to do these things for himself. This is the almost universal experience of occupied invalids.

This bring us to another caution. Never speak to an invalid from behind, nor from the door, nor from any distance from him, nor when he is doing anything.

If we consider these things, which are facts, not fancies, we shall remember that we are doing positive injury by interrupting, by "startling a fanciful" person, as it is called. Alas! it is no fancy.

If the invalid is forced, by his avocations, to continue occupations requiring much thinking, the injury is doubly great. In feeding a patient suffering under delirium or stupor you may suffocate him, by giving him his food suddenly; but if you rub his lips gently with a spoon, and thus attract his attention, he will swallow the food unconsciously, but with perfect safety. Thus it is with the brain. If you offer it a thought, especially one requiring a decision, abruptly, you do it a real not fanciful injury. Never speak to a sick person suddenly; but, at the same time, do not keep his expectation on the tip-toe.

This rule, indeed, applies to the well quite as much as to the sick. I have never known persons who exposed themselves for years to constant interruption who did not muddle away their intellects by it at last. The process with them may be accomplished without pain. With the sick, pain gives warning of the injury.

Do not meet or overtake a patient who is moving about in order to speak to him, or to give him any message or letter. You might just as well give him a box on the ear. I have seen a patient fall flat on the ground who was standing when his nurse came into the room. This was an accident which might have happened to the most careful nurse. But the other is done with intention. A patient in such a state is not going to the East Indies. If you would wait ten seconds, or walk ten yards further, any journey he could make would be over. You do not know the effort it is to a patient to remain standing for even a quarter of a minute to listen to you. If I had not seen the thing done by the kindest nurses and friends, I should have thought this caution quite superfluous.

It is absolutely essential then that a nurse should lay this down as a positive rule to herself, never to speak to any patient who is standing or moving, as long as she exercises so little observation as not to know when a patient cannot bear it. Many of the accidents which happen from feeble patients tumbling down stairs, fainting after getting up, &c., happen solely from the nurse popping out of a door to speak to the patient just at that moment; or from his fearing that she will do so. And if the patient were even left to himself, till he can sit down, such accidents would much seldomer occur. If the nurse accompanies the patient let her not call upon him to speak. It is incredible that nurses cannot picture to themselves the strain upon the heart, the lungs, and the brain, which the act of moving is to any feeble patient.

Patients are often accused of being able to "do much more when nobody is by." It is quite true that they can. Unless nurses can be brought to attend to considerations of the kind of which we have given here but a few specimens, a very weak patient finds it really much less exertion to do things for himself than to ask for them. And he will, in order to do them (very innocently and from instinct), calculate the time his nurse is likely to be absent, from a fear of her "coming in upon" him or speaking to him, just at the moment when he finds it quite as much as he can do to crawl from his bed to his chair, or from one room to another, or down stairs, or out of doors for a few minutes. Some extra call made upon his attention at that moment will quite upset him. In these cases you may be sure that a patient in the state we have described does not make such exertions more than once or twice a day, and probably much about the same hour every day. And it is hard, indeed, if nurse and friends cannot calculate so as to let him make them undisturbed. Remember, that many patients can walk who cannot stand or even sit up. Standing is, of all positions, the most trying to a weak patient.

Everything you do in a patient's room, after he is "put up" for the night, increases tenfold the risk of his having a bad night. But, if you rouse him up after he has fallen asleep, you do not risk, you secure him a bad night.

One hint I would give to all who attend or visit the sick, to all who have to pronounce an opinion upon sickness or its progress.

Come back and look at your patient *after* he has had an hour's lively conversation with you. It is the best test of his real state we know. But never pronounce upon him from merely seeing what he does, or how he looks, during such a conversation. Learn also carefully and exactly, if you can, how he passed the night after it.

People rarely, if ever, faint while making an exertion. It is after it is over. Indeed, almost every effect of over-exertion appears after, not during such exertion. It is the highest folly to judge of the sick, as is so often done, when you see them merely during a period of excitement. People have sometimes died of that which, it has been proclaimed at the time, has "done them no harm."

As an old experienced nurse, I do most earnestly remonstrate against all such careless words. I have known patients delirious all night, after seeing a visitor who called them "better," thought they "only wanted a little amusement," and who came again, saying, "I hope you were not the worse for my visit," neither waiting for an answer, nor even looking at the case. No real patient will ever say, "Yes, but I was a great deal the worse."

It is not, however, either death or delirium of which there is ever most danger to the patient. Unperceived consequences are far more likely to ensue. *You* will not suffer by knowing what you have done—the poor patient will, although *he* may not know either. It will not be directly traceable to its real cause, except by a very careful observant nurse. The patient will often not even mention what has done him most harm.

What most frequently happens is this: that a patient never sits up again after some shock; that a patient is never able to read or write again after some unusual exertion forced upon him; that a patient is never able to go out again after some unreasonable call upon him; that he is obliged to give up his work or his only amusement for ever; and because he does not fall down suddenly and die on the spot, as if he were shot, these unreasonable people, who have "taken it out" of him, think he has "had no harm." They had better have "taken" his life "out of" him. Above all, I would say this of all evening conversations and visits to the invalid.[4]

Remember never to lean against, sit upon, or unnecessarily shake, or even touch the bed in which a patient lies. This is invariably a painful annoyance. If you shake the chair on which he sits, he has a point by which to steady himself, in his feet. But on a bed or sofa, he is entirely at your mercy, and he feels every jar you give him all through him.

In all that we have said, both here and elsewhere, let it be distinctly understood that we are not speaking of would-be invalids. To distinguish between real and fancied disease is an important thing for a nurse to be able to do. To manage fancy patients is an important part of her duties. But the nursing which real and that which fancied patients require is of different, or rather of opposite, character. And the latter will not be spoken of here. Indeed, many of the symptoms which are here mentioned are those which distinguish real from fancied disease.

It is true that would-be invalids very often do that behind a nurse's back which they would not do before her face. Many such I have had as patients who scarcely ate anything at their regular meals, but if you concealed food for them in a drawer, they would take it at night or in secret. But this is quite from a different motive. They do it from the wish to conceal. Whereas the real patient will often boast to his nurse or doctor, if these do not shake their heads at him, of how much he has done, or eaten, or walked. To return to real disease.

Conciseness and decision are above all things necessary with the sick. Let what you say to them be concisely and decidedly expressed. What doubt and hesitation there may be in your own mind must never be communicated to theirs, not even (I would rather say especially not) in little things. Let your doubt be to yourself, your decision to them. People who think outside their heads, who tell everything that led them towards this conclusion and away from that, ought never to be with the sick.

I have been told by women who had difficult confinements, that their strength depended upon the firmness of doctor and nurse. If either had betrayed that there was anything unusual or doubtful in the case, they felt it would have been "all over" with them.

I have observed the same thing in acute cases, when the scale was trembling between life and death. If the doctor betrayed any want of decision, if the nurse lost any portion of her calmness or self-possession, it just turned the scale in favour of death.

Irresolution is what all patients most dread. Rather than meet this in others, they will collect all their data, and make up their minds for themselves. A change of mind in others, whether it is regarding an operation, or re-writing a letter, always injures the patient more than the being called upon to make up his mind to the most dreaded or difficult decision. Farther than this, in very many cases, the imagination in disease is far more active and lively than it is in health. If you proposed to the patient change of air to one place one hour, and to another the next, he has, in each case, immediately constituted himself in imagination the tenant of the place, gone over the whole premises in idea, and you have tired him as much by displacing his imagination, as if you had actually carried him over both places.

Above all, leave the sick room quickly and come into it quickly, not suddenly, not with a rush. But don't let the patient be wearily waiting for when you will be out of the room or when you will be in it. Conciseness and decision in your movements, as well as your words, are necessary in the sick room, as necessary as absence of hurry and bustle. To possess yourself entirely will ensure you from either failing—either loitering or hurrying.

If a patient has to see not only to his own, but also to his nurse's punctuality, or perseverance, or readiness, or calmness, to any or all of these things, he is far better without that nurse than with her—however valuable and handy her services may otherwise be to him, and however incapable he may be of rendering them to himself.

With regard to reading aloud in the sick room, my experience is, that when the sick are too ill to read to themselves, they can seldom bear to be read to. Children, eye-patients, and uneducated persons are exceptions, or where there is any mechanical difficulty in reading. People who like to be read to, have generally not much the matter with them; while in fevers, or where there is much irritability of brain, the effort of listening to reading aloud has often brought on delirium. I speak with great diffidence; because it is an almost universal belief that it is *sparing* the sick to read aloud to them. But two things are certain: —

(1.) If there is some matter which *must* be read to a sick person, do it slowly. People often think that the way to get it over with least fatigue to him is to get it over in least time. They gabble; they plunge and gallop through the reading. There never was a greater mistake. Houdin, the conjuror, says that the way to make a story seem short is to tell it slowly. So it is with reading to the sick. I have often heard a patient say

to such a mistaken reader, "Don't read it to me; tell it me."
Sick children, if not too shy to speak, will always express this
wish. They invariably prefer a story to be *told* to them, rather
than read to them. Unconsciously they are aware that this will
regulate the plunging, the reading with unequal paces, slurring
over one part, instead of leaving it out altogether, if it is unimportant, and mumbling another. If the reader lets his own
attention wander, and then stops to read up to himself, or finds
he has read the wrong bit, then it is all over with the poor
patient's chance of not suffering. Very few people know how
to read to the sick; very few read aloud as pleasantly even as
they speak. In reading they sing, they hesitate, they stammer,
they hurry, they mumble; when in speaking they do none of
these things. Reading aloud to the sick ought always to be
rather slow, and exceedingly distinct, but not mouthing—rather
monotonous, but not sing-song—rather loud, but not noisy—and
above all, not too long. Be very sure of what your patient can
bear.

(2.) The extraordinary habit of reading to one's self in a sick
room, and reading aloud to the patient any bits which will amuse
him, or more often the reader, is unaccountably thoughtless.
What *do* you think the patient is thinking of during your gaps of
non-reading? Do you think that he amuses himself upon what
you have read for precisely the time it pleases you to go on reading to yourself, and that his attention is ready for something else
at precisely the time it pleases you to begin reading again?

One thing more:—From the flimsy manner in which most
modern houses are built, where every step on the stairs, and
along the floors, is felt all over the house; the higher the story
the greater the vibration. It is surprising how much the sick
suffer by having anybody overhead. In the solidly built old
houses, which, fortunately, most hospitals are, the noise and
shaking is comparatively trifling. But it is a serious cause of
suffering, in lightly built houses, and with the irritability peculiar
to some diseases. Better far put such patients at the top of the
house, even with the additional fatigue of stairs, if you cannot
secure the room above them being untenanted; you may otherwise bring on a state of restlessness which no opiate will subdue.
Do not neglect the warning, when a patient tells you that he
"feels every step above him to cross his heart." Remember that
every noise a patient cannot *see* partakes of the character of

suddeness to him; and I am persuaded that patients with these peculiarly irritable nerves, are positively less injured by having persons in the same room with them than overhead, or than separated by only a thin compartment. Any sacrifice to secure silence for these cases is worth while, because no air, however good, no attendance, however careful, will do anything for such cases without quiet.

V.— VARIETY.

To any but an old nurse, or an old invalid, the degree would be quite inconceivable to which the nerves of the sick suffer from seeing the same walls, the same ceiling, the same surroundings during a long confinement to one or two rooms.

Persons suffering severe paroxysms of pain are much more cheerful than persons suffering from nervous weakness. This has often been remarked upon, and attributed to the enjoyment by the former of their intervals of respite. I incline to think that the majority of cheerful cases is to be found among those patients who are not confined to one room, whatever their suffering, and that the majority of depressed cases will be seen among those subjected to a long monotony of objects about them.

The nervous frame really suffers as much from this as the digestion does from long monotony of diet.

The effect in sickness of beautiful objects, of variety of objects, and especially of brilliancy of colour, is hardly at all appreciated.

Such cravings are usually called the "fancies" of patients. And often, doubtless, patients have "fancies," as, *e.g.* when they desire two contradictions. But much more often, their (so-called) "fancies" are most valuable signs of what is necessary for their recovery. And it would be well if nurses would watch these (so-called) "fancies" closely.

I have seen, in fevers (and felt, when I was a fever-patient myself), the most acute suffering produced from the patient (in a hut) not being able to see out of window, and the knots in the wood being the only view. I shall never forget the rapture of fever-patients over a bunch of bright-coloured flowers. I remember (in my own case) a nosegay of wild flowers being sent me, and from that moment recovery becoming more rapid.

People say the effect is only on the mind. It is no such thing.

The effect is on the body, too. Little as we know about the way in which we are affected by form, by colour, and light, we do know this, that they have an actual bodily effect.

Variety of form and brilliancy of colour in the objects presented to patients, are actual means of recovery.

But it must be *slow* variety, *e.g.*, if you show a patient ten or twelve pictures successively, ten to one that he does not become cold and faint, or feverish, or even sick; but hang one up opposite him, one on each successive day, or week, or month, and he will delight in the variety.

The folly and ignorance which are too often supreme over the sick room, cannot be better shown than by this. While the nurse will leave the patient stewing in a corrupting atmosphere, she will deny him, on the plea of unhealthiness, a glass of cut-flowers, or a growing plant. Now, no one ever saw "over-crowding" by plants in a room or ward. And the carbonic acid they give off at nights would not poison a fly. Nay, in over-crowded rooms, they actually absorb carbonic acid, and give off oxygen. Cut-flowers also decompose water, and produce oxygen gas. It is true there are certain flowers, *e.g.* lilies, the smell of which is said to depress the nervous system. These are easily known by the smell, and can be avoided.

A very great deal is now written and spoken as to the effect of the mind upon the body. Much of it is true. But I wish a little more was thought of the effect of the body on the mind. You who believe yourselves overwhelmed with cares, but are able every day to walk up the street, or out in the country, to take your meals with others in other rooms, &c., &c., you little know how much your anxieties are thereby lightened; you little know how intense they become to those who can have no change; how the very walls of their sick rooms seem hung with their cares; how the ghosts of their troubles haunt their beds; how impossible it is for them to escape from a pursuing thought without some help from variety.

It is a matter of painful wonder to the sick themselves, how much more they think of painful things than of pleasant ones; they reason with themselves, they think themselves ungrateful; it is all of no use. The fact is, that these painful ideas are far better dismissed by amusing the invalid, or by showing him something pretty, than by arguing with him. I have mentioned the cruelty of letting him stare at a dead wall. In many diseases, especially in recovery from fever, that wall will appear to make all sorts of faces at him; now flowers never do this.

A patient can just as much move his leg when it is broken, as change his thoughts when no help from variety is given him. This is, indeed, one of the main sufferings of sickness; just as the fixed posture is one of the main sufferings of the broken limb.

It is a constant wonder to me to see people, who call themselves nurses, acting thus. They vary their own objects, their own employments, many times a day; and while nursing (!) some bedridden sufferer, they let him lie there with no view at all but the flies on the ceiling; without any change of object to enable him to vary his thoughts; and it never even occurs to them, at least to move his bed so that he can look out of window. No, the bed is to be always left in the darkest, dullest, closest part of the room.

I remember a case in point. A man received an injury to the spine, from an accident, which, after a long confinement, ended in death. He was a workman—he did not care about "nature," he said—but he was desperate to "see once more out of window." His nurse, who was the woman of the house where he lodged, actually got him on her back, and managed to perch him up at the window for an instant, "to see out." The consequence to the poor woman was a serious illness, which nearly proved fatal. The man never knew it; but a great many other people did. Yet they none of them thought, so far as I know, that the craving for variety in the starving eye is just as desperate as that for food in the starving stomach, and tempts the famishing creature, in either case, to steal for its satisfaction. No other word will express it but "desperation." And it is just as stupid not to provide the sick bed with a "view," or with variety of some kind, as if you did not provide the house with a kitchen.

And in no case does the considerate person meet with the same success as he does with the sick. People write poetry about the "charms of nature." I question whether the intensest pleasure ever felt in nature is not that of the sick man raising a forest tree, six inches high, from an acorn or a horse-chestnut, in a London back-court.

It is a very common error among the well to think that, "with a little more self-control," the sick might, if they choose, "dismiss painful thoughts," which "aggravate their disease," &c. Believe me, almost *any* sick person, who behaves decently well, exercises more self-control every moment of his day than you will ever know till you are sick yourself. Almost every step that crosses his room is painful to him; almost every thought that crosses his brain is painful to him; and if he can speak without being savage, and look without being unpleasant, he is exercising self-control.

Suppose you have been up all night, and instead of being allowed to have your cup of tea, you were to be told that you ought to "exercise self-control," what should you say? Now, the nerves of the sick are always in the state that yours are in after you have been up all night.

We will suppose the diet of the sick to be cared for. Then, this state of nerves is most frequently to be relieved by care in affording them a pleasant view, a variety of flowers, and pretty things. Light by itself will often relieve it. The craving for "the return of day," which the sick so constantly show, is generally nothing but the desire for light, for the relief which a variety of objects before the eye affords to the harassed sick mind.

Again, every man and every woman has some amount of work with the hands, excepting a few fine ladies, who do not even dress themselves, and who are really, as to nerves, very like the sick. Now, you can have no idea of the relief which such manual labour is to you—of the degree to which the being without it increases the peculiar irritability from which many invalids suffer.

A little needlework, a little writing, a little cleaning, would be the greatest relief the sick could have, if they could do it; these *are* the greatest relief to you, though you do not know it. Reading, though it is often the only thing the sick can do, is not this relief. Bearing this in mind, bearing in mind that you have all these varieties of employment which the sick cannot have, bear also in mind to obtain for them all the varieties which they can enjoy.

I need hardly say, that too much needlework, or writing, or any other continued employment, will produce the same irritability that too little produces in the sick.

VI.— TAKING FOOD.

EVERY careful observer of the sick will agree in this, that thousands of patients are annually starved in the midst of plenty, from want of attention to the ways which alone make it possible for them to take food. This want of attention is as remarkable in those who urge upon the sick to do what is quite impossible to them, as in the sick themselves, who will not make the effort to take what is perfectly possible to them.

For instance, to most very weak patients it is quite impossible to take any solid food before 11 a.m., nor then, if their strength is still further exhausted by fasting till that hour. For weak patients have generally feverish nights and, in the morning, dry mouths; and, if they could eat with those dry mouths, it would be the worse for them. A spoonful of beef-tea, of arrowroot and wine, of egg-flip, every hour, will give them the requisite nourishment, and prevent them from being too much exhausted to take at a later hour the solid food which is necessary for their recovery. And every patient who can swallow at all can swallow these liquid things, if he chooses. But how often do we hear a mutton-chop, an egg, a bit of bacon, ordered to a patient for breakfast, to whom (as a moment's consideration would show us) it must be quite impossible to take such things at that hour.

Again, a nurse is ordered to give a patient a teacupful of some article of food every three hours. The patient's stomach rejects it. If so, try a tablespoonful every hour; if this will not do, a teaspoonful every quarter of an hour.

More patients are lost by want of care and ingenuity in these things in private nursing than in public hospitals. And there is more of making common cause to assist one another's hands between the doctor and his head nurse in the hospital than between the doctor and the patient's friends in the private house.

If we did but know the consequences which may ensue, in very weak patients, from ten minutes' fasting or repletion (I call it repletion when they are obliged to leave too small an interval between taking food and some other exertion, owing to the nurse's unpunctuality), we should be more careful never to let this occur. In very weak patients there is often a nervous difficulty of swallowing, which is so much increased by any other call upon their strength that, unless they have their food punctually at the minute, which minute again must be arranged so as to fall in with no other minute's occupation, they can take nothing till the next respite occurs—so that an unpunctuality or delay of ten minutes may very well turn out to be one of two or three hours. And why is it not as easy to be punctual to a minute? Life often literally hangs upon these minutes.

In acute cases where life or death is to be determined in a few hours, these matters are very generally attended to, especially in hospitals; and the number of cases is large where the patient is, as it were, brought back to life by exceeding care on the part of the doctor or nurse, or both, in ordering and giving nourishment with exact punctuality and choice.

But, in chronic cases, lasting over months and years, where death is often determined at last by mere protracted starvation, I had rather not tell the instances which I have known where a little ingenuity, and a great deal of perseverance, might, in all probability, have averted the result. The consulting the hours when the patient can take food, the observation of the times, often varying, when he is most faint, the altering seasons of taking food, in order to prevent such times—all this, which requires observation, ingenuity, and perseverance (and these really consti-tute the good nurse), might save more lives than we wot of.*

To leave the patient's untasted food by his side, from meal to meal, in hopes that he will eat it in the interval, is simply to pre-vent him from taking any food at all. Patients have been literally made incapable of taking one article of food after another, by this piece of ignorance. Let the food come at the right time, and be taken away, eaten or uneaten, at the right time; but never let a patient have "something always standing" by him, if you don't wish to disgust him of everything.

On the other hand, a poor woman's life has been saved (she was sinking for want of food) by the simple question put to her by the doctor, "But is there no hour when you feel you could eat?" "Oh, yes," she said, "I could always take something at—o'clock, and—o'clock." The thing was tried and succeeded. Patients very seldom, however, can tell this; it is for you to watch and find it out.

A patient should, if possible, not see or smell either the food of others, or a greater amount of food than he himself can consume at one time, or even hear food talked about or see it in the raw state. I know of no exception to the above rule. The breaking of it always brings on more or less dislike to taking food.

In hospital wards it is of course impossible to observe all this; and in rooms, where a patient must be closely watched, it is

* NOTE.—Exhaustion from a half-starvation is one of the most frequent causes of loss of sleep. Many a patient will sleep exactly in proportion as he can eat. Any one who has seen a famine will remember the constant cry, "We cannot sleep;" and "sleep seems the only thing which would do us any good." And the constant cry to the doctor is, "Give us something to make us sleep."

often impossible to relieve the nurse, so that her own meals can be taken out of the room. But it is not the less true that, in such cases, even where the patient is not himself aware of it, he is prevented from taking food by seeing the nurse eating her meals. In some cases the sick are aware of it and complain. A poor woman, supposed to be insensible, who complained of it to me as soon as able, to speak, is now in my mind.

Remember, however, that the extreme punctuality in well-ordered hospitals, the rule that nothing shall be done in the ward while the patients are having their meals, go far to counterbalance what unavoidable evil there is in having patients together. The private nurse may be often seen dusting or fidgeting about in a sick room all the while the patient is eating, or trying to eat.

That the more alone an invalid can be when taking food, the better, is unquestionable; and, even if he must be fed, the nurse should not allow him to talk, or talk to him, especially about food, while eating.

When a person is compelled, by the pressure of occupation, to continue his business while sick, it ought to be a rule WITH OUT ANY EXCEPTION WHATEVER, that no one shall bring business to him or talk to him while he is taking food, nor go on talking to him on interesting subjects up to the last moment before his meals, nor make an engagement with him immediately after, so that there be any hurry of mind while taking them.

Upon the observance of these rules, especially the first, often depends the patient's taking food at all, or, if he is amiable, and forces himself to take food, deriving any nourishment from it.

A nurse should never put before a patient milk that is sour, meat or soup that is turned, an egg that is bad, or vegetables underdone. Yet often these things are brought to the sick in a state loathsome to every nose or eye except the nurse's. It is here that the clever nurse appears; she will not bring in the bad article, but not to disappoint the patient, she will whip up something else in a few minutes. Remember that sick cookery should half do the work of your poor patient's weak digestion. But if you further impair it with your bad articles, I know not what is to become of him or of it.

If the nurse is an intelligent being, and not a mere carrier of diets to and from the patient, let her exercise her intelligence in these things. How often have we known a patient eat nothing at all in the day, because one meal was left untasted (at that time he was incapable of eating), at another the milk was sour, the third was spoiled by some other accident. And it never occurred to the nurse to find out some expedient,—it never occurred to her that as he had had no solid food that day, he might eat a bit of toast (say) with his tea in the evening, or he might have some meal an hour earlier. A patient who cannot touch his dinner at two, will often take it gladly, if brought to him at seven. But somehow nurses never "think of these things." One would imagine they did not consider themselves bound to exercise their judgment; they leave it to the patient. Now I am quite sure that it is better for a patient rather to suffer these neglects than to try to teach his nurse to nurse him, if she does not know how. It ruffles him, and if he is ill he is in no condition to teach, especially upon himself. The above remarks apply much more to private nursing than to hospitals.

I would say to the nurse, have a rule of thought about your patient's diet; consider, remember how much he has had, and how much he ought to have to-day. Generally, the only rule of the private patient's diet is what the nurse has to give. It is true she cannot give him what she has not got; but his stomach docs not wait for her convenience, or even her necessity. If it is used to having its food or drink at one hour to-day, and to-morrow it does not have it, because she has failed in getting it, he will suffer. She must be always exercising her ingenuity to supply defects, and to remedy accidents which will happen among the best contrivers, but from which the patient does not suffer the less, "because they cannot be helped."

Why, because the nurse has not got some food to-day which the patient takes, can the patient wait four hours for it to-day who could not wait two hours yesterday? Yet this is the only excuse one generally hears. On the other hand, the opposite course, viz., of the nurse giving the patient a thing because she *has* got it, is almost equally bad. If she happens to have fresh jelly, or fresh fruit, she will frequently give it to the patient half-an-hour after his dinner, or at his dinner, when he cannot possibly eat that and the broth too—or, worse still, leave it by his bed-side till he is so sickened with the sight of it, that he cannot eat it at all.

One very small caution,—take care not to spill into your patient's saucer,—in other words, take care that the outside bottom rim of his cup is quite dry and clean; if, every time he lift his cup to his lips, he has to carry the saucer with it, or else to drop the food upon and to soil his sheet, or his bed-gown, or pillow, or, if he is sitting up, his dress, you have no idea what a difference this small want of care on your part makes to his comfort and even to his willingness for food.

VII.— WHAT FOOD?

I will mention one or two of the most common errors among women in charge of sick respecting sick diet. One is the belief that beef-tea is the most nourishing of all articles. Now, just try and boil down a lb. of beef into beef-tea, evaporate your beef-tea, and see what is left of your beef. You will find that there is barely a teaspoonful of solid nourishment to half-a-pint of water in beef-tea. It is quite true that, by mincing the beef and then stewing it, you can get a larger quantity of solid in the liquor; but then it is not beef-tea, and there are many patients who could not take it. There is a certain restoring quality in beef-tea, we do not know what, as there is in tea; it may safely be given in almost any inflammatory disease, but is little to be depended upon with the healthy or convalescent where much nourishment is required. Again, it is an ever-ready saw that an egg is equi-valent to a lb. of meat; whereas it is not at all so. Also, it is seldom noticed with how many patients, particularly of nervous or bilious temperament, eggs disagree. All puddings made with eggs are distasteful to them in consequence. An egg, whipped up with wine, is often the only form in which they can take this kind of nourishment. Again, if the patient is able to eat meat, it is supposed that to give him meat is the only thing needful for his recovery; whereas scorbutic sores have been actually known to appear among sick persons living in the midst of plenty in England, which could be traced to no other source than this, viz.: that the nurse, depending on meat alone, had allowed the patient to be without vegetables for a considerable time, these latter being so badly cooked that he always left them untouched. Arrowroot is another grand dependence of the nurse. To mix the patient's wine in, being as it is quickly prepared, it is all very well. But it is nothing but starch and water. Flour is both more nutritive, and less liable to ferment, and is preferable wherever it can be used.

Again, milk and the preparations from milk, are a most important article of food for the sick. Butter is the lightest kind of animal fat, and though it wants some of the things which there are in milk, yet it is most valuable both in itself and in enabling the patient to eat more bread. Flour, oats, groats, rice, barley, and their kind, are, as we have already said, preferable in all their preparations to all the preparations of arrowroot, sago, tapioca, and their kind. Cream, in many long chronic diseases, is quite irreplaceable by any other article whatever. It seems to act in the same manner as beef-tea, and to most it is much easier of digestion than milk. In fact, it seldom disagrees. Cheese is not usually digestible by the sick, but it has great nourishment in it, and I have seen sick, and not a few either, whose craving for cheese showed how much it was needed by them.*

But if fresh milk is so valuable a food for the sick, the least change or sourness in it makes it of all articles, perhaps, the most injurious; diarrhoea is a common result of fresh milk allowed to become at all sour. The nurse, therefore, ought to exercise her utmost care in this. In large institutions for the sick, even the poorest, the utmost care is exercised. Ice is used for this express purpose every summer, while the sick person at home, perhaps, never tastes a drop of milk that is not sour, all through the hot weather, so little does the home nurse understand the necessity of such care. Yet, if you consider that the only drop of real nourishment in your patient's tea is the drop of milk, and how much almost all English patients depend upon their tea, you will see the great importance of not depriving your patient of this drop of milk. Buttermilk, a totally different thing, is often very useful, especially in fevers.

Almost all patients in England, young and old, male and female, rich and poor, hospital and private, dislike sweet things, — and while I have never known a person take to sweets when he was ill who disliked them when he was well, I have known many fond of them when in health, who in sickness would leave off anything sweet, even to sugar in tea,—sweet puddings, sweet drinks, are their aversion; the furred tongue almost always likes

---

*In the diseases produced by bad food, such as scorbutic dysentery and diarrhoea, the patient's stomach often craves for and digests things, some of which certainly would never have been ordered for sick, and especially not for such sick. These are fruit, pickles, jams, gingerbread, fat of ham or of bacon, suet, cheese, butter, milk. These cases I have seen not by ones, nor by tens, but by hundreds. And the patient's stomach was right.

what is sharp or pungent. Scorbutic patients are an exception, they often crave for sweetmeats and jams.

Jelly is another article of diet in great favour with nurses and friends of the sick; even if it could be eaten solid, it would not nourish, but it is simply the height of folly to take 1/8 oz. of gelatine and make it into a certain bulk by dissolving it in water and then to give it to the sick, as if the mere bulk represented nourishment. It is now known that jelly does not nourish, that it has a tendency to produce diarrhoea,—and to trust to it to repair the waste of a diseased constitution is simply to starve the sick under the disguise of feeding them. If one hundred spoonfuls of jelly were given in the course of the day, you would have given one spoonful of gelatine, which spoonful has no nutritive power whatever.

Dr. Christison says that "every one will be struck with the readiness with which" certain classes of "patients will often take diluted meat juice or beef-tea repeatedly, when they refuse all other kinds of food." This is particularly remarkable in "cases of gastric fever, in which," he says, "little or nothing else besides beef-tea or diluted meat juice" has been taken for weeks or even months; "and yet a pint of beef tea contains scarcely 1/4 oz. of anything but water."

A small quantity of beef-tea added to other articles of food makes them more nourishing.

The reason why beef-tea should be nourishing and jelly not so to the sick, is a secret yet undiscovered, but it clearly shows that careful observation of the sick is the only clue to the best dietary.

Again, the nourishing power of milk and of the preparations from milk, is very much undervalued; there is nearly as much nourishment in half a pint of milk as there is in a quarter of a lb. of meat. But this is not the whole question or nearly the whole. The main question is, what the patient's stomach can derive nourishment from, and of this the patient's stomach is the sole judge. Chemistry cannot tell this. The patient's stomach must be its own chemist. The diet which will keep the healthy man healthy, will kill the sick one. The same beef which is the most nutritive of all meat, and which nourishes the healthy man, is the least nourishing of all food to the sick man, whose half-dead stomach can *assimilate* no part of it, that is, make no food out of it. On a diet of beef-tea healthy men, on the other hand, speedily lose their strength.

I have known patients live for many months without touching bread, because they could not eat baker's bread. These were mostly country patients, but not all. Home-made bread or brown bread is a most important article of diet for many patients. The use of aperients may be entirely superseded by it. Oat cake is another.

To watch for the opinions, then, which the patient's stomach gives, rather than to read books about "foods," is the business of all those who have to settle what the patient is to eat—perhaps the most important thing to be provided for him after the air he is to breathe.

Now the medical man who sees the patient only once a day, or even only once or twice a weak, cannot possibly tell this without the assistance of the patient himself, or of those who are in constant observation of the patient. The utmost the medical man can tell is, whether the patient is weaker or stronger at this visit than he was at the last visit. I should therefore say, that incomparably the most important office of the nurse, after she has taken care of the patient's air, is to take care to observe the effect of his food, and report it to the doctor.

A great deal too much against tea is said by wise people, and a great deal too much of tea is given to the sick by foolish people. When you see the natural and almost universal craving in English sick for their "tea," you cannot but feel that nature knows what she is about. But a little tea or coffee restores them quite as much as a great deal, and a great deal of tea and especially of coffee impairs the little power of digestion they have. Yet a nurse, because she sees how one or two cups of tea or coffee restore her patient, thinks that three or four cups will do twice as much. This is not the case at all; it is however certain that there is nothing yet discovered which is a substitute to the English patient for his cup of tea; he can take it when he can take nothing else, and he often can't take anything else if he has it not. I should be very glad if any of the abusers of tea would point out what to give to an English patient after a sleepless night, instead of tea. If you give it at five or six o'clock in the morning, he may even sometimes fall asleep after it, and get perhaps his only two or three hours' sleep during the twenty-four. At the same time you never should give tea or coffee to the sick, as a rule, after five o'clock in the afternoon. Sleeplessness in the early night is from excitement generally, and is increased by tea or coffee; sleeplessness which continues to the early morning is from exhaustion often, and is relieved by tea. The only English patients I have ever known refuse tea, have been typhus cases, and the first sign of their getting better was their craving again for tea. In general, the dry and dirty tongue always prefers tea to coffee, and will quite decline milk, unless with tea. Coffee is a better restorative than tea, but a greater impairer of the digestion. Let the patient's taste decide. You will say that, in cases of great thirst, the patient's craving decides that it will drink *a great deal* of tea, and that you cannot help it. But in these cases be sure that the patient requires diluents for quite other purposes than quenching the thirst; he wants a great deal of some drink, not only of tea, and the doctor will order what he is to have, barley-water or lemonade, or soda-water and milk, as the case may be.

It is often recommended to persons about to go through great fatigue, either from the kind of work, or from their being not in a state fit for it, to eat a piece of bread before they go. I wish the recommenders would themselves try the experiment of taking a piece of bread instead of a cup of tea or coffee as a refresher. They would find it very poor comfort. When men have to set out fasting on fatiguing duty, when nurses have to go fasting in to their patients, it is a hot restorative they want, and ought to have, before they go, not a cold bit of bread. If they can take a bit of bread *with* the hot cup of tea, so much the better, but not *instead* of it. The fact that there is more nourishment in bread than in almost anything else has probably induced the mistake. That it is a mistake there is no doubt.

English men and women who have undergone great fatigue, such as taking a long journey without stopping, or sitting up for several nights in succession, almost always say that they can do it best upon a cup of tea. It is also the best refreshment before going out to a long day's work.

In making coffee for the sick, you should always buy it in the berry, and grind it at home. Otherwise you may reckon upon its containing a certain amount of chicory, *at least*. This is not a question of the taste or of the wholesomeness of chicory. It is that chicory has nothing at all of the properties for which you give coffee. And therefore you may as well not give it.

Again, all laundresses, mistresses of dairy-farms, head nurses (I speak of the good old sort only—women who do both a good deal of hard hand-labour, and also the head-work necessary for arranging the day's business, so that none of it shall tread upon the heels of something else) set great value, I have observed, upon having a high-priced tea. This is called extravagant. But these women are "extravagant" in nothing else. And they are right in this. Real tea-leaf tea alone contains the restorative they want; which is not to be found in sloe-leaf tea.

The mistresses of houses, who cannot even go over their own house once a-day, are incapable of judging for these women, for they are incapable themselves, to all appearance, of the spirit of arrangement (no small task) necessary for managing a large ward or dairy.

Cocoa is often recommended to the sick instead of tea or coffee. But independently of the fact that English sick very generally dislike cocoa, it has quite a different effect from tea or coffee. It is an oily starchy nut, having no restorative power at all, but simply increasing fat. It is pure mockery of the sick, therefore, to call it a substitute for tea. For any refreshment it is of, you might just as well offer them chestnuts instead of tea.

An almost universal error among nurses is in the bulk of the food, and especially the drinks, they offer to their patients. Suppose a patient ordered four oz. brandy during the day, how is he to take this if you make it into four pints with diluting it? The same with tea and beef-tea, with arrowroot, milk, &c. You have not increased the nourishment, you have not increased the renovating power of these articles, by increasing their bulk—you have very likely diminished both by giving the patient's digestion more to do, and, most likely of all, the patient will leave half of what he has been ordered to take, because he cannot swallow the bulk with which you have been pleased to invest it. It requires very nice observation and care (and meets with hardly any) to determine what will not be too thick or strong for the patient to take, while giving him no more than the bulk which he is able to swallow.[5]

VIII.— BED AND BEDDING.

A few words upon bedsteads and bedding; and principally as regards patients who are entirely, or almost entirely, prisoners to bed.

Feverishness is generally supposed to be a symptom of fever— in nine cases out of ten it is a symptom of bedding.

The patient has had re-introduced into the body the perspiration from himself which day after day and week after week soaks into his unaired bedding. How can it be otherwise? Look at the ordinary bed in which a patient lies.

If I were looking out for an example in order to show what *not* to do, I should take the specimen of an ordinary bed in a private house: a wooden bedstead, two or even three mattresses piled up to above the height of a table; a vallance fastened to the frame— nothing but a miracle could ever thoroughly dry or air such a bed and bedding. The patient must choose between cold damp after his bed is made, and warm damp before, both from his own perspiration; and this from the time the mattresses are put under him till the time they are picked to pieces, if this is ever done!

For the same reason, if, after washing a patient, you must put the same night-dress on him again, always give it a warm first, at the fire. The night-gown he has worn must be, to a certain extent, damp. It has now got cold from having been off him for a few minutes. The fire will dry and at the same time air it. This is much more important than with clean things.

If you consider that a grown up man in health exhales by the lungs and skin in the twenty-four hours three pints at least of moisture, loaded with matter ready to putrefy; that in sickness the quantity is often greatly increased, the quality is always more hurtful—just ask yourself next where does all this moisture go to? Chiefly into the bedding, because it cannot go anywhere else. And it stays there; because, except perhaps a weekly change of sheets, scarcely any other airing is attempted. A nurse will be careful to fidgetiness about airing the clean sheets from clean damp, but airing the dirty sheets from dirty damp will never even occur to her. Besides this, the most dangerous effluvia we know of are from the excretions of the sick—these are placed, at least for a time, where they must throw their effluvia into the under side of the bed, and the space under the bed is never aired; it cannot be, with our arrangements. Must not such a bed be always saturated, and be always the means of re-introducing into the unfortunate patient who lies in it, that matter to get out which from the body nature had appointed the disease?

My heart always sinks within me when I hear the good house-wife, of every class, say, "I assure you the bed has been well slept in," and one can only hope it is not true. What? is the bed already saturated with somebody else's damp before my patient comes to exhale into it his own damp? Has it not had a single chance to be aired? No, not one. "It has been slept in every night."

The best bedding, either for sick or well, is an *iron* bedstead, (no vallance, of course,) and hair mattress. Whenever you can, hang up the whole of the bedding to air for a few hours.

On no account whatever should a sick person's bed ever be higher than a sofa. Otherwise the patient can get at nothing for himself: he can move nothing for himself. A patient's bed should never have its side against the wall. The nurse must be able to get easily to both sides of the bed, and to reach easily every part of the patient without stretching—a thing impossible if the bed be either too wide, or too high, or in a corner.

When I see a patient in a room nine or ten feet high, upon a bed between four and five feet high, with his head, when he is sitting up in bed, actually within three or four feet of the ceiling, I ask myself, is this to make him feel as if the walls and ceiling were closing in upon him? If, over and above this, the window stops short of the ceiling, then the patient's head may literally be *above* the fresh air, even when the window is open. The heads of sleepers or of sick in ordinary bed-rooms should never be higher than the throat of the chimney, which ensures their being in the current of best air. And we will not suppose it possible that you have closed your chimney with a chimney-board.

If a bed is higher than a sofa, the fatigue of getting in and out of bed will just make the difference, very often, to the patient (who can get in and out of bed at all) of being able to take a few minutes' exercise, either in the open air or in another room.

A patient's bed should always be in the lightest spot in the room; and he should be able to see out of window.

I need scarcely say that the old four-post bed with curtains is bad, whether for sick or well. I wish we might never see another! Never use a feather bed, either for sick or well.[6] A careful woman will air her whole bedding, at least once a week, either by hanging it out in fine weather in the sun and air, or by toasting it before a hot fire. This is especially necessary for children's bedding; especially necessary where the whole family lives in one room.

Not a few cases of scrofula among children proceed from the habit of sleeping with the head under the bed-clothes, and so breathing air already breathed, and full of perspiration from the skin. The same with sick. A good nurse will be careful to attend to this. It is an important part, so to speak, of ventilation.

Consumptive patients often put their heads under the bed-clothes, because it relieves a fit of coughing, brought on by a change of wind or by damp. Of all places to take warm air from, one's own body is certainly the worst. And perhaps, if nurses do encourage this practice, we need no longer wonder at the "rapid decline" of some consumptive patients. A folded silk handker-chief, lightly laid over the mouth, or merely breathing the steam from a basin of boiling water, will relieve the fit of coughing without such danger. But this last must be carefully managed, so as not to make the patient damp.

It may be worth while to remark that, where there is any danger of bed-sores, a blanket should never be placed *under* the patient. It retains damp, and acts like a poultice.

Never use anything but light Witney blankets as bed covering for the sick. The heavy cotton counterpane is bad, for the very reason that it keeps in the perspiration from the sick person, while the blanket allows it to pass through. Weak patients are always distressed by a great weight of bed-clothes, which often prevents their getting any sound sleep whatever.

I once told a "very good nurse" that the way in which her patient's room was kept was quite enough to account for his sleep-lessness; and she answered, with perfect good-humour, that she was not at all surprised at it—as if the state of the room were, like the state of the weather, entirely out of her power. Now, in what sense was this woman to be called a "nurse?"

A true nurse will always make her patient's bed carefully her-self. Consider the importance of sleep to the sick, the necessity of a well-made bed to give them sleep. But a careless nurse doubles the blankets over the patient's chest, instead of leaving the lightest weight there—she puts a thick blanket under him—she does not turn his mattress *every* way every day; and the patient would rather than not that his bed were made by any body else.

One word about pillows. Every weak patient, be his illness what it may, suffers more or less from difficulty in breathing. (1.) To take the weight of the body off the poor chest, which is hardly up to its work as it is, ought therefore to be the object of the nurse in arranging his pillows. Now what *does* she do, and what are the consequences? She piles the pillows one a-top of the other like a wall of bricks. The head is thrown upon the chest, and the shoulders are pushed forward, so as not to allow the lungs room to expand. The pillows, in fact, lean upon the patient, not the patient upon the pillows. It is impossible to give a rule for this, because it must vary with the figure of the patient. But the object is to support, with the pillows, the back *below* the breathing apparatus, to allow the shoulders room to fall back, and to support the head, without throwing it forward. The suffering of dying patients is immensely increased by neglect of these points. And many an invalid, too weak to drag about his pillows himself, slips his book or anything at hand behind the lower part of his back to support it. (2.) Tall patients suffer much more than short ones, because of the *drag* of the long limbs upon the waist. Something to press the feet against is a relief to all.

Having said this about the two principles to be observed for giving ease to patients in bed, I must add that they apply equally to them when up. I scarcely ever saw an invalid chair which did not *increase* the drag of the limbs upon the waist, and throw too much of the weight upon the spine, thereby preventing any relief to the chest. An ordinary *low* well-stuffed arm-chair, with pillows and a footstool, is the best—not too high, nor too deep in the seat, but supporting the legs and feet so as to raise the knees, generally a great relief to invalids sitting up. To support the patient's frame, at as many points as possible, is the thing. And this is what invalid chairs do *not* do; and when the patient is in, he cannot get out.

IX.— LIGHT.

IT is the result of all experience with the sick, that second only to their need of fresh air is their need of light; that, after a close room, what hurts them most is a dark room, and that it is not only light but direct sun-light they want. You had better carry your patient about after the sun, according to the aspect of the rooms, if circumstances permit, than let him linger in a room when the sun is off. People think the effect is upon the spirits only. This is by no means the case. The sun is a painter. He does the photograph. Light has quite as real effects upon the human body. But this is not all. Who has not observed the purifying effect of light, and especially of direct sun-light, upon the air of a room? Here is an observation within everybody's experience. Go into a room where the shutters are always shut (in a sick room or a bed-room there should never be shutters shut), and though the room be uninhabited, though the air has never been polluted by the breathing of human beings, you will observe a close, musty smell of corrupt air, of air, *i.e.*, unpurified by the effect of the sun's rays. The mustiness of dark rooms and corners, indeed, is proverbial. The cheerfulness of a room, the usefulness of light, is all-important.

Healthy people never remember the difference between *bed*-rooms and *sick*-rooms, in making arrangements for the sick. To a sleeper in health it does not signify what the view is from his bed. He ought never to be in it excepting when asleep, and at night. Aspect does not very much signify either (provided the sun reach his bed-room some time in every day, to purify the air, although sunny rooms are always the best), because he ought never to be in his bed-room except during the hours when there is no sun. But the case is exactly reversed with the sick, even should they be as many hours out of their beds as you are in yours, which probably they are not. Therefore, that they should be able, without raising themselves or turning in bed, to see out of a window from their beds, to see sky and sun-light at least, if you can show them nothing else, I assert to be, if not of the very first importance for recovery, at least something very near it. And you should therefore look to the position of the beds of your sick one of the very first things. If they can see out of two windows instead of one, so much the better. Again, the morning sun and the mid-day sun—the hours when they are quite certain not to be up, are of more importance to them, if a choice must be made, than the afternoon sun. Perhaps you can take them out of bed in the afternoon and set them by the window, where they can see the sun. Give them as much direct sun-light as possible from the moment he rises till the moment he sets.

Another great difference between the *bed*-room and the *sick*-room is, that the *sleeper* has a very large balance of fresh air to begin with, when he begins the night, if his room has been open all day as it ought to be; the *sick* man has not, because all day he has been breathing the air in the same room, and dirtying it by the emanations from himself. Far more care is therefore necessary to keep up a constant change of air in the sick-room.

It is hardly necessary to add that there are acute cases (particularly a few eye cases, and diseases where the eye is morbidly sensitive), where a subdued light is necessary. But a dark north room is inadmissible even for these. You can always moderate the light by blinds and curtains.

Heavy, thick, dark window or bed curtains should, however, hardly ever be used for any kind of sick in this country. A light white curtain at the head of the bed is, in general, all that is necessary, and a green blind to the window, to be drawn down only when necessary.

Where is the shady side of deep valleys, there idiots grow. Where are cellars and the unsunned sides of narrow streets, there are the weakly of the human race—mind and body equally degenerating. Put the pale withering plant and human being to live in the sun, and, if not too far gone, each will recover health and vigour in time.

It is a curious thing to observe how almost all patients lie with their faces turned to the light exactly as plants always make their way towards the light; a patient will even complain that it gives him pain "lying on that side." "Then why *do* you lie on that side?" He does not know—but we do. It is because it is the side towards the window. Walk through the wards of a hospital, remember the bed sides of patients you have seen, and count how many sick you ever saw lying with their faces towards the wall.

X.— CLEANLINESS OF ROOMS AND WALLS.

It cannot be necessary to tell a nurse that she should be clean or that she should keep her patient clean,—seeing that the greater part of nursing consists in preserving cleanliness. No ventilation can freshen a room or house where the most scrupulous cleanliness is not oberved. Unless the wind be blowing through the windows at the rate of twenty miles an hour, dusty carpets, dirty wainscots, musty curtains and furniture, will always give off a close smell. I have lived in a large London house, where I had two very lofty rooms, with opposite windows, to myself, and yet, owing to the above-mentioned dirty circumstances, no opening of windows could ever keep those rooms free from closeness; but the carpet and curtains having been turned out of the rooms altogether, they became as fresh as could be wished. It is pure nonsense to say that in London a room cannot be kept clean. Many of our hospitals show the exact reverse.

But no particle of dust is ever or can ever be removed or really got rid of by the present way of dusting. Dusting in these days means nothing but flapping the dust from one part of a room on to another with doors and windows closed. What you do it for, I cannot think. You had much better leave the dust alone if you are not going to take it away altogether. For from the time a room begins to be a room, up to the time when it ceases to be one, no one atom of dust can ever actually leave it thus. Tidying a room means nothing now but removing a thing from one place, which it has kept clean for itself, on to another and a dirtier one. Flapping by way of cleaning is only admissible in the case of pictures, or anything made of paper. The only way I know to *remove* dust, the plague of all lovers of fresh air, is to wipe everything with a damp cloth. And all furniture ought to be so made as that it may be wiped with a damp cloth without injury to itself, and so polished as that it may be damped without injury to others. To "dust," as it is now practised, really means to distribute dust more equally over a room.

If you like to clean your furniture by laying out your clean clothes upon your dirty chairs or sofa, this is one way certainly of doing it. From the chairs, tables, or sofa, upon which the "things" have lain, during the night, and which are therefore clean from dust or blacks, the *"things"* having "caught" it, you then remove them to other chairs, tables, sofas, upon which you could write your name with your finger in the dust or blacks. The *other* side of the "things" is therefore now evenly dirtied or dusted. The woman then flaps everything or some things, not out of her reach, with a thing called a duster—the dust flies up, then re-settles more equally than it lay before. This is called "putting the room to rights."

As to floors, the only really clean floor I know is the old-fashioned polished oak floor, which is wet rubbed and dry rubbed every morning to remove the dust.

For a sick room, a carpet is perhaps the worst invention which could by any possibility have been made. If you must have a carpet, the only safety is to take it up two or three times a year, instead of once. A dirty carpet literally infects the room. And if you consider the enormous quantity of dirt from the feet of people coming in, which must saturate it, this is by no means surprising.

Washing floors of sick-rooms is most objectionable, for this reason. In any school-room or ward, much inhabited, you may smell a smell, while the floor is being scoured, quite different from that of soap and water. It is the exhalation from the animal matter which has soaked into the floor from the feet and breath of the inhabitants.

Dry dirt is comparatively safe dirt. Wet dirt becomes dangerous.

Uncleansed towns in dry climates have been made pestilential by having a water supply.

Doctors have forbidden scrubbing in hospitals. And nurses have done it in the earliest morning, so as not to be detected.

What is to be done?

In the sick-room, the doctor should always be asked whether and at what hour he chooses the floor to be washed. If a patient can be moved, it will probably be best to wash the floor only when he can be taken into another room, and his own room dried by fire and opened windows before he returns. A dry day and not a damp one is, therefore, necessary.

But a private sick-room (where there is not the same going to and fro as in a hospital ward) has been kept perfectly clean by wiping the floor with a damp cloth, and drying it with a floor-brush.

All the furniture was wiped in the same way with, a cloth wrung out of hot water—thus freeing the room from dust.

In more than one house the purpose has been answered by planing the floors, saturating them with "drying" linseed oil, well rubbed in, staining them (for the sake of appearance merely), and using beeswax and turpentine.

The floor was cleaned by using a brush with a cloth tied over it. And if anything offensive was spilt, it was washed off immediately with soap and water and the placed dried.

I hope the day will come in England when other floors will cease to be ever used, whether in school-rooms, lunatic asylums, hospitals, or houses.

As for walls, the worst is the papered wall; the next worst is plaster. But the plaster can be made safe by frequent lime-washing and occasional scraping; the paper requires frequent renewing. A glazed paper gets rid of a good deal of the danger. But the ordinary bed-room paper is all that it ought *not* to be.

A person who has accustomed her senses to compare rooms proper and improper, for the sick and for children, could tell, blindfold, the difference of the air in old painted and in old papered rooms. The latter will always be musty, even, with all the windows open.

The close connection between ventilation and cleanliness is shown in this. An ordinary light paper will last clean much longer if there is an Arnott's ventilator in the chimney than it otherwise would.

The best wall now extant is oil paint. From this you can wash the animal matters.*

These are what make a room musty.

Air can be soiled just like water. If you blow into water you will soil it with the animal matter from your breath. So it is with air. Air is always soiled in a room where walls and carpets are saturated with animal exhalations.

Want of cleanliness, then, in rooms and wards which you have to guard against, may arise in three ways: —

1. Dirty air coming in from without, soiled by sewer emanations, the evaporation from dirty streets, smoke, bits of unburnt fuel, bits of straw, bits of horse-dung.

If people would but cover the outside walls of their houses with tiles, what an incalculable improvement would there be in light, cleanliness, dryness, warmth, and consequently economy. The play of a fire-engine would then effectually wash the outside of a house. This kind of *walling* would stand next to paving in improving the health of towns.

2. Dirty air coming from within, from dust which you often displace, but never remove. And this recalls what ought to be a *sine quâ non*. Have as few ledges in your room or ward as possible. And under no pretence have any ledge whatever out of sight. Dust lies there, and will never be wiped off. This is a certain way to soil the air. Besides this, the animal exhalations from your inmates saturate your furniture. And if you never

* I never can imagine why people suppose that their walls do not require washing, but that their floors do. They say, "Oh! because our floors are walked upon." Not everywhere: not under the beds and tables: yet you scour there. Scour your walls in the same way.

If you like to wipe your dirty door, or some portion of your dirty wall, by hanging up your clean gown or shawl against it on a peg, this is one way certainly, and the most usual way, and generally the only way of cleaning either door or wall in a bed-room.

clean your furniture properly, how can your rooms or wards be anything but musty? Ventilate as you please, the rooms will never be sweet. Besides this, there is a constant *degradation*, as it is called, taking place from everything except polished or glazed articles—*e.g.*, in colouring certain green papers arsenic is used. Now in the very dust even, which is lying about in rooms hung with this kind of green paper, arsenic has been distinctly detected. You see your dust is anything but harmless; yet you will let such dust lie about your ledges for months, your rooms for ever.

Again, the fire fills the room with coal-dust.

3. Dirty air coming from the carpet. Above all, take care of the carpets that the animal dirt left there by the feet of visitors does not stay there. Floors, unless the grain is filled up and polished, are just as bad. The smell, already mentioned, from the floor of a school-room or ward, when any moisture brings out the organic matter by which it is saturated, might alone be enough to warn us of the mischief that is going on.

The outer air, then, can only be kept clean by sanitary improvements, and by consuming smoke. The expense in soap, which this single improvement would save, is quite incalculable.

The inside air can only be kept clean by excessive care in the ways mentioned above,—to rid the walls, carpets, furniture, ledges, &c., of the organic matter and dust—dust consisting greatly of this organic matter,—with which they become saturated, and which is what really makes the room musty.

Without cleanliness, you cannot have all the effect of ventilation; without ventilation, you can have no thorough cleanliness.

Very few people, be they of what class they may, have any idea of the exquisite cleanliness required in the sick-room. For much of what is here said applies less to the hospital than to the private sick-room. The smoky chimney, the dusty furniture, the utensils emptied but once a day, often keep the air of the sick constantly dirty in the best private houses.

The well have a curious habit of forgetting that what is to them but a trifling inconvenience, to be patiently "put up" with, is to the sick a source of suffering, delaying recovery, if not actually hastening death. The well are scarcely ever more than eight hours, at most, in the same room. Some change they can always make, if only for a few minutes. Even during these eight hours, they can change their posture or their position in the room. But the sick man who never leaves his bed, who cannot change by any movement of his own his air, or his light, or his warmth; who cannot obtain quiet, or get out of the smoke, or the smell, or the dust; he is really poisoned or depressed by what is to you the merest trifle.

"What can't be cured must be endured," is the very worst and most dangerous maxim for a nurse which ever was made. Patience and resignation in her are but other words for carelessness or indifference—contemptible, if in regard to herself; culpable, if in regard to her sick.

XI.— PERSONAL CLEANLINESS.

In almost all diseases, the cleanliness of the skin is most important. And this is particularly the case with children. But the perspiration, which comes from the skin, is left there, unless removed by washing or by the clothes. Every nurse should keep this fact constantly in mind—for, if she allow her sick to remain unwashed, or their clothing to remain on them after being saturated with perspiration or other excretion, she is interfering with the process of health just as effectually as if she were to give the patient a dose of slow poison by the mouth. Poisoning by the skin is no less certain than poisoning by the mouth—only it is slower in its operation.

Country people are much more afraid of water than town people; poor people than rich people. Many a good, active, cleanly, country housewife has told me with pride that she has never had her children's feet washed in all their lives, nor let one of them ever touch himself with cold water. Many a collier and labouring man still boasts that he has never washed anything below his face, except his hands. In districts where the water-cure is established, in towns where baths and wash-houses are well known, these extraordinary prejudices are dying out. But there is still many a school where the greatest difficulty is found in getting the children to have their feet washed. All schools ought to have baths and washing-places attached to them.

Even in remote country villages, however, people are getting wiser. An excellent old grandmother, who had never washed her own children, began, in her old age, to wash her delicate little orphan grandchild all over every day, and found him grow up a stout boy. An old lady began to wash herself all over with cold water, for the first time after eighty years of age, and lived ten good years afterwards.

The amount of relief and comfort experienced by sick after the skin has been carefully washed and dried, is one of the commonest observations made at a sick bed. But it must not be forgotten that the comfort and relief so obtained are not all. They are, in fact, nothing more than a sign that the powers of life have been relieved by removing something that was oppressing them. The nurse, therefore, must never put off attending to the personal cleanliness of her patient under the plea that all that is to be gained is a little relief, which can be quite as well given later.

In all well-regulated hospitals this ought to be, and generally is, attended to. But it is very generally neglected with sick at home.

Just as it is necessary to renew the air round a sick person frequently, to carry off sickly vapours from the lungs and skin, by maintaining free ventilation, so is it necessary to keep the pores of the skin free from all obstructing excretions. The object, both of ventilation and of skin-cleanliness, is pretty much the same,—to wit, removing hurtful matter from the body as rapidly as possible.

Care should be taken in all sponging, washing, and cleansing the skin, not to expose too great a surface at once, so as to check the perspiration, which would renew the evil in another form.

The various ways of washing the sick need not here be specified — the less so as the doctors ought to say which is to be used.

Where the skin is hard and harsh, the relief afforded by washing with a great deal of soft soap is incalculable. In other cases, sponging with tepid soap and water, then with tepid water, and drying with a hot towel will be ordered.

Every nurse ought to be careful to wash her hands very frequently during the day. If her face, too, so much the better.

One word as to cleanliness merely as cleanliness.

Compare the dirtiness of the water in which you have washed when it is cold without soap, cold with soap, hot with soap. You will find the first has hardly removed any dirt at all, the second a little more, the third a great deal more. But hold your hand over a cup of hot water for a minute or two, and then, by merely rubbing with the finger, you will bring off flakes of dirt or dirty skin. After a vapour bath you may peel your whole self clean in this way. What I mean is, that by simply washing or sponging with water you do not really clean your skin. Take a rough towel, dip one corner in very hot water—if a little spirit be added to it it will be more effectual—and then rub as if you were rubbing the towel into your skin with your finger. The black flakes which will come off will convince you that you were not clean before, however much soap and water you have used. These flakes are what require removing. And you can really keep yourself cleaner with a tumbler of hot water and a rough towel and rubbing, than with a whole apparatus of bath and soap and sponge, without rubbing. It is quite nonsense to say that anybody need be dirty. Patients have been kept as clean by these means on a long voyage, when a basin full of water could not be afforded, and when they could not be moved out of their berths, as if all the appurtenances of home had been at hand.

Washing, however, with a large quantity of water has quite other effects than those of mere cleanliness. The skin absorbs the water, and becomes softer and more perspirable. To wash with soap and soft water is, therefore, desirable from other points of view than that of cleanliness.

You ought to use fresh water as freely for the skin as fresh air for the lungs. But the water must be soft. People very little think of this. They think mainly of hard water as chapping their hands, not as being a promoter of drunkenness, uncleanliness, indigestion. "Water-dressings," used to sores, have absolutely the opposite effect, viz., poisoning the sore, when made with very hard water, to what they have, viz., cleansing and healing the sore, when the water is soft. When water is hard, it is worth while to have distilled water for every water-dressing. For all washing of the sick, it is worth while to collect rain-water, or to condense steam from a boiler, or to boil water, which will often remove from one-half to three-fourths of the hardness. Soap and *hard* water actually dirty your patient's skin. The oil in the soap, the perspiration from the skin, and the lime in the water, unite to form a kind of varnish upon the skin, which comes off in the above-mentioned black flakes when rubbed.

The use of soft or filtered water for making tea or drinks, boiling vegetables, or mixing medicines, is very important. A careless nurse sometimes takes the water from the wash-hand stand for this last purpose. She had often as well not give the medicine at all.

XII.— CHATTERING HOPES AND ADVICES.

THE invalid to his advisers: —

"My advisers! Their name is Legion. * * * Somehow or other, every man, woman, and child considers him, her, or itself, privileged especially to advise me. Why? That is precisely what I want to know." And this is what I have to say to them. I have been advised to go to every place in and out of England—to take every kind of exercise by every kind of cart, carriage -yes, and even swing (!) and dumb-bell (!) in existence; to drink every different kind of stimulus that ever has been invented. And this when those *best* fitted to know, viz., medical men, had declared any journey out of the question, had forbidden any kind of motion whatever, had closely laid down the diet and drink. What would my advisers say, were they the medical attendants, and I, the patient, left their advice, and took the casual adviser's? But the singularity in Legion's mind is this: it never occurs to him that everybody else is doing the same thing, and that I, the patient, *must* say in self-defence, "I could not do with all."

"Chattering Hopes" may seem an odd heading. But I really believe there is scarcely a greater worry which invalids have to endure than the incurable hopes of their friends. There is no one practice against which I can speak more strongly from actual personal experience, wide and long, of its effects during sickness observed both upon others and upon myself. I would appeal most seriously to all friends, visitors, and .attendants of the sick to leave off this practice of attempting to "cheer" the sick by making light of their danger and by exaggerating their probabilities of recovery.

Far more now than formerly does the medical attendant tell the truth to the sick who are really desirous to hear it about their own state.

But then it must be the truth.

I mean that there are physician fatalists and Patient fatalists — physician fatalists, who will consider the case of a patient with organic disease hopeless; fatalist Patients, who, if told by the doctor that they have organic disease, that they must give up work, &c., consider themselves as much doomed to death as if they were on their way to be hung; and the very sentence that they *have* organic disease does doom them to death. They are never told, nor do they consider, how they might avoid, or at least delay, the fatal end. The very sentence hurries it.

I need hardly say that this is *not* telling them the truth.

Also, in the case of sick infants, no telling of hopelessness can, of course, affect the poor little sufferer, but it may the nurse. The more devoted the nurse, the better for poor baby; and a really efficient nurse is generally a woman of deep feeling. I have heard such an one cry out, "Oh! he should not have told me there was no hope. I shan't be able to do all that can be done, if I have no hope!" She does "do all that can be done" till the end; but still it was scarcely true, scarcely wise, to give her no hope. Children do make such wonderful recoveries, if all that can be done is done for them "till the end." And, on the other hand, so trifling a neglect will turn the scale of life to death! "While there is life, there *is* hope," is true, and while there is hope, there is life, is also true—in children's cases pre-eminently.

But, leaving well-founded hopes, to return to "chattering" hopes —

How intense is the folly, then, to say the least of it, of the friend, be he even a medical man, who thinks that his opinion, given after a cursory observation, will weigh with the patient, against the opinion of the medical attendant, given, perhaps, after years of observation, after using every help afforded by the stethoscope, the examination of pulse, tongue, &c., and certainly after much more observation than the friend can possibly have had.

Supposing the patient to be possessed of common sense—how can the "favourable" opinion, if it is to be called an opinion at all, of the casual visitor "cheer" him—when different from that of the experienced attendants. Unquestionably the latter may, and often does, turn out to be wrong. But which is most likely to be wrong?

The fact is, that the patient* is not "cheered" at all by these

---

* There are, of course, cases, as in first confinements, when an assurance from the doctor or experienced nurse to the frightened suffering woman that there is nothing unusual in her case, that she has nothing to fear but a few hours' pain, may

well-meaning, most tiresome friends. On the contrary, he is depressed and wearied. If, on the one hand, he exerts himself to tell everybody, one after the other, why he does not think as they do—in what respect he is worse—what symptoms exist that they know nothing of—he is fatigued instead of "cheered," and his attention is fixed upon himself. In general, patients who are really ill do not want to talk about themselves. Would-be invalids do; but again I say we are not on the subject of would-be invalids.

If, on the other hand, and which is much more frequently the case, the patient says nothing but "Oh!" and "Ah!" in order to escape from the conversation about himself the sooner, he is depressed by want of sympathy. He feels isolated in the midst of friends. He feels what a convenience it would be, if there were any single person to whom he could speak simply and openly, without pulling the string upon himself of this shower-bath of silly hopes and encouragements; to whom he could express his wishes and directions without that person persisting in saying, "I hope that it will please God yet to give you twenty years," or "You have a long life of activity before you." How often we see at the end of biographies, or of cases recorded in papers, "after a long illness A. died rather suddenly," or "unexpectedly, both to himself and to others." "Unexpectedly" to others, perhaps, who did not see, because they did not look; but by no means "unexpectedly to himself," as I feel entitled to believe, both from the internal evidence in such stories, and from watching similar cases: there was every reason to expect that A.

cheer her most, effectually. This is advice of quite another order. It is the advice of experience to utter inexperience. But the advice we have been referring to is the advice of inexperience to bitter experience; and, in general, amounts to nothing more than this, that *you* think I *shall* recover from consumption, because somebody knows somebody somewhere who has recovered from fever.

I have heard a doctor condemned whose patient did not, alas! recover, because another doctor's patient of a *different* sex, of a different age, recovered from a *different* disease, in a *different* place. Yes, this is really true. If people who make these comparisons did but know (only they do not care to know) the care and preciseness with which such comparisons require to be made (and are made), in order to be of any value whatever, they would spare their tongues. In comparing the deaths of one hospital with those of another, any statistics are justify considered absolutely valueless which do not give the ages, the sexes, and the diseases of all the cases. It does not seem necessary to mention this. It does not seem necessary to say that there can be no comparison between old men with dropsies and young women with consumptions. Yet the cleverest men and the cleverest women are often heard making such comparisons, ignoring entirely sex, age, disease, place—in fact, *all* the conditions essential to the question. It is the merest *gossip*.

would die, and he knew it; but he found it useless to insist upon his knowledge to his friends.

On the other hand, there is nobody so credulous as a credulous invalid, except, perhaps, the credulous friends of a credulous invalid. How often does it happen that, no sooner have the doctor and nurse come to a perfect understanding as to what must be done, than the nurse is surprised by having an opinion given her as to what ought to be done from somebody she never heard of before. It is sometimes an old friend or an old school-fellow who suddenly finds out that everybody, patient, doctor, nurse, has been wrong, and that such and such other management would answer better; and everything is upset, confidence is destroyed or disturbed, everybody is annoyed, but only one person is injured, and that is the patient. This kind of interference is mostly out of mere officiousness or wilfulness. But it does more mischief than the mischief-maker at all knows of.

The credulity of patients or of friends often leads to quackery of a much more dangerous kind. There is a morbid dislike to calling in the regular doctor, or he is too expensive. And there is a morbid craving after the advice of any quack who will adver-tise himself most impudently. "Bone-setters," and others such are the scourge of the poor. Life is too precious to be played with in such a game. Confidence should be placed in both doctor and nurse till there is very good reason for taking it away. But it should certainly never be given to quacks, either male or female.

So also as to all the advice showered so profusely upon the sick, to leave off some occupation, to try some other doctor, some other house, pill, powder, or specific; I say nothing of the incon-sistency, for these advisers are sure to be the same persons who exhorted the sick man not to believe his own doctor, because "doctors are always mistaken," but to believe some other doctor, because "this doctor is always right."

Wonderful is the face with which friends will come in and worry the patient with recommendations to do something or other, having just as little knowledge as to its being feasible, or even safe for him, as if they were to recommend a man to take exercise, not knowing he had broken his leg. What would the friend say, if *he* were the medical attendant, and if the patient, because some *other* friend had come in, because somebody, anybody, nobody, had recommended something, anything, nothing, were to disregard *his* orders, and take that other body's recommendation? But people never think of this.

If such friends and acquaintances would but consider for one moment, that it is probable the patient has heard such advice at least fifty times before, and that had it been practicable, it would have been practised long ago. But of such consideration there appears to be no chance.

To me these commonplaces, leaving their smear upon the cheerful, single-hearted, constant devotion to duty, which is so often seen in the decline of such sufferers, recall the slimy trail left by the snail on the sunny southern garden-wall loaded with fruit.

No mockery in the world is so hollow as the advice showered upon the sick. It is of no use for the sick to say anything, for what the adviser wants is, *not* to know the truth about the state of the patient, but to turn whatever the sick may say to the support of his own argument, set forth, it must be repeated, without any inquiry whatever into the patient's real condition.

To nurses I say—these are the visitors who do your patient harm. When you hear him told:— 1. That he has nothing the matter with him, and that he wants cheering. 2. That he is killing himself, and that he wants preventing. 3. That he is the tool of somebody who makes use of him for a purpose. 4. That he will listen to nobody, but is obstinately bent upon his own way; and 5. That he ought to be called to the sense of duty, and is flying in the face of Providence;—then know that your patient is receiving all the injury that he can receive from a visitor.

How little the real sufferings of illness are known or understood. How little does any one in good health fancy him or even *herself* into the life of a sick person!

Do, you who are about the sick, or who visit the sick, try and give them pleasure, remember to tell them what will do so. How often in such visits the sick person has to do the whole conversation, while you would take the visitor, absorbed m his own anxieties, for the sick person. "Oh! my dear, I have so much to think of, I really quite forgot to tell him that; besides, I thought he would know it," says the visitor to another friend. How could "he know it?" Depend upon it, the people who say this are really those who have little "to think of." There are many burthened with business who always manage to keep a corner in their minds, full of things to tell the "invalid."

I do not say, don't tell him your anxieties—I believe it to be good for him and good for you too; but if you tell him what is anxious, surely you can remember to tell him what is pleasant too.

A sick person does so enjoy hearing good news:—for instance, of a love and courtship, while in progress to a good ending. If you tell him only when the marriage takes place, he loses half the pleasure, which God knows he has little enough of; and ten to one but you have told him of some love-making with a bad ending.

A sick person also intensely enjoys hearing of any *material* good, any positive or practical success of the right. He has so much of books and fiction, of principles, and precepts, and theories; do, instead of advising him with advice he has heard at least fifty times before, tell him of one benevolent act which has really succeeded practically,—it is like a day's health to him.*

You have no idea what the craving of sick with undiminished power of thinking, but little power of doing, is to hear of good practical action, when they can no longer partake in it.

Do observe these things, especially with invalids. Do remember how their life is to them disappointed and incomplete. You see them lying there with miserable disappointments, from which they can have no escape but death, and you can't remember to tell them of what would give them so much pleasure, or at least an hour's variety.

They don't want you to be whining with them, they like you to be fresh and active and interested, but they cannot bear absence of mind, and they are so tired of the advice and preaching they receive from every body, no matter whom it is, they see.

There is no better society than babies and sick people for one another. Of course you must manage this so that neither shall suffer from it, which is perfectly possible. If you think the "air of the sick room" bad for the baby, why it is bad for the invalid too, and, therefore, you will of course correct it for both. It freshens up a sick person's whole mind to see "the baby." And a very young child, if unspoiled, will generally adapt itself won-

---

* A small pet animal is often an excellent companion for the sick, for long chronic cases especially. A bird in a cage is sometimes the only pleasure of an invalid confined for years to the same room. If he can feed and clean the animal himself, he ought always to be encouraged and assisted to do so. An invalid, in giving an account of his nursing by a nurse and a dog, infinitely preferred that of the dog; "above all, it did not *talk*."

derfully to the ways of a sick person, if the time they spend together is not too long.

If you knew how unreasonably sick people suffer from reasonable causes of distress, you would take more pains about all these things. An infant laid upon the sick bed will do the sick person thus suffering, more good than all your eloquence. A piece of good news will do the same.

It has been very justly said that sick and invalids are like children in this, there is no *proportion* in events to them. Now it is your business as their visitor to restore this right proportion for them—to show them what the rest of the world is doing. How can they find it out otherwise? You will find them far more open to conviction than children in this. And you will find that their unreasonable intensity of suffering from unkindness, from want of sympathy, &c., will disappear with their freshened interest in the big world's events. But then you must be able to give them real interests, not gossip.

And oh! how much might be spared to the dying! If anxious friends would but not ask the dying man to "give a sign;" to assure them of his "eternal salvation;" of his being "happy;" to say "farewell;" how much they would spare him!

Don't distress the dying father with, "What will become of us when you are gone?" Nor the dying child with the mother's longings to keep it. I have heard a child say, "Oh, mother, don'tee wish so! I can't die easy while thou'rt wishing!"[7]

So also with making a will, family arrangements and the hundred other things which are often crowded into the few hours or even minutes before death, when, too, the dying are weakened by disease, confused by medicines, and either in a state of half torpor or unnatural excitement.

The sooner you settle all the affairs of life, the better. The stronger you are when you are doing it, the better, and the more chance of recovery you give yourself when you *are* ill.

It is the last straw that breaks the camel's back.

Many a last chance of life has been lost by putting off business to the last moment; most of all, the highest business of salvation. Many a so-called "miracle" has been worked by the mind, calm and freed from these anxieties, allowing the body to make the needful effort to live.

This is one of the commonest experiences of God's ways to those who have watched many death-beds. All classes are nearly alike. But small farmers and shopkeepers are perhaps most prone to put off the business of life until death.

The physical difference of death-beds by different diseases, is little observed. Patients who die of consumption very frequently die in a state of seraphic joy and peace; the countenance almost expresses rapture. Patients who die of cholera, peritonitis, &c., on the contrary, often die in a state approaching despair. The countenance expresses horror.

In dysentery, diarrhoea, or fever, the patient often dies in a state of indifference.

Again, in some cases, even of consumption and peritonitis, there are alternations almost of ecstasy, and of despondency. In the lives of the "Saints," and in religious biographies, we often find such death-beds described truly enough. But then the patient and friends make unwise exertions to bring back the state of rapture, quite unaware that it may be only a physical state. And if it does not return, both may perhaps consider that its absence is a token of a state of "reprobation," or "backsliding."

Friends, in all these cases, are apt to judge most unfairly of the spiritual state of the sick from the physical state.

XIII.—OBSERVATION OF THE SICK.

THE most important practical lesson that can be given to nurses is to teach them what to observe—how to observe—what symptoms indicate improvement—what the reverse—which are of importance—which are of none—which are the evidence of neglect — and of what kind of neglect.

All this is what ought to make part, and an essential part, of the training of every nurse. At present how few there are, either professional or unprofessional, who really know at all whether any sick person they may be with is better or worse.

I can record but a very few specimens of the answers which I have heard made by friends and nurses, and accepted by physicians and surgeons at the very bed-side of the patient, who could have contradicted every word but did not—sometimes from amiability, often from shyness, oftenest from languor!

"How often have the bowels acted, nurse?" "Once, sir." This generally means that the utensil has been emptied once, it having been used perhaps seven or eight times.

"Do you think the patient is much weaker than he was six weeks ago?" "Oh no, sir; you know it is very long since he has been up and dressed, and he can get across the room now." This means that the nurse has not observed that whereas six weeks ago he sat up and occupied himself in bed, he now lies still doing nothing; that, although he can "get across the room," he cannot stand for five seconds.

Another patient who is eating well, recovering steadily although slowly, from fever, but cannot walk or stand, is represented to the doctor as making no progress at all.

It is a much more difficult thing to speak the truth than people commonly imagine. There is first the man who gives, in answer to a question asked about a thing that has been before his eyes perhaps for years, information exceedingly imperfect, or says he does not know. He has never observed. And people simply think him stupid.

The second has observed just as little, but he describes the whole thing from imagination merely, being perfectly convinced all the while that he has seen or heard it; or he will repeat a whole conversation, as if it were information which had been addressed to him; whereas it is merely what he has himself said to somebody else. This is the commonest of all. These people do not even observe that they have *not* observed nor remember that they have forgotten.

Courts of justice seem to think that anybody can speak the "whole truth and nothing but the truth," if he does but intend it. It requires many faculties combined of observation and memory to speak "the whole truth" and to say "nothing but the truth."

"I knows I fibs dreadful: but believe me, Miss, I never finds out I have fibbed until they tells me so," was a remark actually made. It is also one of much more extended application than most people have the least idea of.

I have heard thirteen persons "concur" in declaring that a fourteenth who had never left his bed, went to a distant chapel every morning at seven o'clock.

I have heard persons in perfect good faith declare, that a man came to dine every day at the house where they lived, who had never dined there once; that a person had never taken the sacrament, by whose side they had twice at least knelt at Communion; that but one meal a day came out of a hospital kitchen, which for six weeks they had seen provide from three to five and six meals a day. Such instances might be multiplied *ad infinitum* if necessary.

Questions as asked now (but too generally) of, or about patients, would obtain no information at all about them, even if the person asked of had every information to give. The question is generally a leading question; and it is singular that people never think what must be the answer to this question before they ask it; for instance, "Has he had a good night?" Now, one patient will think he has a bad night if he has not slept ten hours without waking. Another does not think he has a bad night if he has had intervals of dozing occasionally. The same answer has actually been given as regarded two patients—one who had been entirely sleepless for five times twenty-four hours, and died of it, and another who had not slept the sleep of a regular night, without waking. Why cannot the question be asked, How many hours' sleep has —— had? and at what hours of the night? This is important, because on this depends what the remedy will be. If a patient sleeps two or three hours early in the night, and then does not sleep again at all, ten to one it is not a sleeping dose he wants, but food or stimulus, or perhaps only warmth. If, on the other hand, he is restless, and awake all night, and is drowsy in the morning, he probably wants sedatives, either quiet, coolness, or medicine, a lighter diet, or all four. Now the doctor should be told this; or how can he judge what to give?

How few there are who, by five or six pointed questions, can elicit the whole case and get accurately to know and to be able to report *where* the patient is.

I knew a very clever physician, of large dispensary and hospital practice, who invariably began his examination of each patient with "Put your finger where you *be* bad." That man would never waste his time with collecting inaccurate information from nurse or patient. Leading questions always collect inaccurate information.

At a recent celebrated trial, the following leading question was put successively to nine distinguished medical men. "Can you attribute these symptoms to anything else but poison?" And out of the nine, eight answered "No!" without any qualification whatever. It appeared, upon cross-examination:—1. That none of them had ever seen a case of the kind of poisoning supposed. 2. That none of them had ever seen a case of the kind of disease to which the death, if not to poison, was attributable. 3. That none of them were even aware of the main fact of the disease and condition to which the death was attributable.

Surely nothing stronger can be adduced to prove what little use leading questions are of, and what they lead to.

I had rather not say how many instances I have known, where, owing to this system of leading questions, the patient has died, and the attendants have been actually unaware of the principal feature of the case.

It is useless to go through all the particulars, besides sleep, in which people have a peculiar talent for gleaning inaccurate information. As to food, for instance, I often think that that most common question, How is your appetite? can only be put because the questioner believes the questioned has really nothing the matter with him, which is very often the case. But where there is, the remark holds good which has been made about sleep. The *same* answer will often be made as regards a patient who cannot take two ounces of solid food per diem, and a patient who does not enjoy five meals a day as much as usual.

Again, the question, How is your appetite? is often put when How is your digestion? is the question meant. No doubt the two things often depend on one another. But they are quite different. Many a patient can eat, if you can only "tempt his appetite." The fault lies in your not having got him the thing that he fancies. But many another patient does not care between grapes and turnips,—everything is equally distasteful to him. He would try to eat anything which would do him good; but everything "makes him worse." The fault here generally lies in the cooking. It is not his "appetite" which requires "tempting;" it is his digestion, which requires sparing. And good sick cookery will save the digestion half its work.

There may be four different causes, any one of which will produce the same result, viz., the patient slowly starving to death from want of nutrition.

1. Defect in cooking;
2. Defect in choice of diet;
3. Defect in choice of hours for taking diet;
4. Defect of appetite in patient.

Yet all these are generally comprehended in the one sweeping assertion that the patient has "no appetite."

Surely many lives might be saved by drawing a closer distinction; for the remedies are as diverse as the causes. The remedy for the first is, to cook better; for the second, to choose other articles of diet; for the third, to watch for the hours when the patient is in want of food; for the fourth, to show him what he likes, and sometimes unexpectedly. But no one of these remedies will do for any other of the defects not corresponding with it.

It cannot too often be repeated that patients are generally either too languid to observe these things, or too shy to speak about them; nor is it well that they should be made to observe them, it fixes their attention upon themselves,

Again, I say, what *is* the nurse, or friend there for except to take note of these things, instead of the patient doing so?

It is commonly supposed that the nurse is there to spare the patient from making physical exertion for himself—I would rather say, that she ought to be there to spare him from taking thought for himself. And I am quite sure, that if the patient were spared all thought for himself and *not* spared all physical exertion, he would be the gainer. The reverse is generally the case in the private house. In the hospital it is the relief from all anxiety, afforded by the rules of a well-regulated institution, which has often such a beneficial effect upon the patient.

"Can I do anything for you?" says the thoughtless nurse— and the uncivil patient invariably answers "no"—the civil patient, "no thank you." The fact is, that a real patient will rather go without almost anything than make the exertion of thinking *what* the nurse has left undone. And surely it is for her, not for him, to make this exertion. Such a question is, on her part, a mere piece of laziness, under the guise of being "obliging." She wishes to throw the trouble on the patient of nursing himself.

Again, the question is sometimes put, Is there diarrhoea? And the answer will be the same, whether it is just merging into cholera, whether it is a trifling degree brought on by some trifling indiscretion, which will cease the moment the cause is removed, or whether there is no diarrhoea at all, but simply relaxed bowels.

It is useless to multiply instances of this kind. As long as observation is so little cultivated as it is now, I do believe that it is better for the physician *not* to see the friends of the patient at all. They will oftener mislead him than not. And as often by making the patient out worse as better than he really is.

In the case of infants, *everything* must depend upon the accurate observation of the nurse or mother who has to report. And how seldom is this condition of accuracy fulfilled!

It is the real test of a nurse whether she can nurse a sick infant. Of *it* she can never ask, "Can I do anything for you?"

A celebrated man, though celebrated only for foolish things, has told us that one of his main objects in the education of his son, was to give him a ready habit of accurate observation, a certainty of perception, and that for this purpose one of his means was a month's course as follows:—he took the boy rapidly past a toy-shop; the father and son then described to each other as many of the objects as they could, which they had seen in passing the windows, noting them down with pencil and paper, and returning afterwards to verify their own accuracy. The boy always succeeded best, *e.g.*, if the father described 30 objects, the boy did 40, and scarcely ever made a mistake.

How wise a piece of education this would be for much higher objects; and in our calling of nurses the thing itself is essential. For it may safely be said, not that the habit of ready and correct observation will by itself make us useful nurses, but that without it we shall be useless with all our devotion.

One nurse in charge of a set of wards not only carries in her head all the little varieties in the diets which each patient is allowed to fix for himself, but also exactly what each patient has taken during each day. Another nurse, in charge of one single patient, takes away his meals day after day all but untouched, and never knows it.

If you find it helps you to note down such things on a bit of paper, in pencil, by all means do so. Perhaps it more often lames than strengthens the memory and observation. But if you cannot get the habit of observation one way or other, you had better give up the being a nurse, for it is not your calling, however kind and anxious you may be.

Surely you can learn at least to judge with the eye how much an oz. of solid food is, how much an oz. of liquid. You will find this helps your observation and memory very much, you will then say to yourself "A. took about an oz. of his meat to-day;" "B. took three times in 24 hours about 1/4 pint of beef tea;" instead of saying "B. has taken nothing all day," or "I gave A. his dinner as usual."

I have known several of our real old-fashioned hospital "sisters" who could, as accurately as a measuring glass, measure out all their patient's wine and medicine by the eye, and never be wrong. I do not recommend this,—one must be very sure of one's self to do it. I only mention it, because if a nurse can by practice measure medicine by the eye, surely she is no nurse who cannot measure by the eye about how much food (in oz.) her patient has taken. In hospitals those who cut up the diets give with quite sufficient accuracy, to each patient, his 12 oz. or his 6 oz. of meat without weighing. Yet a nurse will often have patients loathing all food and incapable of any will to get well, who just tumble over the contents of the plate or dip the spoon in the cup to deceive the nurse, and she will take it away without ever seeing that there is just the same quantity of food as when she brought it, and she will tell the doctor, too, that the patient has eaten all his diets as usual, when all she ought to have meant is that she has taken away his diets as usual.

Now what kind of a nurse is this?

There are two causes for mistakes of inadvertence. 1. A want of ready attention; only part of a patient's request is heard at all. 2. A want of the habit of observation.

To a nurse I would add, take care that you always put the same things in the same places; you don't know how suddenly you may be called on some day to find something, and may not be able to remember in your haste where you yourself had put it, if your memory is not in the habit of seeing the thing there always.

Good nursing consists simply in observing little things which are common to all sick, and those which are particular to each sick individual.

Some people have a curious power over animals. They can collect wild birds round them in a wood. This, once thought witchcraft, is now supposed to be some peculiar power, which we can't see into, like the calculating boy's. It is nothing at all but the minute observation of the habits and instincts of birds.

So the "peculiar power" of one nurse, and the want of power of another over her patient, is nothing at all but minute observation in the former of what affects him, and want of observation in the latter.

In nothing is this more remarkable than in inducing patients to take food. A patient is sinking for want of it under one nurse; you put him under another, and he takes it directly. How is this? People say, oh! she has a command over her patients. It is no command. It is the way she feeds him, or the way she pillows his head, so that he can swallow comfortably. Opening the window will enable one patient to take his food; washing his face and hands another; merely passing a wet towel over the back of the neck, a third; a fourth, who is a depressed suicide, requires a little cheering to give him spirit to eat. The nurse amuses him with giving some variety to his ideas. I remember that, when very ill, the way in which one nurse put the spoon into my mouth enabled me to swallow, when I could not if I was fed by any one else.

It is just the observation of all these little things, no unintelligible "influence," which enables one woman to save life; it is the want of such observation which prevents another from finding the means to do so.

Even delirium, which seems to place the patient so out of the reach of all human relief, that he is shrieking and calling for you, and you cannot make him understand that you are there by him, is often increased by an awkward noise or touch, and yet the nurse who does so never perceives it.

Again, few things press so heavily on one suffering from long and incurable illness, as the necessity of telling his nurse, from time to time, who will not otherwise see, that he cannot do this or that, which he could do a month or a year ago. What is a nurse there for, if she cannot observe these things for herself? Yet I have known more accidents (fatal, slowly or rapidly) arising from this want of observation among nurses than from almost anything else. Because a patient could get out of a warm bath alone a month ago—because a patient could walk as far as his door, or call so as to be heard a week ago,[8] the nurse concludes that he can do so now. She has never observed the change; and the patient is lost from being left in a helpless state of exhaustion, till some one accidentally comes in. And this not from any unexpected apoplectic, paralytic, or fainting fit (though even these could be expected far more, at least, than they are now, if we did but *observe*). No, from the expected, or to be expected, inevitable, visible, calculable, uninterrupted increase of weakness, which none need fail to observe.

Again, a patient not usually confined to bed, is compelled, by an attack of diarrhoea, vomiting, or other accident, to keep his bed for a few days; he gets up for the first time, and the nurse lets him go into another room, without coming in, a few minutes afterwards, to look after him. It never occurs to her that he is quite certain to be faint, or cold, or to want something. She says, as her excuse, Oh, he does not like to be fidgeted after. Yes, he said so some weeks ago; but he never said he did not like to be "fidgeted after," when he is in the state he is in now; and if he did, you ought to make some excuse to go to him. More patients have been lost in this way than is at all generally known, viz., from relapses brought on by being left for an hour or two, faint, or cold, or hungry, after getting up for the first time.

You do not know how small is the power of resistance in a weak patient—how he will succumb to habits of the nurse, which occasion him positive pain for the time, and total prostration for the whole day, rather than remonstrate. A good nurse gets the patient into a good habit, such as washing and dressing at different times so as to spare his strength. A bad nurse succeeds, and the patient adopts her bad ways without a struggle. *Patients do what they are expected to do.* This is equally important to be remembered, for good as well as for bad.

There are two habits of mind often equally misleading: — (1.) a want of observation of conditions, and (2.) a habit of taking averages.

1. Men whose profession, like that of medical men, leads them to observe only, or chiefly, palpable and permanent organic changes are often just as wrong in their opinion of the result as those who do not observe at all. For instance, there is a cancer or a broken leg; the surgeon has only to look at it once to know; it will not be different if he sees it in the morning to what it would have been had he seen it in the evening. In whatever conditions the broken leg is, or is likely to be, there will still be the broken leg until it is united. The same with many organic diseases. An experienced physician has but to feel the pulse once, and he knows that there is aneurism which will kill some time or other.

But with the great majority of cases, there is nothing of the kind; and the power of forming any correct opinion as to the result must entirely depend upon an inquiry into all the conditions in which the patient lives. In a complicated state of society in large towns, death, as every one of great experience knows, is far less often produced by any one organic disease, than by some illness, after many other diseases, producing just the sum of exhaustion necessary for death.

There is nothing so absurd, nothing so misleading as the verdict one so often hears: So-and-so has no organic disease,—there is no reason why he should not live to extreme old age; sometimes the clause is added, sometimes not: Provided he has quiet, good food, good air, &c., &c., &c.; the verdict is repeated by ignorant people *without* the latter clause; or there is no possibility of the conditions of the latter clause being obtained; and this, the *only* essential part of the whole, is made of no effect.

I have known two cases, the one of a man who intentionally and repeatedly displaced a dislocation, and was kept and petted by all the surgeons; the other of one who was pronounced to have nothing the matter with him, there being no organic change perceptible, but who died within the week. In both these cases, it was the nurse who, by accurately pointing out what she had accurately observed to the doctors, saved the one case from persevering in a fraud, the other from being discharged when actually in a dying state.

But one may even go further and say, that in diseases which have their origin in the feeble or irregular action of some function, and not in organic change, it is quite an accident if the doctor who sees the case only once a day, and generally at the same time, can form any but a negative idea of its real condition. In the middle of the day, when such a patient has been refreshed by light and air, by his tea, his beef tea, and his brandy, by hot bottles to his feet, by being washed and by clean linen, you can scarcely believe that he is the same person as he lay with a rapid fluttering pulse, with puffed eyelids, with short breath, cold limbs, and unsteady hands, this morning. Now what is a nurse to do in such a case? Not cry, "Lord bless you, sir, why, you'd have thought he were a dying all night." This may be true, but it, is not the way to impress with the truth a doctor, more capable of forming a judgment from the facts, if he did but know them, than you are. What he wants is not your opinion, however respectfully given, but your facts. In all diseases it is important, but in diseases which do not run a distinct and fixed course, it is not only important, it is essential, that the facts the nurse alone can observe, should be accurately observed and accurately reported to the doctor.

The nurse's attention should be directed to the extreme variation there is not unfrequently in the pulse of such patients during the day. A very common case is this: Between 3 and 4 A.M. the pulse becomes quick, perhaps 130, and so thready it is not like a pulse at all, but like a string vibrating just underneath the skin. After this the patient gets no more sleep. About midday the pulse has come down to 80; and though feeble and compressible, is a very respectable pulse. At night, if the patient has had a day of excitement, it is almost imperceptible. But if the patient has had a good day, it is stronger and steadier and not quicker than at midday. This is a common history of a common pulse; and others, equally varying during the day, might be given. Now, in inflammation, which may almost always be detected by the pulse, in typhoid fever, which is accompanied by the low pulse that nothing will raise, there is no such great variation. And doctors and nurses become accustomed not to look for it. The doctor indeed cannot. But the variation is in itself an important feature.

Cases like the above often "go off rather suddenly," as it is called, from some trifling ailment of a few days, which just makes up the sum of exhaustion necessary to produce death. And everybody cries, Who would have thought it?—except the observing nurse, if there is one, who had always expected the exhaustion to come, from which there would be no rally, because she knew the patient had no capital in strength on which to draw, if he failed for a few days to make his barely daily income in sleep and nutrition.

Really good nurses are often distressed, because they cannot impress the doctor with the real danger of their patient; and quite provoked because the patient "will look," either "so much better," or "so much worse," than he really is "when the doctor is there." The distress is very legitimate, but it generally arises from the nurse not having the power of laying clearly and shortly before the doctor the facts from which she derives her opinion, or from the doctor being hasty and inexperienced, and not capable of eliciting them. A man who really cares for his patients, will soon learn to ask for and appreciate the information of a nurse, who is at once a careful observer and a clear reporter.

In Life Insurance and such like societies, were they instead of having the persons examined by a medical man, to have the houses, conditions, ways of life, of these persons examined, at how much truer results would they arrive! W. Smith appears a fine hale man, but it might be known that the next cholera epidemic he runs a bad chance. Mr. and Mrs. J. are a strong healthy couple, but it might be known that they live in such a house, in such a part of London, so near the river, that they will kill four-fifths of their children; which of the children will be the ones to survive might also be known.

2. Averages again do not lead to minute observation. "Average mortalities" merely tell that so many per cent die in this town, and so many in that, per annum. But whether A. or B. will be among these, the "average rate" of course does not tell. We know, say, that from 22 to 24 per 1,000 will die in London next year. But minute inquiries into conditions enable us to know that in such a district, nay, in such a street—or even on one side of that street, in such a particular house, or even on one floor of that particular house, will be the excess of mortality; that is, the person will die who ought not to have died before old age.

Now, would it not very materially alter the opinion of whoever were endeavouring to form one, if he knew that from that floor of that house of that street the man came? And would you not avoid that floor and that house?

It is well known that the same names may be seen constantly recurring on workhouse books for generations. That is, the persons were born and brought up, and will be born and brought up, generation after generation, in the conditions which make paupers. Death and disease are like the workhouse; they take from the same family, the same house, or, in other words, the same conditions. Why will we not observe what these are, and how to prevent them?

The close observer may safely predict that such a family, whether its members marry or not, will become extinct; that such another will degenerate morally and physically. But who learns the lesson? On the contrary, it may be well known that the children die in such a house at the rate of 8 out of 10; one would think that nothing more need be said; for how could Providence speak more distinctly?—yet nobody listens, the family goes on living there till it dies out, and then some other family takes it. Neither would they listen "if one rose from the dead."

XIV.—CONVALESCENCE.

MANY, indeed most, of the hints given for sickness will not do for convalescence; for instance, the *patient's* fancies about diet are often valuable indications to follow—the *convalescent's* often the reverse.

When convalescence has fairly set in, the patient very often has longings, especially for articles of food, which, if incautiously indulged, may lead to violent reaction, or even to relapse. The medical attendant is, of course, the best judge of the food and regimen required; but during convalescence he is not there day by day, very often not above once or twice a week; and the nurse, at one of the most important periods of her patient's life, is left almost to herself—she has to be doctor and nurse too.

It has happened that a single well-meant but ill-directed indulgence has ended in death.

The nurse has often to deal not only with the patient's appetite, but with the officiousness of his friends. Some unwholesome, perhaps poisonous, delicacy is one of the first offerings generally made by them.

On the other hand, it may be that the main difficulty in the recovery is the patient's *want* of appetite, most likely to occur where he has no change of air. In such cases the nurse must exercise the same care in regard to diet and the times at which it is to be given, as is indicated for sickness at Chap. VI.

There are other indulgences besides those of the stomach which require to be kept under check. Some patients are apt to overexert themselves in various ways, to incur unnecessary exposure and fatigue, perhaps to be followed by sitting in a draught. Friends often carry on long and exhausting conversations, or prolonged readings, at one time, which are followed by a loss of power to the patient, requiring some time for its recovery. Errors in too much or too little clothing have also to be guarded against; but as a rule convalescents require warm clothing.

In all these things, a convalescent is, so to speak, like a child; neither mind nor body has recovered its proper tone, and for a certain time differing in different diseases, the nurse has to guide him by her own experience.

Change, a change of air, is of the very first importance as soon as the disease has "taken a turn." Everybody must have remarked how a person recovering remains sometimes for weeks without making any progress, yet with apparently nothing the matter with him. The change from a ground-floor to an upstairs room will sometimes hasten a patient's recovery. The mere move will give him a fillip. Change is essential. He must go

to another place, or even only to another room. Then he immediately begins to "pick up." This is every-day experience. But,
with the poor, "change of air" is next to impossible. A place
with the most careful nursing and every comfort, *together with
country air*, would save many lives from being spent in the Union
Workhouse, many from requiring poor-law relief at all, many from
giving birth to unhealthy families, and many premature deaths.

There are those to whom this subject appears unimportant;
such people say, when a sick man is convalescing, he is doing
well, and there is an end of it. They never consider that convalescence has its degrees and its course the same as disease.
And you may have a very long convalescence instead of a short
one, or perhaps no convalescence at all, by simply entertaining
the habit of thought that "there is an end of it."

Such people do not see "why convalescents are to be *nursed* at
all." And yet persons who have taken the pains to watch are
perfectly well aware that many cases would be irretrievably lost
but for careful nursing. Some would become permanent invalids;
others burdens to themselves and their friends for the rest of
their days. There may be return to *life*; but return to health
and usefulness depends upon the *after*-nursing in almost all cases.
Careful nursing has done in a few weeks what uncareful medical
observation has declared it impossible to do in less than two years.
Long convalescence ending in relapse or death is by no means
unfrequent among the poor.

Follow these people to their homes, and what do you find?
A straightened household, overtaxed to the utmost by a long
illness of its head or support, receiving back, perhaps from
expected death, its head (not to be a *support* but) to be a further
call upon it for nursing, clothing, and above all for suitable food
and comforts. There can be no doubt that these defective recoveries, gone through in bad air and in the absence of almost
every requisite, eventually go to swell the Death List; nor that
apparently hopeless cases would recover, if sick poor were enabled
by their richer neighbours to have change of air.

XV.—WHAT IS A NURSE?

THE very alphabet of a nurse is to be able to read every change
which comes over a patient's countenance, without causing him
the exertion of saying what he feels. What would many a nurse
do otherwise than she does, if her patient were a valuable piece

of furniture or a sick cow? I do not know. Yet a nurse must be something more than a lift or a broom. A patient is not merely a piece of furniture, to be kept clean and ranged against the wall, and saved from injury or breakage—though to judge from what many a nurse does and does not do you would say he was. But watch a good old-fashioned monthly nurse with the infant; she is firmly convinced, not only that she understands everything it "says," and that no one else can understand it, but also that it understands everything she says, and understands no one else.

Now a nurse *ought* to understand in the same way every change of her patient's face, every change of his attitude, every change of his voice. And she ought to study them till she feels sure that no one else understands them so well. She may make mistakes, but she is *on the way* to being a good nurse. Whereas the nurse who never observes her patient's countenance at all, and never expects to see any variation, any more than if she had the charge of delicate china, is on the way to nothing at all. She never will be a nurse.

"He hates to be watched," is the excuse of every careless nurse. Very true. All sick people and all children "hate to be watched." But find a nurse who really knows and understands her children and her patients, and see whether these are aware that they have been "watched." It is not the staring at a patient which tells the really observant nurse the little things she ought to know.

People often talk of a nurse who has been ten or fifteen years with the sick, as being an "experienced nurse." But it is observation only which makes experience; and a woman who does not observe might be fifty or sixty years with the sick and never be the wiser.

Nay more, experience sometimes tells in the opposite direction. A farmer "who practises the blunders of his predecessors," is often said to be "a practical man;" and she who perpetuates the "blunders of her predecessors" is often called an experienced nurse. The friends of a patient have been known to recommend the lodging in which he fell ill, just for the very reason which made him ill. A nurse has alleged as her reason for doing the things by which her predecessor ruined her own and her patient's health, that her predecessor "had always done them." People have taken a house because it had been emptied by death of all its occupants. These are they whom *no* experience will teach—viz., those who cannot see or understand the practical results of what they and others do. Now it is *no* reason that A did it for B to do it. It would be a reason if the results of A's doing it had been proved to be good.

What strikes one most with many women, who call themselves nurses, is that they have not learnt this A B C of a nurse's education. The A of a nurse ought to be to know what a sick human being is. The B to know how to behave to a sick human being. The C to know that her patient is a sick human being and not an animal.

What is it to feel a *calling* for any thing? Is it not to do your work in it to satisfy your own high idea of what is the *right*, the *best*, and not because you will be "found out" if you don't do it? This is the "enthusiasm" which every one, from a shoemaker to a sculptor, must have, in order to follow his "calling" properly. Now the nurse has to do, not with shoes, or with chisel and marble, but with human beings; and if she, for her own satisfaction, does not look after her patients, no *telling* will make her capable of doing so.

A nurse who has such a "calling" will, for her own satisfaction and interest in her patient, inform herself as to the state of his pulse, which can be quite well done without disturbing him. She will have observed the state of the secretions, whether told to do so or not. Nay, the very appearance of them, a slight difference in colour, will betray to her observing eye that the utensil has not been emptied after each motion.

She will, in like manner, have observed the state of the skin, whether there is dryness or perspiration—the effect of the diet, of the medicines, the stimulants. And it is remarkable how often the doctor is deceived in private practice by not being told that the patient has just had his meal or his brandy. She will most carefully have watched any redness or soreness of the skin, always on her guard against bed-sores. Any loss of flesh will never take place unknown to her. Nor will she ever mistake puffing or swelling for gaining in flesh. She will be well acquainted with the different eruptions of fevers, measles, &c., and premonitory symptoms. She will know the shiver which betrays that matter is forming—that which shows the unconscious patient's desire to pass water—that which precedes fever. She will observe the changes of animal heat in her patient, and whether periodical, and not consider him as a piece of wood or stone, in keeping him warm or cool.

A nurse who has such a "calling" will look at all the medicine bottles delivered to her for her patients, smell each of them, and, if not satisfied, taste each. Nine hundred and ninety-nine times there will be no mistake, but the thousandth time there may be a serious mistake detected by her means. But if she does not do this for her own satisfaction, it is no use telling her, because you may be sure that she will use neither smell nor taste to any purpose.

A nurse who has *not* such a "calling," will never be able to learn the sound of her patient's bell from that of others.

She will, when called to for hot brandy-and-water for her fainting patient, offer the weekly "Punch" (fact). Or she will wait to bring the cordial till she brings his tea (fact).

Under such a nurse, the patient never gets a hot drink. She pours out his tea, then she makes a journey to the larder for the butter, then she remembers that she has forgotten the toast, and has another journey to the kitchen fire to make the toast, then she fills a hot water bottle, and last of all she takes him his tea.

Such a nurse will never know whether her patient is awake or asleep. She will rouse him up to ask him "if he wants anything," and leave him uncared for when he *is* up.

She will make the room like an oven when he is feverish at night, and let out the fire when he is cold in the morning.

Such a nurse seems to have neither eyes, nor ears, nor hands.

She never touches anything without a crash or an upset.

She does not shut the door, but pulls it after her, so that it always bursts open again.

She cannot rub in an embrocation without making a sore, which, in too many cases, never heals during the patient's life.

She catches up a cup and saucer in one hand, and pokes the fire with the other. Both of course come to "grief." Or she carries in a tray in one hand, and a coal scuttle in the other. Both of course tip out their contents. And she, in stooping to pick them up, knocks over the bedside table upon the patient with her head (fact).

Tables are made for things to stand upon—beds for patients to lie in.

But such a nurse puts down a heavy flower-pot upon the bed, or a large book or bolster which has rolled upon the floor.

Yet these things are not done by drinking old females, but by respectable women.

Yet we are often told that a nurse needs only to be "devoted and obedient."

This definition would do just as well for a porter. It might even do for a horse. It would not do for a policeman. Consider how many women there are who have nothing to devote—neither intelligence, nor eyes, nor ears, nor hands. They will sit up all night by the patient, it is true; but their attendance is worth nothing to him, nor their observations to the doctor.

Cases have been known where the patient was cold before the nurse had observed he was dead—and yet she was not asleep—many cases where she supposed him comfortably sleeping, and he was insensible—very many where she never knew he was dying, unless he told her so himself.

But let no woman suppose that obedience to the doctor is not absolutely necessary. Only, neither doctor nor nurse lay suffi- cient stress upon *intelligent* obedience, upon the fact that obedience alone is a very poor thing.

I have known an obedient nurse, told not to disturb a very sick patient as usual at ten o'clock with some customary service which she used to perform for him then, actually leave him in the dark all night, alleging this order as her reason for not carrying in his night-light as usual.

Everybody has known the window left open in heavy fog or rain, or shut when the patient was fainting, by such obedient nurses.

There seems to be no medium for them between a furnace of a fire and no fire at all; and one is actually obliged in this variable climate to divide the year into two parts, and tell them—"Now no fire," "Now fire;" as if they were volunteer riflemen. You cannot trust them to make a *small* fire, although in England it is a question whether, except when the air without is hotter than the air within, patients are not always the better of some fire, if only to promote ventilation. But no; such nurses make it impossible.

The elements of a nurse's duty are to observe the state of the pulse; the effect of the diet,—of sleep, whether it has been dis- turbed; whether there have been startings up in bed—a common mark of fatal disease; whether it has been a heavy, dull sleep, with stertorous breathing; whether there has been twitching of the bed-clothes,—to observe the state of the expectoration, the rusty expectoration of pneumonia, the frothy expectoration of pleurisy, the viscid mucous expectoration of bronchitis, the blood-streaked, dense, heavy expectoration which often occurs in consumption,—the nature of the cough itself by which the expectoration is expelled,—to observe the state of the secretions (yet nine-tenths of all nurses know nothing about these), whether the motions are costive or relaxed, and what is their colour, or whether there are alternations every few days of diarrhoea, and of no action of the bowels at all; whether the urine is high-coloured or pale, excessive or scanty, muddy or clear, or whether it is high-coloured when the bowels do not act, and pale when there is diarrhoea; whether there is ever blood in the motions, — in children, whether there are worms. All these things most nurses do not appear to consider it their business to observe.

The condition of the breathing and the position in which the patient breathes most easily, is another thing essential for the nurse to observe. In heart complaints life is often extinguished by the patient "accidentally" falling into a position in which he cannot breathe—and life is preserved by an "accidental" change of position. Now, what a thing it is to have to say of a nurse that it was not through her means, but through an "accident" that her patient was able to breathe.

Another essential duty of the nurse is, to observe the action of medicine; as, for instance, that of quinine. The sore throat, the deafness, the tight feeling in the head, are well known effects of quinine. But the loss of memory it often occasions, is seldom known except to a very observant nurse. Indeed, she has often not memory enough herself to remember that the patient has forgotten.

A good nurse scarcely ever asks a patient a question—neither as to what he feels nor as to what he wants. But she does not take for granted, either to herself or to others, that she knows what he feels and wants, without the most careful observation and testing of her own observations.

But why, for instance, should a nurse ask a patient every day, "Shall I bring your coffee?" or "your broth?" or whatever it is—when she has every day brought it to him at that hour. One would think she did it for the sake of making the patient speak. Now, what the patient most wants is, never to be called upon to speak about such things.

Remember, every nurse should be one who is to be depended upon; in other words, capable of being a "confidential" nurse. She does not know how soon she may find herself placed in such a situation; she must be no gossip, no vain talker; she should never answer questions about her sick except to those who have a right to ask them; she must, I need not say, be strictly sober and honest; but more than this, she must be a religious and devoted woman; she must have a respect for her own calling, because God's precious gift of life is often literally placed in her hands; she must be a sound, and close, and quick observer; and she must be a woman of delicate and decent feeling.

XVI.—"MINDING BABY."

AND now, girls, I have a word for you. You and I have all had a great deal to do with "minding baby," though "baby" was not our own baby. And we would all of us do a great deal for baby, which we would not do for ourselves.

Now, all that I have said about nursing grown-up people applies a great deal more to nursing baby. For instance, baby will suffer from a close room when you don't feel that it is close. If baby sleeps even for a few hours, much more if it is for nights and nights—in foul air, baby will, without any doubt whatever, be puny and sickly, and most likely have measles or scarlatina, and not get through it well.

Baby will feel want of fresh air more than you. Baby will feel cold much sooner than you. Above all, baby will suffer more from not being kept clean (only see how it enjoys being washed in nice luke-warm water). Baby will want its clothes and its bed clothes changed oftener than you. Baby will suffer more from a dirty house than you. Baby *must* have a cot to itself; else it runs the risk of being over-laid or suffocated. Baby must not be covered up too much in bed, nor too little. The same when it is up. And you must look after these things. Mother is perhaps too busy to see whether baby is too much muffled up or too little.

You must take care that baby is not startled by loud sudden noises; all the more you must not wake it in this way out of its sleep. Noises which would not frighten you, frighten baby.

And many a sick baby has been killed in this way.

You must be very careful about its food; about being strict to the minute for feeding it; not giving it too much at a time (if baby is sick after its food, you *have* given it too much). Neither must it be under fed. Above all, never give it any unwholesome food, nor anything at all to make it sleep, unless the doctor orders it.

If you knew how many, even well-to-do, babies I have known who have died from having had something given to make them sleep, and "keep them quiet,"—not the first time, nor the second, nor the tenth time perhaps,—but at last.

I could tell you many true stories, which have all happened within my own knowledge, of mischief to babies from their nurses neglecting these things.

Here are a few.

1. Baby, who is weaned, requires to be fed often, regularly, and not too much at a time.

I knew a mother whose baby was in great danger one day from convulsions. It was about a year old. She said she had wished to go to church; and so, before going, had given it its three meals in one. Was it any wonder that the poor little thing had convulsions?

I have known (in Scotland) a little girl, not more than five years old, whose mother had to go great distances every day, and who was trusted to feed and take care of her little brother, under a year old. And she always did it right. She always did what mother told her. A stranger, coming into the hut one day (it was no better than a hut), said "You will burn baby's mouth." "Oh no," she said, "I always burn my own mouth first."

2. When I say, be careful of baby, I don't mean have it always in your arms. If the baby is old enough, and the weather warm enough for it to have some heat in itself, it is much better for a child to be crawling about than to be always in its little nurse's arms. And it is much better for it to amuse itself than to have her always making noises to it.

The healthiest, happiest, liveliest, most beautiful baby I ever saw was the only child of a busy laundress. She washed all day in a room with the door open upon a larger room, where she put the child. It sat or crawled upon the floor all day with no other play-fellow than a kitten, which it used to hug. Its mother kept it beautifully clean, and fed it with perfect regularity. The child was never frightened at anything. The room where it sat was the house-place; and it always gave notice to its mother when any body came in, not by a cry, but by a crow. I lived for many months within hearing of that child, and never heard it cry day or night.

I think there is a great deal too much of amusing children now; and not enough of letting them amuse themselves.

Never distract a child's attention. If it is looking at one thing, don't show it another; and so on.

3. At the same time, dulness and especially want of light, is worse for children than it is for you.

A child was once brought up quite alone in a dark room, by persons who wished to conceal its being alive. It never saw any one, except when it was fed; and though it was treated perfectly kindly, it grew up an idiot. This you will easily guess.

Plenty of light, and sun-light particularly, is necessary to make a child active, and merry, and clever. But, of all things, don't burn baby's brains out by letting the sun bake its head when out, especially in its little cart, on a hot summer's day.

Never leave a child in the dark; and let the room it lives in be *always* as light as possible, and as sunny. Except, of course, when the doctor tells you to darken the room, which he will do in some children's illnesses.

4. Do you know that one-half of all the nurses in service are girls of from five to twenty years old? You see you are very important little people. Then there are all the girls who are nursing mother's baby at home; and, in all these cases, it seems pretty nearly to come to this, that baby's health for its whole life depends upon you, girls, more than upon anything else.

I need hardly say to you, What a charge! For I believe that you, all of you, or nearly all, care about baby too much not to feel this nearly as much as I do. You, all of you, want to make baby grow up well and happy, if you knew how.

So I say again, —

5. The main want of baby is always to have fresh air.

You can make baby ill by keeping the room where it sleeps tight shut up, even for a few hours.

You can kill baby when it *is* ill by keeping it in a hot room, with several people in it, and all the doors and windows shut.

The doctor who looks after the Queen's children says so.

This is the case most particularly when the child has something the matter with its lungs and its breathing.

I found a poor child dying in a small room, tight shut up, with a large fire, and four or five people round it to see it die. Its breathing was short and hurried; and it could not cough up what was choking its lungs and throat—*mucus* it is called. The doctor, who was a very clever man, came in, set open door and window, turned everybody out but one, and stayed two hours to keep the room clear and fresh. He gave the child no medicine; and it was cured simply by his fresh air.

A few hours will do for baby, both in killing and curing it, what days will not do for a grown-up person.

Another doctor found a child (it was a rich one) dying in a splendid close room, nearly breathless from throat-complaint. He walked straight to the window and pulled it open; "for," he said, "when people can breathe very little air, they want that little good." The mother said he would kill the child. But, on the contrary, the child recovered.

But, —

6. Take you care not to let a draught blow upon a child, especially a sick child.

Perhaps you will say to me, "I don't know what you would have me do. You puzzle me so. You tell me, don't feed the child too much, and don't feed it too little; don't keep the room shut up, and don't let there be a draught; don't let the child be dull, and don't amuse it too much." Dear little nurse, you must learn to *manage*. Some people never do learn management. I have felt all these difficulties myself; and I can tell you that it is not from reading my book that you will learn to mind baby well, but from practising yourself how best to manage to do what other good nurses (and my book, if you like it,) tell you.

But about the draughts.

It is all nonsense what some old nurses say, that you can't give baby fresh air without giving it a chill; and, on the other hand, you may give baby a chill which will kill it (by letting a draught blow upon it when it is being washed, for instance, and chilling its whole body, though only for a moment), without giving it fresh air at all; and depend upon this, the less fresh air you give to its lungs, and the less water you give to its skin, the more liable it will be to colds and chills.

If you can keep baby's air always fresh in doors and out of doors, and never chill baby, you are a good nurse.

A sick baby's skin is often cold, even when the room is quite close. Then you must air the room, and put hot flannels or hot bottles (not too hot) next baby's body, and give it its warm food.

But I have often seen nurse doing just the contrary; namely, shutting up every chink and throwing a great weight of bed-clothes over the child, which makes it colder, as it has no heat in itself.

You would just kill a feverish child by doing this.

A children's doctor, very famous in London, says that when a sick child dies, it is just as often an *accident* as not; that is, people kill it by some foolish act of this kind, just as much as if they threw it out of window. And he says, too, that when a sick child dies suddenly, it is almost always an accident. It might have been prevented. It was *not* that the child was ill, and so its death could not be helped, as people say.

He tells us what brings on these sudden deaths in sick children:—Startling noises; chilling the child's body; wakening it suddenly; feeding it too much or too quickly; altering its posture suddenly, or shaking it roughly; frightening it. And to this you may add (more than anything else, too), *keeping it in foul air, especially when asleep, especially at night*, even for a few hours, and even when you don't feel it yourself. This is, most of all, what kills babies.

Baby's breathing is so tender, so easily put out of order. Sometimes you see a sick baby who seems to be obliged to attend to every breath it draws, and to "breathe carefully," in order to breathe at all; and if you disturb it rudely, it is all over with baby. Anything which calls upon it for breath may stop it alto-gether.

7. *Remember to keep baby clean.* I can remember when mothers boasted that *their* "children's feet had never been touched by water; no, nor any part of them but faces and hands;" that somebody's "child had had its feet washed, and it never lived to grow up, &c."

But we know better now. And I dare say you know that to keep every spot of baby's body always clean, and never to let any pore of its tender skin be stopped up by dirt or unwashed per-spiration is the only way to keep baby happy and well.

It is a great deal of trouble; but it is a great deal more trouble to have baby sick.

The safest thing is to wash baby all over once or twice a day;

and to wash it besides whenever it has had an accidental wetting. You know how easily its tender skin gets chafed.

There may be danger in washing a child's feet and legs only. There never can be in washing it all over. Its clothes should be changed oftener than yours, because of the greater quantity baby perspires. If you clothe baby in filth, what can you expect but that it will be ill? Its clothes must never be tight, but light and warm. Baby, if not properly clothed, feels sudden changes in the weather much more than you do. Baby's bed-clothes must be clean oftener than yours.

Now, can you remember the things you have to mind for baby? There is—

1. Fresh air.

2. Proper warmth.

3. Cleanliness for its little body, its clothes, its bed, its room, and house.

4. Feeding it with proper food, at regular times.

5. Not startling it or shaking either its little body or its little nerves.

6. Light and cheerfulness.

7. Proper clothes in bed and up.

And management in *all* these things.

I would add one thing. It is as easy to put out a sick baby's life as it is to put out the flame of a candle. Ten minutes' delay in giving it food may make the difference.

CONCLUSION.

THE whole of the preceding remarks apply even more to children and to women in childbed, than to patients in general. They also apply to the nursing of surgical, quite as much as to that of medical cases. Indeed, if it be possible, accidents require such care even more than sick. The nurse must be ever on the watch, ever on her guard, against want of cleanliness, foul air, want of light, and of warmth.

During recovery from an accident the patient may be, and ought to be, in perfect health. And it is often the fault of the nurse if he is not. Let no one think that because *sanitary* nursing is the subject of these notes, therefore what may be called the handicraft of nursing is to be undervalued. A patient may be left to bleed to death in a sanitary palace. Another, who cannot move himself, may die of bed-sores, because the nurse does not know how to change and clean him, while he has every requisite of air, light, and quiet. But nursing, as a handicraft, has not been treated of here for three reasons: 1. that these notes do not pretend to be a manual for nursing, any more than for cooking for the sick; 2. that the writer, who has herself seen more of what may be called surgical nursing, *i.e.*, practical manual nursing, than perhaps any one in Europe, honestly believes that it is impossible to learn it from any book, and that it can only be thoroughly learnt in the wards of a hospital; 3. while thousands die of foul air, &c., who have this surgical nursing to perfection, the converse is comparatively rare.

To sum up:—the answer to two of the commonest objections urged against the desirableness of sanitary knowledge for women, with a caution, comprises the whole argument for the art of nursing.

(1.) It is often said that it is unwise to teach women anything about these laws of health, because they will take to physicking, — that there is a great deal too much of amateur physicking as it is, which is indeed true. One eminent physician told me that he had known more calomel given, both at a pinch and for a continuance, by mothers, governesses, and nurses, to children than he had ever heard of a physician prescribing in all his experience. Another says, that women's only idea in medicine is calomel and aperients. This is undeniably too often the case. There is nothing ever seen in any professional practice like the reckless physicking by amateur females. Many women, having once obtained a "bottle" from a druggist, or a pill from a quack, will give and take it for anything and everything—with what effect may be supposed. The doctor, being informed of it, substitutes for it some proper medicine. The woman complains that it "does not suit her half so well."

If women will take or give physic, by far the safest plan is to send for "the doctor" every time. There are those who both give and take physic, who will not take pains to learn the names of the commonest medicines, and confound, *e.g.*, colocynth with colchicum. This *is* playing with sharp-edged tools "with a vengeance."

There are also excellent women who will write to London to their physician that there is much sickness in their neighbourhood in the country, and ask for some prescription from him, which they "used to like" themselves, and then give it to all their friends and to all their poorer neighbours who will take it. Now, instead of giving medicine, of which you cannot possibly know the exact and proper application, nor all its consequences, would it not be better if you were to persuade and help your poorer neighbours to remove the dunghill from before the door, to put in a window which opens, or an Arnott's ventilator, or to drain, cleanse, and lime-wash their cottages? Of these things the benefits are sure. The benefits of the inexperienced administration of medicines are by no means so sure.

An almost universal error amongst women is the supposition that everybody *must* have the bowels opened once in every twenty-four hours, or must fly immediately to aperients. The reverse is the conclusion of experience.

This is a doctor's subject, and I will not enter more into it; but will simply repeat, do not go on taking or giving to your children your abominable "courses of aperients," without calling in the doctor.

It is very seldom indeed, that by choosing your diet, you cannot regulate your own bowels; and every woman may watch herself to know what kind of diet will do this; deficiency of meat produces constipation, quite as often as deficiency of vegetables; baker's bread much oftener than either. Home-made brown bread will oftener cure it than anything else.

A really experienced and observing nurse neither physics herself nor others. And to cultivate in things pertaining to health observation and experience in women who are mothers, governesses, or nurses, is just the way to do away with amateur physicking, and, if the doctors did but know it, to make the nurses obedient to them,—helps to them instead of hindrances. Such education in women would indeed diminish the doctor's work — but no one really believes that doctors wish that there should be more illness, in order to have more work.

(2.) Nothing but observation and experience will teach us the ways to maintain or to bring back the state of health. It is often thought that medicine is the curative process. It is no such thing; medicine is the surgery of functions, as surgery proper is that of limbs and organs. Neither can do anything but remove obstructions; neither can cure; nature alone cures. Surgery removes the bullet out of the limb, which is an obstruction to cure, but nature heals the wound. So it is with medicine; the function of an organ becomes obstructed; medicine, so far as we know, assists nature to remove the obstruction, but does nothing more. And what nursing has to do in either case, is to put the patient in the best condition for nature to act upon him. Generally, just the contrary is done. You think fresh air, and quiet and cleanliness extravagant, perhaps dangerous, luxuries, which should be given to the patient only when quite convenient, and medicine the panacea. If I have succeeded in any measure in dispelling this illusion, and in showing what true nursing is, and what it is not, my object will have been answered.

Now for the caution:

(3.) It seems a commonly received idea among men, and even among women themselves, that it requires nothing but a loving heart, the want of an object, a general disgust or incapacity for other things, to turn a woman into a good nurse.

This reminds one of the parish where a stupid old man was set to be schoolmaster, because he was "past keeping the pigs."

Apply the above receipt for making a good nurse to making a good servant. And the receipt will be found to fail.

What cruel mistakes are sometimes made by benevolent men and women in matters of business about which they can know nothing, and think they know a great deal.

The everyday management of a sick room, let alone of a house —the knowing what are the laws of life and death for men, and what the laws of health for houses—(and houses are healthy or unhealthy, mainly according to the knowledge or ignorance of the woman)—are not these matters of sufficient importance and difficulty to require learning by experience and careful inquiry, just as much as any other art? They do not come by inspiration to the loving heart, nor to the poor drudge hard-up for a livelihood.

And terrible is the injury which has followed to the sick from such wild notions.

APPENDIX ON METHOD OF TRAINING NURSES UNDER THE NIGHTINGALE FUND AT SAINT THOMAS'S HOSPITAL, LONDON.[9]

To women desirous of devoting themselves to nursing, the following information regarding the training of nurses in this Hospital, where a school was established in 1860, under the auspices of the Committee of the Nightingale Fund, may be of service.

We require that a woman be sober, honest, truthful, without which there is no foundation on which to build.

We train then in habits of punctuality, quietness, trustworthiness, personal neatness. We teach her how to manage the concerns of a large ward or establishment.

We train her in dressing wounds and other injuries, and in performing all those minor operations which nurses are called upon day and night to undertake.

We teach her how to manage helpless patients in regard to moving, changing, feeding, temperature, and the prevention of bed-sores.

She has to make and apply bandages, line splints for fractures, and the like. She must know how to make beds with as little disturbance as possible to their inmates. She is instructed how to wait at operations, and as to the kind of aid the surgeon requires at her hands. She is taught cooking for sick; the principles on which sick wards ought to be cleansed, aired, and warmed; the management of convalescents; and how to observe sick and maimed patients, so as to give an intelligent and truthful account to the physician or surgeon in regard to the progress of cases in the intervals between visits—a much more difficult thing than is generally supposed.[10]

We do not seek to make "medical women," but simply nurses acquainted with the *principles* which they are required constantly to apply at the bed-side.

For the future superintendent is added instruction in the administration of a hospital, including, of course, the linen arrangements, and what else is necessary for a matron to be conversant with.

In the process of training the following are the steps:

Every candidate applying for admission is required to fill up a Form of Application, which will be supplied to her by the matron of St. Thomas's Hospital, London, S.E.

The age considered desirable for candidates is from 25 to 35. The period of training is a complete year. Board, lodging, and washing, and a certain quantity of outer clothing, are provided free, besides a salary of £10 for the year.

After being received on a month's trial and trained for a month, if the probationer shows sufficient aptitude and character, and is herself desirous to complete her training, she is required to come under an obligation binding her to take service as a nurse for the sick poor,* for at least four years. This is the only recompense the Committee exact for the costs and advantages of training.

A list of "Duties" is put into the hands of every probationer on entering the service, as a general instruction for her guidance.

Once admitted to St. Thomas's Hospital, the probationer is placed under a head nurse (ward "sister") having charge of a ward, and performs the duties of an assistant nurse.

The ward training of the probationers is thus carried out under the ward "sisters" and matron. [The probationers are, whether on or off duty, entirely under the moral control of the matron.][11]

Instruction is also given by the Resident Medical Officer on duties of a medical and surgical character.

A record is kept of the conduct and qualifications of each probationer; and the character the nurse receives at the end of the year is made to correspond as nearly as may be with the results of the training.

The regulations and previous information required may be obtained by writing to the Secretary of the Nightingale Fund, H. Bonham-Carter, Esq., 91, Gloucester Terrace, Hyde Park, London, W.

Before admission, personal application should be made to Mrs. Wardroper, St. Thomas's Hospital, London, S.E.

It has occurred to me to suggest whether, among the large Union Schools, a number of girls might not be found willing and suitable to be trained as nurses.

These girls are usually put out to service between the ages of 14 and 16.

This is quite too young to put them at once into any kind of infirmary or hospital to take their chance altogether with the other probationers, especially in the men's wards.

But it is not at all too young, where arrangements and provision can be made under a proper female head, for them to learn sick cookery, cleaning, needlework, orderly habits, all that is learnt in a servants' training school, and to take their turn in doing what they can be taught to do in children's sick wards, and

*The obligation is at present limited to service in Hospitals or Infirmaries.

in female sick wards, till the full-blown hospital nurse is developed out of them.

Girls of from 14 to 16 years of age are not at all too young to choose between domestic service or hospital nursing, under the restrictions mentioned above.

These girls, if trained into good hospital nurses, would earn higher wages than girls who enter domestic service at 14 or 15 years of age ever would do.

The position as well as the wages of nurses in many hospitals and workhouse infirmaries, and also in civil life, has been very much improved of late years. Women of the age of 25 and upwards, sometimes younger, may, if duly qualified, readily obtain from £20 to £30 a-year, with everything "found;" hospital, *i.e.*, ward "sisters," in some London hospitals £50, with like advantages; and matrons or superintendents in provincial hospitals from £60 to £100, with board and lodging; in some London Hospitals, more.

The salaries given to a nursing staff, which we have sent to Sydney, New South Wales, were on a more liberal scale.

Editor's Notes

1. In her "Answers to Written Questions ... Affecting the Sanitary Condition of the Army," in *Notes on Hospitals* (1859), p. 64, Nightingale comments,

   > Our grandfathers' lofty fire-places are the greatest loss in modern house architecture. The little low fire-places of this date bring the best current of air below the stratum in which we are breathing. With our system, to breathe the best air, we must not be more than six years old, or we must lie down.

2. This reference to the reformer Edwin Chadwick is F.N.'s acknowledgement of his specialist contribution to the 1861 edition. See the Introduction.
3. New material to be added here in a proposed 1875 edition is in Part Four.
4. In 1861 this last sentence reads, "to all evening conversations."
5. New material to be added here in a proposed 1875 edition is in Part Four.
6. Nightingale comments on beds under the heading of "Defective Ward Furniture" in *Notes on Hospitals* (1859), p. 16:

   > Hospital bedsteads should always be of iron, the rest of the furniture of oak. Hair is the only material yet discovered fit for hospital mattresses. It is not hard nor cold. It is easily washed. It does not retain miasma. Straw has the advantage of being easily renewed, but it is not desirable. It is too hard and too cold not to render necessary the use of a blanket *under* the patient, which use is likely to encourage bed-sores. I speak from actual experience of the fatal effect of using the paillasse with patients much reduced. It may lower their vital energy beyond repair.

7. This usage of "wishing" is explained in Mrs. Elizabeth Gaskell's novel *Mary Barton: A Tale of Manchester Life* (1848), ch. vii:

   > 'donno' ye know what "wishing" means? There's none can die in the arms of those who are wishing them sore to stay on earth. The soul o' them as holds them won't let the dying soul go free; so it has a hard struggle for the quiet of death. We mun get him away fra' his mother, or he'll have a hard death.

8. The rationale for this revision is explained above, in the Introduction to *Notes on Nursing for the Labouring Classes.*
9. This is discussed in the Introduction, above, p. 31.
10. This problem is treated in "Observation of the Sick." In the Library Standard Edition, this falls under the heading "Want of truth the result of want of observation."
11. This sentence is placed in square brackets in the original.

Part
Four

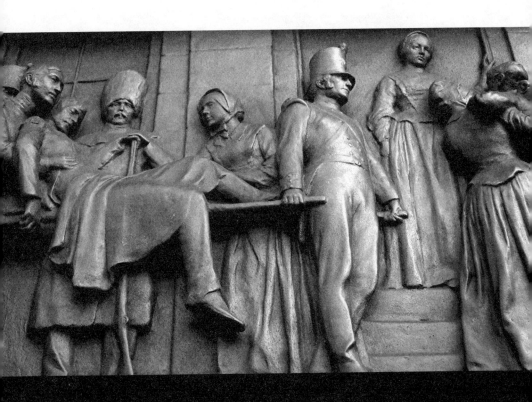

1875 Additions

1875: THIS MANUSCRIPT ADDITION IS HEADED 'BABY'S FOOD'.[1]

AMONG the causes of Baby Deaths, has any body ever thought that bad, weak, watered milk may be one? —that poor baby may have been starved & defrauded out of the very life's food by the rascal milk seller?

In 'minding baby', take good heed of the dairyman, — & 'mind' *him* too.

Under the new 'Adulteration Laws' poor Baby will have a better chance of getting beyond babyhood than now, we hope.[2]

In India, two dear little children I knew were made ill by the milk of a creature fed on dung: milk bad as it was, made worse by being watered by the seller so as to be of hardly any use as milk. One of the two little children died: &, what is yet sadder, this brought about that the mother & infant she was nursing died too: one poor motherless child only was left.

The number of cases of this kind in India are Legion. It is one cause of the enormous Death-rate among children in India.

But we need not go so far as India: We need go no farther than Lancashire: nor the present moment (1875): when it is to be feared things are rather worse than better. What else do you think can be said of this?

A Lancashire factory child between 13 & 15 years of age who had milk, real milk, night & morning, grew 15 lbs a year. One in exactly the same circumstances who had tea or coffee instead of milk grew 4 lbs a year.

Perhaps you will say this was only in one instance[.] No such thing.

During 14 years' experience in a large factory town of factory children between 13 & 15 years of age it was found that those who had milk twice a day grew on an average nearly 4 times as fast as those who had tea or coffee. And now a days people in some towns rear (or do not rear) their children, as soon as they are weaned, on tea or coffee. In fact many children are fed on tea three times a day.

There are other weak bad things, besides weak bad milk, of which Baby may die. There are all sorts of 'prepared' flour & foods sold in packets for Baby—& also for sick people—in which the 'preparing' has been nothing more nor less than washing out nearly all the nourishment, & selling the remaining starch at a high price. A good Mother or Nurse will have nothing to do with such things: And Government ought to make a law that the composition of all these pretended foods be printed on each packet: if indeed they ought to be sold at all.

We are by degrees getting to know about the causes of high baby death-rates. The wonder is that poor Baby escapes at all out of the hands of Soothing Syrups: & then bad milk: —& starch instead of nourishing food.

How few do escape might be shown by some figures: in Glasgow & other large towns.

But enough of this has been said in the Preface.[3]

Editor's Notes

1. This is discussed in the Introduction, p. 33 onwards.
2. The New Sale of Food and Drugs Act of 1875 replaced and strengthened the Adulteration of Food Act (1872), but it was weakened by Disraeli's insistence on permissive legislation, and "did not render it compulsory on local authorities to appoint the analysts who alone could make the measure effective" (P. Smith, *Disraelian Conservatism and Social Reform* [London, 1967], pp. 223–224, and note 3, "Not until 1879 was the appointment of analysts made compulsory.")
3. The "Preface" seems not to have survived.

1875: IN THIS MANUSCRIPT ADDITION NIGHTINGALE DESCRIBES THE RELATIONSHIP BETWEEN AIR FROM SEWERS AND DISEASE, AND SUGGESTS THE REMEDY.[1]

TYPHOID fever is more especially bound up with filth[.]

In camps, when there is Filth outside, such as horse dung: & when this is added to overcrowding: then, Typhoid Fever is known to grow out of simple Fever.

In Schools, what are called "unaccountable" out-breaks of Typhoid Fever are often to be traced from Sewer Air: aye, and in grand houses too. And we know that the Prince of Wales was at death's door from this cause: & he was rescued by good Nursing. We all remember the Thanksgiving at St. Paul's for his recovery. But to the Schools first:

I could tell you many facts: I will tell you one about what happened at one great School I knew: to find out how the Air from certain Sewers came in, a handkerchief was held: & was instantly blown up out of the drain by a blast of Sewer Air. The necessary works were done: & the Fever immediately ceased. But till the present hour the "Sanitary authority" has never been known to think or say: "We neglected our sewers, fever came: our neglects were repaired, fever went away[".]

Now for the great houses: people who live in grand houses do not like to think that there has been foulness under all the grandeur: tho, in many large houses, the water-closet pipes run down behind the fine drawing room paper:

And they prefer to trace their Typhoid Fever to some distant country farm-yard instead of to the cess-pits under their own house & to bad drainage[.]

But we must not suppose that the farm-yard is always healthy, altho' foolish people sometimes take sick children to it for benefit. The filth & foul drainage get into the air & water: & then we have Typhoid in a fine open country: And the first thing the foolish do is:—not to cleanse the place & purify the well but—to examine where in the world the Fever could have been 'brought from', for, say they: "it is impossible to suppose it has sprung up in so healthy a country".

But Typhoid Fever may become as much a home-made Article on a filthy farm as cheese.

If one hears of a "fatal outbreak" of Scarlet Fever, does one not always hear of "remedies adopted" to "prevent the disease from spreading"—these "remedies" always being: *not* removing the causes but—shutting up the well children & not allowing them to play with other children, or to go to School?

But an energetic Registrar says, speaking of an "outbreak" of "Scarlatina"—"the Patients actually dying as it were from an overdose of the poison": —"To a number of houses where the disease occurred I noticed bad privies discharging into open pits in the yards to the rear".

421

Would we know about Sewer Air coming into our own dwellings—how it comes—as exemplified too often, alas! —or—in Colleges at our splendid Universities or—in large public Schools—or in any of the numberless instances of Typhoid and Typhus, and Scarlet Fever among children— the best tests of Sanitary condition—even among noble-men's children, —we must seek the cause in bad sewers and drains.

Would we know—not only how Sewer Air comes in but— how it is to be prevented, we must find out what a great work has to be done by individual householders, by School Masters, by employers, even before the Law can be usefully appealed to—but also what we should attempt to introduce as Legislation: for there are accumulations of filth against which any single householder is helpless.

We cannot get any reply that will cover all our cases, just as we could not get a Medical opinion or treatment that would cover every case of illness. That would be quackery.

Sewer air comes from sewers. And if Sewers are made so that it can get into our houses it will do mischief—And it can be kept out by certain engineering details.

I know a house in what is called the healthiest suburb in London where Invalids are always ordered for health[.] Which is literally a trap for Sewer Air. This has saturated the whole house, between floor & ceiling, & in every part: so that not only the sewerage & drainage but the house itself must be taken up, & pulled down, & rebuilt, & relaid, if any good is to be done.

It may happen that the sewerage & drainage of districts may have to be relaid.

The whole question of the best arrangement of drainage for a large city is one which depends on the perfect execution of an enormous number of details[.]

Sewer air come essentially from *bad* sewers: The "cases" of bad sewers would fill volumes. In my own street one of the main causes is half a mile away. In other words, the cause of the Sewer air must be sought in the bad construction of sewers & drains:

The rules "as under" are embodies in "suggestions" published by the Local Government Board, which it is evident local authorizes do not sufficiently attend to: —

"Main sewers are underground conduits for sewage to flow down, and if they are not fully ventilated at regular intervals along the crown by fixed openings communicating with the external air, they become flues up which sewage gases will rise and pass through the drains to the connected houses.

"Ordinary main sewer ventilation should be provided for on all sewers at intervals not greater than one hundred yards apart.

"The upper or dead ends of all sewers and drains should have means provided for dull ventilation continues beyond the drain junction of the last house.

"House drains should not pass direct from sewers to the inside of houses, but all drains should end at an outside wall. House drains, sink pipes, and soil popes should have amole means of external ventilation.

"Where drains must traverse a basement they should be bedded and covered in concrete, and have external ventilation back and front.["]

Openings from the drains within the basement should not be allowed, as no form of trap will be safe.

These rules have been in print some years and have been acted upon in many places; but they have been neglected in many places, and that neglect may continue.[2]

The day *may* come when people will have *time* to attend to the facts, & will become aware that other people will pay them a sum large enough to cover all their rates & taxes for the refuse of their houses which they are now very heavily taxed to throw into the river with most direful effects.

So far as concerns out house itself: all house drain-pipes should be cut off from the street sewer by efficient trapping: & all house drain-pipes should be ventilated by pipes carried about the roof, & all cistern overflow pipes cut off from the water-closet pipes.

The cause of the Prince of Wales' attack was sewer air: but how it got there no one seems to know to this day. The case of a famous College is a muddle of the same kind, & for the same reason.

At this very moment, September 1875, the great War Office of this great country is in a state which puts the perils of "the Office" in sickness & death almost on a par with the perils of war. This is owing to the basement of an overcrowded building, supplying Sewer Air & gas, "reinforced on each floor by the exhalations from the closets," for the breathing of every man in the place, from the Comander-in-Chief downwards, so that it may be said that from the highest to the lowest 'Men share the perils of War' Offices.

Yet nothing has been done.

In a large public School, gastric fever had existed for 10 years: the disease was traced to Sewer air from foul sewers. The sewers were ventilated, & the water pipes cut off from them: And since then there has been not gastric Fever. But no one seemed to think that this was the result of a cause: nor the Fever of another. They would not allow the sewers to be relaid, because this would have condemned other authorizes. And without this one would be loth to certify that the place was safe: What do you say to having 30 cases of Scarlet Fever and 4 Deaths in one year in it?

As to a nobleman's house, where was terrible Fever among the children: I dare say it is neither better nor worse than others in fine London squares. They ought all to be carefully examined.

The only way to prevent such calamities is to enable Local Boards to examine & certify the plans of all House Drainage & Water supply, in order to be sure that no drains are carried down inner walls: that they are all trapped and ventilated: & that the water-cisterns have no direct connection with the soil pipes.

All other Death-rates, compared with that of Fever, may almost be called insignificant in England. And it takes all ranks, from Prince to pauper. For every Fever *death* may be reckoned too at least six bad illnesses. And the way in which the whole vitality is lowered of those who do not die or are not seriously ill, & their power to work diminished, cannot be reckoned. Yet the causes of Fever are almost entirely under our control.

They are: bad Drainage & bad water. Would we had Mr. Plimsole for Fevers as well as for unseaworthy ships[!][3]

Editor's Notes

1. This passage is discussed in the Introduction, p. 33.
2. Robert Rawlinson, "Typhoid Fever and House Drains," a letter to the editor, *The Times* (July 31, 1875), p. 16. Nightingale has marked up a clipping with Rawlinson's letter, indicating that this material is to be inserted directly from it. Rawlinson had served with Nightingale's colleague Dr. John Sutherland as Sanitary Commissioner during the Crimean War (Cook, *Life of Florence Nightingale*, i. 220). On October 8, 1860, she asked him to write notes on the drainage of "Cottage Property" that she could append "to a Cottage Edition of the Nursing book, for which I have been asked over and over again" (cited in L. A. Montiero, ed., *Letters of Florence Nightingale in the History of Nursing Archive, Special Collections, Boston University Libraries* [Boston, 1974], p.11).
3. Samuel Plimsoll, 1824–1898, agitated for legislation against dangerous and decaying ships. Nightingale's spelling is not the usual one.

1875: THIS MANUSCRIPT ADDITION IS ENTITLED 'STEADY DEGENERATION'.[1]

In the Chapter on Health of Houses, something has been said as to the house habits which make a race degenerate. Something more must needs be said as to the stomach habits which make our race degenerate. And it is an awful fact that a steady degeneration seems going on among our Factory population in certain large factory towns.

That boys & girls do grow on milk & don't grow on tea and coffee we know.

But this is not all.

Factory boys often smoke or chew tobacco or both. In one factory town I know at least one half of the boys between 12 and 20 years of age who worked in the Mills either smoked or chewed tobacco or both. And, bad as this is for grown men, it is found, as might be expected, that it is far worse for growing boys. It stunts them, mind & body.

Is there any wonder that, between smoking and drinking, boys & girls (who are going to be fathers & mothers) destroy their own constitutions: give these same destroyed constitutions to their children: & then finish the work of destruction by the way they bring them up on tea & Soothing Syrups & all kinds of trumpery, worth nothing for food & nourishment.

You think this is romancing perhaps. It is a frightful fact.

In the five years, 1869, 1870, 1871, 1872, 1873, quite one half the children who came before the 'Certifying Surgeon' under the Factory Accts of one large factory town, were perfectly unfit to work full time[.] The number increased year by year; & is increasing still.

Will you not cry, as they do in Parliament, 'Hear, hear'?

And do not say: it is all the fault of the Mills: the mills are more healthy to work in now than they ever were before.

It is the fault of drinking: it is the fault of tobacco: it is the fault of mothers going to the mills instead of stopping at home to nurse their children & make their homes comfortable: it is the fault of mothers not caring or not knowing how to make their homes healthy or comfortable: it is the fault of mothers not caring or not knowing how to rear or to manage or to feed their children: but how to drug them—indeed they know very well. They do not know what is to come of what they do: nor how sure it is to come.

You see children in the mills who have not grown a single ounce in half a year, but have instead lost weight.

And have you ever thought that sound common sense, for which English & Scotch workmen used to be famous, depends upon a sound state of the body? that a nation or town of weak bodies generally means a nation or town of weak brains? —have you ever thought that a workman cannot judge of machinery, a better thing—cannot, in one word, "think as well as work", if his weak brains are farther stupefied by tobacco or drink?—or even if his body, stunted and feeble, makes his mind feeble & his spirits unsteady?

What do weak foolish brains naturally run to? A "fool's Paradise".

What do weak stunted bodies naturally run to? More drink: less work: employing leisure again in drinking.

What do we mean by a "fool's Paradise"? is it not when such workmen, having deprived themselves of their common sense, becoming a prey to "Agitators", & think that, by driving trade & manufactures away from England, where it will not so soon return, they can raise wages? get a higher wage for shorter hours of work?

Bodily strength, grounded upon wholesome habits, is the foundation of other strength: especially of strong common sense: as a rule.

England is strong—let us not be obliged to say: *has* been strong—in trade & manufactures & common sense, because her labouring & artisan classes were wont to be, —let us not be obliged to say: *have* been—strong in a sober life, in a sober understanding. A sober strength can in no way stand upon an *in*sober life.

A great School Master of the Middle Ages was wont to say it was useless to attempt to educate the mind, if the body were neglected: and, he said, anything unnecessary or irregular in eating & sleeping (& had he lived in these days, he would have added, drinking & smoking) &

personal bad habits & self-indulgence, "were the first fertile sources of the moral & physical disorders of youth".

Shall we be behind the Middle Ages?

Note

1. This is discussed in the Introduction, p. 33.

FLORENCE NIGHTINGALE'S
NOTES ON NURSING

FIRST EDITION—GUIDE TO IDENTIFICATION

The first edition of *Notes on Nursing*—that is, the first version of the book as it was printed from the original setting of type—was published in the first week of January 1860, remaining in print till 1901, and possibly longer. Early copies are much sought after, fetching several thousand dollars. It has been difficult to prove which copies are earlier than others because the book was never dated on the first page, the title page, where the date of publication is commonly to be found. It is the purpose of this guide to make accurate identification possible in three easy steps.

Every copy of the first edition of *Notes on Nursing* has its own distinctive combination of three elements: (1) the end-papers, (2) the bindings, and (3) the typographical characteristics. The "End-papers" are sheets of paper, half of which are stuck down as a lining for the inside of the front and back covers, the other half becoming the first and last leaves in the book. These are the fly-leaves, found in the front before the text begins at the title page, and at the back after the text ends. "Bindings" is a word that describes the covers of the book, in this case identifiable from one another by variations in the pattern of the border. "Typographical characteristics" are the peculiar ways in which the type-face has left its imprint upon the page, whether a letter is too high, or has fallen out, or is in the wrong case (too large or too small, or in italic or gothic instead of roman), or whether the spelling or spacing between words is one way or another. The original setting of the type is described as the first state, and any further changes as second state, and so on.

My detailed examination of these three aspects in a large number of copies is described in "Florence Nightingale's *Notes on Nursing: The First Version and Edition*."[1] This study reveals that during the more than 41 years of production the end-papers, the bindings, and the typographical characteristics occur in 32 different combinations, which I call Groups. By tracing the development of the typographical characteristics throughout the book, including breakage and replacement of letters and punctuation, and alterations to spelling and spacing, and then relating these to the end-papers and the bindings of the copies in which they occur, I have identified the chronological sequence in which the 32 groups occur. By following this guide, anybody should be able to find the correct group, and therefore the place within the history of the book, of any copy of the first edition of *Notes on Nursing*.

Step 1: Compare the End-Papers

Although a few copies have nothing printed inside the front and back covers (on the end-papers), most have publisher's advertisements with dates printed in them. I have noted 16 variations in the end-papers, though there may be others. In the first 25 groups the only year mentioned is 1860. Advertisements in later copies refer to January 1864 (Group 26), and then to 1873 (Group 27), 1883 (Group 28), 1891 (Group 29), 1897 (Group 30).

With the exception of Groups 13 and 15, where the binding is in charcoal fine bead-cloth, all copies in Groups 1 to 29 (1891) are bound in charcoal medium-fine bead-cloth over pliable cardboard. Beginning with Group 30 (1897) the binding changes to a dark blue medium-fine bead-cloth on thick hard cardboard. Group 31 has an undated advertisement that begins, "The health of/the Prairie is/brought to the/Sick-Room by/LEMCO", but Group 32 has nothing at all on the end-papers. At the foot of the title page, however, where in Groups 1 to 30 the publisher styles himself "HARRISON, 59, PALL MALL, / BOOKSELLER TO THE QUEEN.", in Groups 31 and 32 he calls himself "HARRISON & SONS, 59, PALL MALL, / BOOKSELLERS TO HIS MAJESTY THE KING." Groups 31 and 32 are therefore published after the death of Queen Victoria on January 22, 1901.

As Groups 26 to 32 can be dated by their end-papers or bindings, no further detail about them is needed in this guide. The copies that present a problem are those which are earlier, those in Groups 1 to 25. These are charcoal-coloured and either have blank end-papers or have advertisements containing the date 1860. Normally, copies with blank end-papers are in Groups 1 and 2, but later specimens with blank end-papers do exist.

Opening your copy, compare the end-papers pasted inside the front cover with the following nine descriptions. Although in many examples the colors have faded so that pale pink and pale yellow may be indistinguishable, by comparing the typographical features you should be able to find one or two end-papers that fit with yours. Now note the groups in which those end-papers are found.

The development of the end-papers begins by neatly coinciding with the chronological order of the groups, but this soon gets scrambled because the binders randomly picked up earlier or later printings from the heaps given to them. Thus, End-papers 3 can fall anywhere in Groups 7 to 20.

Descriptions of the Front End-Papers Inside the Front Cover

1   –pale yellow
    –no printing
    –found in Groups 1 and 2
2   –pale yellow
    –first setting of type with the first set of advertisements, line 1 reads, "NEW WORKS and NEW EDITIONS, Published by"; large centered heraldic crest of Sir Bernard Burke, Ulster King of Arms, 4.3 × 5 cm; dated 1860
    –found in Groups 3 to 6
3   –pale yellow
    –second setting of type, in the first state: second advertisements, line 1 reads, "LONDON: HARRISON, Bookseller to the Queen, 59, PALL MALL."; on left, a small heraldic crest of Sir Bernard Burke, Ulster King of Arms, 2.1 × 2.55 cm; dated 1860. In line 4, 1860 has

a large case "8". Line 22 reads "Foreign titles . . . British Bri-".

    –found in Groups 7 to 20

4   –bright yellow—otherwise as 3

    –found in Groups 13 and 19

5   –pale yellow

    –second setting of type, in the second state: line 22 is reset to read "Foreign titles . . . British"—otherwise as 3

    –found in Groups 14, 17, 19, and 20

6   –pale pink—otherwise as 5

    –found in Group 20

7   –pale pink

    –second setting of type, in the third state: in line 4, "8" in "1860" is replaced in the correct case—otherwise as 5

    –found in Groups 20, 21, and 25

8   –pale yellow—otherwise as 7

    –found in Group 22

9   –bright yellow—otherwise as 7

    –found in Groups 23 and 24

Having now examined the front end-papers in your copy, and found the groups to which your copy might belong, go to Step 2.

Step 2: Compare the Bindings

The ten bindings described below are prefaced with the numbers of the groups in which they are found. Looking under the groups to which you have already ascertained that your copy might belong, count, and if necessary measure, the lines or "blind rules" that make up the border around the edges of the front cover. These blind rules are pressed into the cover by iron blocks. The external dimensions of the blocks help to distinguish between bindings that appear to be similar.

Description of the Bindings

1 –found in Groups 1 to 7
   –3 blind rules: (beginning at the outermost) 1.5 mm (with 1 mm between), then 4 mm (with 1 mm between), then 1.25 mm
   –size of blind rule block 12.9 × 21.4 cm; copies between 21.9 cm and 22.1 cm tall

2 –found in Group 8
   –2 blind rules: 3 mm (with 2.5 mm between), then 1.5 mm
   –size of blind rule block 12.5 × 20.5 cm; copies between 21.1 and 21.5 cm tall

3 –found in Groups 9 to 11, and 15
   –4 blind rules: 3.5 mm (with 1 mm between), then 1 mm (with 3.5 to 5 mm between, varying on any given copy), then 1.5 mm (with 1 mm between), then 1 mm
   –size of blind rule block 12.8 to 12.95 × 20.9 to 21 cm; copies between 21.3 and 21.5 cm tall

4 –found in Groups 11 to 17, and 19
   –3 blind rules: 3.5 mm (with 2 mm between), then 1 mm (with 2 mm between), then 1 mm
   –size of blind rule block 12.8 × 20.7 cm; copies between 21.4 and 21.7 cm tall

5 –found in Groups 14, and 19 to 20
   –3 blind rules: 3.5 mm (with 2 mm between), then 1 mm (with 2 mm between), then 1 mm. The corners are mitered by a 1 mm wide blind rule cutting diagonally across.
   –size of blind rule block 12.75 × 20.6 cm; copies between 21.4 and 21.7 cm tall

6 –found in Groups 13 and 15
   –2 blind rules: 2.5 mm (with 2.5 mm between), then 1 mm
   –size of blind rule block 12.5 × 20.5 cm; copies between 21.4 and 21.7 cm tall

7 –found in Groups 18, and 20 to 22
   –3 blind rules: 3.5 mm (with 2 mm between), then 1 mm (with 2 mm between), then 1 mm. The corners

are mitered by a 1 mm wide blind rule cutting diagonally across.

–size of blind rule block 12.8 × 21.2 cm (this is a larger
block than in Binding 5 above); copies between 21.25
and 21.7 cm tall

8 –found in Group 23

–2 blind rules: 2 mm (with 1 mm between), then 1 mm

–size of blind rule block 12.5 × 21.2 cm; copies between
21.4 and 21.7 cm tall

9 –found in Group 24

–2 blind rules: 2 mm (with 1 mm between), then
0.5 mm

–size of blind rule block 13 × 20.7 cm; copies between
21.4 and 21.7 cm tall

10 –found in Group 25

–2 blind rules: 2 mm (with 1.5 mm between), then
0.5 mm

–size of blind rule block 12.7 × 20.2 cm; copies between
21.4 and 21.7 cm tall

When you have found your binding and the group or groups
it is in, go on to Step 3 to confirm your identification.

Step 3: Check the Typographical Characteristics

Check the groups you have selected for your copy against
the following list of the characteristics of Groups 1 to 25. As these
accumulate during the development of the book, the group in
which your copy should be placed is the last one with which it
shares any of these characteristics.

Because of the haphazard nature of the process of manufacturing books, earlier states of the pages can sometimes be bound
into later bindings and end-papers. Again, the group to which
such copies belong is the last one with which they share any of
the characteristics.

Group 1
–End-papers 1 (blank) in Binding 1

–There is no translation notice at the foot of the title page.

–At p. 17, note 3, line 3, the "l" in "laws" is 1.75 mm too low, its top being level with the foot of the "a". At p. 78, instead of "60-", the "0" is omitted, printing "6 -".

Group 2

–End-papers 1 (blank) in Binding 1

–There is no translation notice at the foot of the title page.

–At p. 17, note 3, line 3, the top of "l" in "laws" is half-way up the "a".

Group 3

–End-papers 2 (dated 1860) in Binding 1

–There is no translation notice at the foot of the title page.

–On p. 15, lines 24–5, the first words "habit" and "water" print very poorly.

Group 4

–End-papers 2 (dated 1860) in Binding 1

–There is no translation notice at the foot of the title page.

–On p. 15, lines 24–5, with the exception of "r" in "water", "habit" and "water" are perfectly printed.

Group 5

–End-papers 2 (dated 1860) in Binding 1

–There is no translation notice at the foot of the title page.

–At p. 73, note 1, "Summary" is reset with "ummary" moved left to close the gap ("Summary" was originally set with a gap between "S" and "u").

Group 6

–End-papers 2 (dated 1860) in Binding 1

–There is no translation notice at the foot of the title page.

–*A large number of changes are made in the type, the most readily noticeable being:* at p. 17, note 3, line 3, the "l" in "laws", originally below the line, and then halfway up, is now corrected (see above, under Group 1.) Page 47, line 17, originally "ex halations", is now corrected to "exhalations". On p. 48, note, lines 2–5 are moved half a space left and obtrude into the margin. At p. 78, in addition to the "0" dropping out in the original printing (see Group 1) to give "6 -", now the piece of type with "6" comes off its foot, falling sideways against the dash so that the right side of "6" does not print.

Group 7

–End-papers 3 in Binding 1

–There is no translation notice a the foot of the title page.

–At the foot of p. 33, the signature (the capital letter "D"), originally centered slightly left of "o" in "window", is reset in the same place with a rounder case "D" than normal (compare p. 35).

Group 8

–End-papers 3 in Binding 2

–There is no translation notice at the foot of the title page.

Group 9

–End-papers 3 in Binding 3

–There is no translation notice at the foot of the title page.

–In some copies on p. 33 the signature (the capital letter "D") is missing from the foot of the page (see above, Group 7).

FROM THIS POINT ONWARD THE TRANSLATION NOTICE ALWAYS APPEARS AT THE FOOT OF THE TITLE PAGE

Group 10

–End-papers 3 in Binding 3

–At p. 44, at the end of line 1, in addition to the original piece of type with the full-stop being turned upside-down (the point prints above the "e"), now the right side of the "e" is not printing. On p. 78, the page number is missing.

Group 11

–End-papers 3 in Binding 3 and also End-papers 3 in Binding 4

–At p. 35, note 4, line 1, the "t" in "effect" is missing. At p. 44, end of line 1, the full-stop, originally raised above "e" (turned type), is corrected. At p. 74, the end of line 53, "quite as" prints as "quitea s". On p. 78, the missing page number (see above, under Group 10) is added (the numbers are reset level at the base, so the top of "7" is higher than top of "8"). On p. 78, line 4 is reset as "60 –" (see above, under Group 6).

In some copies on p. 4, line 17, the "X" is missing from "APPENDIX"; in others on p. 74, at the end of line 52, the space in "kind of" is misplaced giving "kindof" and a space at the end.

Group 12

–End-papers 3 in Binding 4

–At p. 4, line 17, there is a new "X" in "APPENDIX" (the distance from the beginning of the line to the end of the last set of four points is reduced from 7.9 cm to 7.85 cm). At p. 19, line 22, the original "tke" is corrected to "the". On p. 21, note 7, line 3, the final question mark goes missing.

Group 13

–End-papers 3 or 4 in Binding 4 and also End-papers 3 in Binding 6

–*A major correction of the type occurs here, the most readily noticeable features being:* at p. 35, note 4, line 1 runs along line 51; the "t" in "effect" is replaced (the ascender above the crossbar is straight), but the tip of the second "f" is pushed up (see above, under Group 11). On p. 38, line 46 originally begins "ead", and is now corrected to "had". At p. 45, line 24, "bedding,because" is reset as "bedding, because". Also on p. 45, in line 27, "fidgettiness" is reset as "fidgetiness". On p. 60, line 46, the original "aginative" is reset as "imaginative". At p. 74, lines 52–53, in line 52, "of" is missing, and in line 53, "quitea s" is corrected.

Group 14

-End-papers 3 or 5 in Binding 4 and also End-papers 3 in Binding 5

-At p. 48, note 1, lines 2–5, the left margin is straightened or "justified," and line 2 is level with the tops of the short letters of line 22 (see above, under Group 6).

Group 15

-End-papers 3 in Bindings 3, 4, or 6

-At p. 11, line 25, the original turned "s" in "feverish" is corrected. At p. 14, line 10, the original "slop pail", without the hyphen, is changed to "slop-pail".

Group 16

-End-papers 3 in Binding 4

-At p. 14, line 31, the original "HOUSES*." is reset as "HOUSES.*" (with the asterisk after the full-stop).

Group 17

-End-papers 3 or 5 in Binding 4

-At p. 21, note 7, line 3, the missing question mark is replaced, though the top left end is broken off this piece of type (see above, Group 12). At p. 70, line 5, the full-stop at the end is reset as a question mark; also on p. 70, in line 34 the original "copper," is reset without the comma as "copper".

Group 18

-End-papers 3 in Binding 7

-At p. 30, note 2, line 3, the original "faney" is reset as "fancy".

Group 19

-End-papers 5 in Binding 4 and also End-papers 3 or 4 in Binding 5

-At p. 64, note 2, line 4, the original comma after "of" is removed.

Group 20

-End-papers 3 in Binding 5 and also End-papers 5 or 6 or 7 in Binding 7

-*A major correction of the type occurs here, the most readily noticeable features being:* at p. 4, line 17, a third set of four points replaces the original solid bar.

On p. 33, the first "3" of the page number is corrected from the original italic to roman. At p. 41, line 33, the original gothic 2nd "t" in "nutritive" is reset in roman. On p. 51, lines 44–45, "atmos-/pheres" is reset as "atmo-/spheres". At p. 65, note 3, line 1, "Physionomy" is reset in two lines as "Physiog-/nomy". At p. 73, the original head-title at the top of the page, "OBSERVATION ON THE SICK", is reset as "CONCLUSION"; and on p. 76, the original running-title at the top of the page, "CONCLUSION", is reset as "NOTES ON NURSING".

Group 21

–End-papers 7 or 8 in Binding 7

–*A major correction of the type occurs here, the most readily noticeable features being:* at p. 1 (title page), line 1, the colon after "NURSING" is replaced with one in which the dots are elongated—where originally the bar of the "G" would run through the centre of the top dot, now it would run below the top dot. On p. 2, the verso or back of the title page, originally blank, now has the publisher's name and address in 2 lines centered on the page (line 2 reads "ST,"). On p. 4, the Table of Contents, the original height of the printed area, 11.4 cm, is now reset in 9.9 cm. On p. 5, the dropped head-title above the text, originally 3 mm high and 4.95 cm long, is now reset in type 4 mm high by 4.85 cm long. On p. 32, note 4, originally in 5 lines, is reset in 4 lines. On p. 51, note 6, originally in 5 lines with a turned or upside-down "s" in "clothes", is reset in 4 lines and the "s" corrected. At p. 71, line 46, the original space between "i." and "e." in "i. e." is closed up and a comma is added at the end, but the full-stop after "e" drops out leaving a blank in "i.e ,". On p. 80, the original blank page now has a two-line colophon (printer's name and address) mid-page.

Group 22

–End-papers 8 in Binding 7

–At p. 9, in the bottom line, for "it" there is a blank space. At p. 12, line 50, in "the" in "the damp", the "t" is missing and the "h" is high. At p. 16, note 1, the note is moved 2 spaces right (in relation to notes 2 and 3 which are not moved).

Group 23

–End-papers 9 in Binding 8
–At p. 33, at the foot of the page the signature (the capital letter "D"), absent in Group 9 only, is moved right to a position under the "t" of the first "the".

Group 24

–End-papers 9 in Binding 9

Group 25

–End-papers 7 in Binding 10

If you cannot identify your copy by following these three steps, consult the full study mentioned above. Should your copy turn out to belong to Groups 1 or 2, the chances are that it could be extremely valuable, and you should exercise caution in whom you take advice from about selling it.

Note

1. "Florence Nightingale's *Notes on Nursing: The First Version and Edition*," *The Library*, 6th Ser., xv (1993), 24–46.

Index

Note: Index page numbers are the actual page numbers—where the pages fall in this volume—given at the feet of pages. An n or t following a page number in the index indicates a note or a table, respectively.

A

"Accidental death," 117–118, 247–250, 264–265, 336

Accidents
age and, 31
babies and, 405
breathing and, 400
convalescence from, 269
management and, 117–118, 120–121, 336
observation and, 232, 389
patience and, 134–135, 342–343
recovery from, 406–407

Activities, 151, 351, 402

Adams, Dr., 286n13

Adulteration of Food Act (1872), 419n2

Advice, 200–211, 375–382

Ægineta, Paulus, 286n13

Affectation, 128, 339

Ages of nurses, 282n, 284t, 410

Agitators, 429

Air. See also Ventilation; Wind; Windows
babies and, 401, 403–404, 405
children and, 247, 248, 274, 276, 277
convalescence and, 271–272, 394
dirty, 191, 370
flowers and, 147, 349
importance of, 290n56
light and, 182–183, 364–365, 366
sleep and, 247, 248
surgery and, 245
urban areas and, 274
walls and, 370

Air tests, ix, 78–79, 285n3

Aitken, William, 13, 42n17

Alcohol (intemperance), 33, 78, 311, 330, 427, 428–429

American editions (NN), 5–6, 41n7

American publishers, 12–13

Aneurisms, 239

Angélique of Port Royale, Mère, 256, 293n98

Anglo-Saxons, 267

"Antiseptic Midwifery" (Godson), 43n37

Anxiety, 113–116, 147, 220, 333–335, 349–351, 386

NN = *Notes on Nursing*; NNLC = *Notes on Nursing for the Labouring Classes*

Aperients, 102–103, 104, 166, 250, 252, 329, 408

Apoplexy, 240, 291n83

"Appendix on Method of Training Nurses under the Nightingale Fund at Saint Thomas's Hospital, London," 8, 9, 31–32

Appetite. See Cooking; Digestion; Eating (nutrition); Feeding; Food

Appleton and Company, 13

Approach, 11–12

Aretaeus, 286n13

Arnauld, Jacqueline Marie Angélique, 256, 293n98

Arnold, Matthew, 39

Arnott's ventilator, 190, 251, 320, 370

Arrowroot, 161, 172, 357

Arsenic, 192, 371

Ashpits, 322

Asthma, 294n119

As You Like It (Shakespeare), 290n65

Australia, 412

Averages, 241–242, 390–391, 393. See also Statistics

B

Babies. See also Childbirth; Children; Infant mortality
    basics, 401–406
    communication with, 258, 396
    company, as, 209–210, 380
    hope and, 376
    milk and, 417–418
    observation and, 221, 387
    sudden death of, 13, 247, 292n90, 405

Bacon, 162n, 357n

Barley, 161, 357

Bathing. See also Hygiene, personal
    babies, 401, 404, 405–406
    basics, 195–198, 373–374
    country life and, 372–373
    dressing after, 174, 362
    skin and, 372
    ventilation and, 83, 314
    windows and, 84, 314

Beds and bedding. See also Blankets; Mattresses
    airing, 87, 98, 316, 326
    babies and, 401, 405, 406
    basics, 173–181, 319, 361–365, 413n6
    children and, 247
    infection and, 331
    location of, 183–184, 310, 365
    observing and, 264, 399
    shaking of, 138, 344–345
    uses of, 262
    variety and, 149, 350

Bed sores, 178–179, 364, 397, 407, 413n6

Beef tea, 160, 164–165, 166, 172, 288n41, 356, 358

Beer, 276

Bees-wax, 279–280, 369

Beeton, Isabella, 39–40, 43n46, 285n9

Behavioral determinants of health, ix

Being in charge, 122, 326, 336–337. See also Management

Bindings, 7

Birds, 209n

Birth rates, 105t–106, 330

Blackwell, Elizabeth, 293n100

Blankets, 178–179, 289n54, 363–364, 413n6. See also Beds and bedding

Bleeding (blood-letting), 240, 291n83

Book of Household Management (Beeton), 39–40, 285n9

Bowels. See also Excreta
aperients and, 252, 408
diarrhoea and, 221, 386
observation of, 213, 264, 382, 400

Bracebridge, Selena, 291n72, 292n97

Brain diseases, 227, 240

Brandy, 171, 361

Bread, 166, 169–170, 252, 359, 360, 408

Breathing. See also Air; Ventilation
babies and, 403–404, 405
basics, 400
observation and, 264–265
pillows and, 180, 363–364
remedies, 249
warming and, 308

Brewster, David, 289n55

Bronchitis, 83, 264, 314, 400

Brucellosis, viii

The Builder, 113, 286n15, 289n55, 333

Business, 156, 354, 381–382

Bustling, 132, 140, 341, 345–346

Butter, 161, 162n, 357, 357n

Buttermilk, 163, 357

C

A Calendar of the Letters of Florence Nightingale (Goldie), 43n37

Calling, nurse's, 260, 261, 397–398. See also Professionalism

Calmness, 139, 345, 346

Calomel, 250, 407

Carbon, 165

Carpets, 98, 186, 188, 192, 325, 368–369, 371

Carriages, 91n

Carter, Henry Bonham, 29, 31–32, 42n30

Catarrh, 294n119

Catholic countries, 255

Celts, 267

Cervantes, Miguel, 270, 294n115

Cesspools, 322

Chadwick, Edwin, 5–6, 12–13, 322, 413n2

Chamber pots/privies/water-closets, 87–89, 98, 316–318, 322, 421. See also Excreta

Change, 271, 394–395

Chattering hopes, 200–211, 375–382

"Chattering Hopes and Advices," 30

Cheering the sick, 201–203, 376–377

Cheese, 161–162, 357

Chemistry, 165–166, 358

Chicory, 170, 360

Childbirth, 294n104, 376n, 406. See also Midwifery

Children. See also Babies; Schools
basics, 7, 245, 406
beds and, 178, 363
class issues, 273–274
company, as, 209–210, 380
country life and, 275

Children *(continued)*
  degeneration and, 106, 330
  diseases of, 110, 331
  food and, 427–428
  milk and, 417–418
  morality and, 66–67
  reading aloud and, 141n,
    346, 347
  sanitary nursing and,
    246–248
  ventilation and, 95, 325
  worms and, 264
"Children: their greater suscepti-
    bility to the same things,"
    7
Chills. See Warming
Chimneys. See also Fires
  basics, 96, 320, 325–326
  sleep and, 177
  smoky, 86, 310, 315
Cholera, 266, 322, 382
Christison, Robert, 164, 170,
    288n41, 358
Cisterns, 425
Civilization, 101, 328
Class issues. See also Poverty;
    Young ladies
  air and, 285n10
  basics, 323–324
  children and, 273
  consumption and, 102,
    328–329
  convalescence and, 271–272,
    395
  degeneration and, 101, 104,
    328, 329
  health and, 211n
  hospitals and, 67
  nursing, 262
  servants' quarters, 100,
    327–328

  sewers and, 93–94, 421, 425
  third edition (NNLC) and,
    21–26
  typhoid fever and, 420
  ventilation and warming
    and, 78, 94–95, 311,
    324–325
Cleanliness. See Hygiene
Clothing. See also specific arti-
    cles of clothing
  baby, 406
  children and, 247
  hygiene and, 195
  nurses', 128–129, 130, 339–340
  walls and, 370
  warming and, 270, 277, 314
Clough, Arthur Hugh, 29, 42n31
Coal dust, 192, 371
Cocoa, 171, 361
Coffee, 167–168, 170, 288n46,
    359–360, 418
Colchicum, 251, 407
Colds, 72–73, 307
Collected Works (Stewart),
    294n112
Colocynth, 251, 292n93, 407
Colours, 145–146, 150n, 349, 397
Common sense
  convalescence and, 270–271
  health and, 428–429
  ventilation and warming
    and, 75–76
  visitors and, 201–202, 376
  warming and, 81, 313
  windows and, 309
Communication. See also Speak-
    ing; Whispering
  anxiety and, 115–116, 334,
    341–342
  conciseness, 139, 345
  patients, with, 258, 265

visitors and, 132–133
whispering, 128, 339
Conciseness, 139, 345
"Conclusions" (first and second
versions [NN]), 7–8, 10
Confidential nurses, 243–244,
401
Congestion, 240
Constipation, 408
Construction
children and, 274
factories and, 311
hospitals and, 12, 286n13,
286n15
light and, 183
noise and, 143, 347–348
sewers and, 33, 422–423
ventilation and, 91–94,
274–275, 318–320
Consumption
basics, 101–103, 328–329,
400
coughing remedies, 178, 364
death and, 266–267, 382
expectoration and, 264
rheumatic phthisicky and,
294n119
young ladies and, 23,
101–103, 328–329, 377n
Contagion. See Infection/conta-
gion
Contamination, ix
Contemplation, 3
Convalescence, 268–273,
277–278, 393–395
"Convalescence," 7
Cook, Edward, 16
Cooking, 86, 157, 316, 354. See
also Digestion; Eating
(nutrition); Feeding;
Food

Coughs, 99, 110, 178, 264, 400
Country life, 273–277, 285n7,
321, 323, 372, 421
Cravings, 162n, 357n
Cream, 161, 357
Crimean fever, viii, 287n36
Crimean War, vii, 9, 10n, 21,
41n13
Crinoline fires, 30, 39–40, 130,
287n22, 340
Crinolines, 340
Curtains, 98, 184–185, 186, 367

D

Deafness, 400
Death. See also Infant mortality
"accidental," 117–118,
247–250, 264–265, 336
babies and, 401, 402, 405, 406
causes of, 235, 238, 390–391,
392
class issues, 272
faces and, 266–267
novels and, 204, 278
preparation for, 381–382
sewers and, 425
Decent care, x
Decisions, 139–140, 345–346
Degeneration (degradation)
basics, 427–430
children and, 106, 330
class issues, 101, 104, 242,
328, 329, 392
diet and, 276
light and, 185, 367
Delirium
dreams versus, 267–268
feeding and, 134, 342
management and, 118
noise and, 127, 138, 338–339
observation and, 137, 231, 389

Delirium *(continued)*
    visitors and, 137, 344
    windows and, 73n, 308n
Depression, 203, 228, 230, 239,
        348, 349, 372, 377
Devotion, 262–263, 294n110,
        399, 401
Diarrhoea
    accidents and, 232, 389–390
    basics, 400
    bathing and, 196
    death and, 266, 382
    jelly and, 164, 358
    milk and, 162, 357
    observation and, 221, 264,
        386, 389–390
    ventilation and, 88, 317
Dickens, Charles, 19–20, 21,
        290n64, 294n104
Dictionary of Medicine (Quain),
        43n37
Diet. See Cooking; Digestion;
        Eating (nutrition); Feed-
        ing; Food
Digestion. See also Cooking; Eat-
        ing (nutrition); Feeding;
        Food; specific foods
    aperients and, 329
    appetite versus, 218–219, 269
    cooking and, 157
    degeneracy and, 104
    feeding and, 172
    variety and, 348
    women's, 162n
Diluent, 169, 288n44, 360
Diseases. See also specific dis-
        eases
    basics, 25, 64–65, 82,
        108–109, 313, 332
    convalescence versus, 268
    progression of, 231–233

temperament and, 267
Disinfectants, 90, 318
Disraeli, Benjamin, 419n2
Distortions, 40
Distribution, 39
Doctors
    aperients and, 408
    bathing and, 196, 373
    confidence in, 378, 407
    construction and, 92
    convalescence and, 269
    eating (nutrition) and, 167,
        359
    female, 293n100
    nurses and, 18, 153, 353, 397,
        399, 408
    observation and, 236–237,
        238–239, 260–261, 390,
        391, 392–393
    Sutherland, J., on, 11
    ventilation and warming
        and, 74
Domestic nurses, 19
Don Quixote (Cervantes), 270,
        294n115
Doors
    basics, 85, 262, 315, 398
    draughts and, 83–84
    noise and, 131, 341
    pyaemia and, 98
    sewers and, 324
    ventilation and, 313–314
Doubt, 139, 345
Drains, 94, 321, 322, 324, 421,
        423–324. See also Sewers
Draughts, 82–83, 270, 314, 404
Dreams, 267–268
Dress. See Clothing
Drinks, 168–169, 359–361,
        374–375, 398. See also
        specific drinks

Dry earth systems, 34, 43n41
Dunghills, 322, 420
Dust/dusting, 98, 186–188, 192,
    368, 369, 371
Dysentery, 162n, 196, 266, 357n,
    382

E

Eating (nutrition). See also
    Cooking; Digestion;
    Feeding; Food
  basics, xviii, 152–159, 351–356
  beds and, 176
  children and, 276
  consumption and, 102, 104
  information about, 218–220,
    385–386
  observation and, 222–223,
    387–388, 397
  recovery and, 213, 383
  warming and, 81, 313
  young ladies and, 23,
    102–103, 329
Editions
  1868 edition (NNLC), 29–32
  1875 edition (unpublished),
    xviii, 32–38
  first version (NN), 5–6,
    10–14, 13, 16, 291n72
  identification of, 431–442
  second version (1860 Library
    Standard edition), xvii,
    14–21, 18–19, 26–27
  third version (NNLC), 7–10,
    21–29
Education of nurses
  basics, viii, 3–4, 14, 26–27,
    49–50, 111–112, 303,
    332–333, 397, 398
  Blackwell and, 293n100
  books and, 246

doctors and, 408
experience and, 260
hospitals and, 264
need for, 282–283
Nightingale's era, xvi–xvii
objections to, 407
observation and, 221–223
physicking and, 252–253
Saint Thomas's Hospital
    method, 410–414
schools and, 283
Sutherland, J., on, 11–12, 13
Edwards, Dr., 289n55
Effluvia, 87–89, 316–318
Eggs, 160, 356
1868 edition (NNLC), 29–32
1875 edition (unpublished), xviii,
    32–38
Emaciation, 227
Employers, 78, 311. See also Fac-
    tories
England and Her Soldiers
    (Nightingale), 40n1
Environmental determinants of
    health, ix
Erysipelas, 189, 245
Ethics, 243
European editions (NN), 7, 8, 11,
    40n4, 41nn8
Euthanasia, 42n31
Excreta, 87–89, 174–175, 213,
    264, 317–318, 382, 397.
    See also Bowels; Cham-
    ber pots/privies/water-
    closets; Drains; Sewers
Exercise, 276, 277, 311
Exertion, 137, 343
Expectations
  basics, 115–116
  conciseness and, 140
  exertion and, 134, 342, 343

Expectations *(continued)*
   management and, 334
   noise and, 125, 337
   nurses setting of, 232–233,
      390
   visitors and, 127, 137
Expectoration, 264
Experience, 170, 202n, 259–260,
      264, 376n, 396–397, 408.
      See also Observation
Eyes, 184, 367

F

Faces, 227, 228, 234, 258–259,
      294n113, 382
Factories, 77–78, 79, 311–312,
      427, 428
Facts, 237, 391
Facts Related to Hospital Nurses
      (Flint), 20
Fainting, 228–229, 398, 399
Fancies. See Imagination (fan-
      cies)
Farms, 421. See also Country life
Farr, William, 30–31, 42n35
Fasting, 153, 352
Fat, 162n, 357n
Fatalism, 375–376
Fear, 127–128, 265–266, 275,
      338–339, 340–341
Feeding, 134, 156, 230, 342,
      401–402, 406. See also
      Cooking; Digestion; Eat-
      ing (nutrition); Food
Feminism, 256–257, 262–263,
      286n17, 287n19,
      293n100. See also Sexism;
      Women
Fevers/feverishness. See also spe-
      cific diseases
   babies and, 405

   basics, 109
   bedding and, 173, 361–362
   buttermilk and, 357
   death and, 266, 382
   pulses and, 239
   reading aloud and, 346
   shivers and, 261, 397
   variety and, 146, 148, 348
   warming and, 73
Fires. See also Chimneys
   air and, 192, 413n1
   basics, 399
   clothing and, 340
   crinoline, 30, 39–40, 130,
      287n22, 340
   management and, 337
   ventilation and, 82, 86, 313,
      314, 316
   warmth and, 263
First version (NN), 5–6, 10–14,
      13, 16, 291n72. See also
      Identification of editions
Flannels, 80, 83, 87, 285n6
Flint South, John, 20
Floors. See also Carpets
   air and, 192–193
   basics, 188–190, 326, 368
   drainage and, 321
   polishing, 279–280, 290n62
   pyaemia and, 98
Flour, 161, 357, 418
Flowers, 146, 147, 148, 150, 348,
      349, 350
Fog, 322, 399
Food. See also Cooking; Diges-
      tion; Eating (nutrition);
      Feeding; specific foods
   babies and, 401–402
   basics, 157, 160–172,
      356–361
   bowels and, 252, 408

children and, 247, 277
class issues, 272
convalescence and, 268, 269,
    393–394
education and, 429–430
importance of, 290n56
labor movement and, 33, 429
"prepared," 418, 419n2
Fraser's Magazine, 21, 281, 295
Friends. See Visitors
Fruit, 162n, 357n
Fry, Elizabeth, 256, 293n99
Fumigations, 90, 318
Furniture. See also Beds and bedding
    air and, 325, 370
    dusting, 187, 189, 326, 368,
        369
    odors and, 186, 192, 367
    pyaemia and, 98
Future nursing, x

G

Galen, 286n13
Gamp, Sarah *(Martin Chuzzle-
    wit)* (Dickens), 19, 20, 21,
        294n104
Gangrene, 240, 245
Gaskell, Elizabeth, 285n10
Gastric fever, 38, 164, 358, 425
Gelatine, 164, 358
Gender, 30–31
Gentleness, 127, 138
German editions (NN), 6
Gingerbread, 162n, 357n
Girls, 28–29, 31, 403, 411–412
Global consciousness, 3, 25
Globalization, x
God. See also Religion
    disease and, 82, 313
    hands of, 79–80, 312
    intermarriage and, 278

laws of, 100, 305
natural laws and, 99–100
odors and, 316n
teachings of, 97, 99, 326, 327
Godson, C., 43n37
Godwin, George, 286n15
Goldie, S., 43n37
Good news, 208–209, 210–211,
    380–381
Gossip, 211, 381, 401
Grace, 268
Groats, 161, 357

H

Haemorrhages, 239
Ham, 162n, 357n
Handicraft of nursing, 246
Hands, 227
Handwritten material, 16–17
Harrison and Sons, 12, 13–14,
    29–30
Healing, viii, x
Health and the healthy, ix, 66,
    272, 304, 371–372, 395
"Health of Houses," 30, 33, 34,
    35, 36
Heart disease, 264–265, 400
Heredity, 103, 329
Home, 287n29
Homeopathy, 251–252, 292n95
Honesty, 203. See also Truth
Hooping (whooping) cough, 110,
    286n14, 332
Hopes, 200–211, 375–382
"Hospital Construction"
    (Nightingale), 12
Hospitals. See also *Notes on
    Hospitals* (Nightingale)
    army, 286n13, 288n41; See
        also *Sword and Gown*
        (Lawrence)

Hospitals *(continued)*
    bathing and, 373
    beds and, 177, 179
    class issues, 272
    construction, 12, 286n13,
        286n15
    convalescence and, 273
    Dickens on, 42n27
    eating (nutrition) and,
        153–156, 158, 162, 352,
        353–354, 355, 357
    education of nurses and, 264,
        283, 410–414
    employment of women, 281
    floors and, 189–190, 279,
        280, 290n62, 369
    hygiene and, 186, 189,
        286n13
    light and, 183, 289n55
    lying-in, 43n37
    management and, 117, 335
    need for, 66–68, 304–305
    nurses and, 19–20, 255
    personal hygiene and, 196
    suffering and, 64
    ventilation and, 82–83, 85,
        92, 309, 318
    wages and, 412
Hot water bottles, 81, 313, 405
Houghton, W.E., 289n55
Houses. See also Construction;
        Sewers; specific parts of
        houses
    basics, 91–110, 318–332
    children and, 276
    Sutherland, J., on, 34
    women and, 409
Humor, 23, 148
Hurrying, 132, 140, 156, 345–346
Hygiene. See also Bathing; specific
        issues, locations and objects

    babies and, 401, 405
    children and, 247, 276
    degeneration and, 104, 330
    factories and, 77–78, 311
    houses and, 95, 96, 323,
        325–327
    infant mortality and, 67–68
    medications versus, 251
    nurses, of, 196, 373
    personal, 195–199, 372–375;
        See also Bathing
    rooms, of, 186–194, 367–372
    surgery and, 244–246
    ventilation and, 275
    women and, 283
Hypnotism, 291n80
Hypochondriacs, 138, 203, 345

I

Identification of editions (NN),
        431–442
Idiosyncracies, patient, 229
The Illiad (Homer), 287n29
Imagination (fancies). See also
        Delirium; Mind;
        Thoughts
    convalescence and, 268, 271,
        394
    disease and, 140
    food and, 163, 394
    observation and, 146, 214,
        348, 383
    variety and, 348
Immorality, 21, 311, 430
India, 31
Infant mortality, 66–67, 104–105,
        304, 330, 417, 418. See also
        Babies, sudden death of
Infants. See Babies
Infection/contagion
    basics, 286n13

children and, 332
heredity versus, 103, 329
novels and, 278
sewers and, 421
small pox and, 107–108, 109,
    278–279, 331
Inflammation, 238, 239, 392
Information. See Observation
Ingenuity, 157, 158, 354
Intemperance (alcohol), 33, 78,
    311, 330, 427, 428–429
Intermarriage, 278, 330
International Council of Nurses, x
Interruptions, 133, 134, 342, 403.
    See also Surprises
Invalids, 209, 381
Irresolution, 139–140, 345–346
Irritability. See also Nerves
    noise and, 143–144,
        337–338, 347–348
    variety and, 151, 351

J

Jams, 162n, 163, 357n
Japanese editions (NN), 7
Jargons, 256–257
Jellies, 163–164, 165, 278, 355, 358

K

Kindness/unkindness
    carelessness versus, 86, 315
    light versus, 403
    management versus, 120
    observation versus, 222, 264,
        387
    patience and, 135, 343
    remedies, 211, 381
    second edition (NN), in, 19
    third edition (NNLC), in, 22
King's College Hospital, 32,
    42n37

L

Labor movement, 33, 429
Lady Lushington, 14
"The Latest Decalogue"
    (Clough), 42n31
Laughter, 148
Lawrence, George Alfred, 21,
    292n97
Laws of England, 323. See also
    specific laws
Laws of God, 100, 305
Laws of health, 100, 110, 332,
    407, 409
Laws of nature (life), 68–69, 95,
    286n13, 305, 325, 327,
    409
Lehmann, Julius, 170, 288,
    288n46
Letters of patients, 113, 133, 342
Library Standard edition (second
    version), xvii, 6–7, 14–21,
    18–19, 26–27. See also
    Identification of editions
Life of Florence Nightingale
    (Cook), 16, 287n20
Light
    babies and, 403
    basics, 95, 182–185, 325,
        365–367
    beds and, 177
    children and, 247, 277
    importance of, 290n56
    nerves and, 150–151
    recovery and, 289n55
    surgery and, 245
    variety and, 349, 351
    ventilation and, 288n42
    walls and, 191
Lilies, 147, 349
Liverpool paper, 11, 12
Living conditions, 236–242, 331

London, 66, 273–277, 294n118, 304
Lord Elcho, 37, 38
Lord Melbourne, 39
Love, 292n96. *See also Sword and Gown* (Lawrence)
Lushington, Lady, 14

M

Macaulay, Thomas Babington, 68, 285n2
Macbeth (Shakespeare), 268, 294n114
Malaria, 85
Management, 111–124, 332–337, 404, 409
Manchester, 305n
Manual labour, 151, 351
Marketing, 9
   Notes on Nursing: What It Is, and What It Is Not, 5
Martin Chuzzlewit (Dickens), 19–20, 21, 294n104
Martineau, Harriet, 4, 17, 39, 40n1, 42n25
Mary Barton (Gaskell), 285n10, 413n7
Mattresses, 173, 175, 180, 289n50, 362, 363, 364, 413n6
Measles, 94, 108, 110, 321, 324, 331, 401
Meat, 160–161, 164–165, 252, 276, 356, 358, 408
Medicines, 65–66, 199, 397, 398, 400. *See also* Physicking
   babies and, 402
   basics, 253–254, 408–409
   observation and, 223, 260, 261, 265
   water and, 374–375
Melbourne, Lord, 129

Memoirs (Robert-Houdin), 291n72
Memory, 225, 265, 400
Men, 262
Midwifery, 31–32, 43n37, 282, 294n104. *See also* Childbirth
Military hospitals, 117–119, 286n13. *See also* Soldiers
Milk, 172, 276, 355–356, 357n, 358
   basics, 161, 162–163, 166, 356, 357, 358
   children and, 276, 427
   diluted, 33, 172, 361, 417
   infants and, 417–418
   Sutherland on, 34
   typhus patients and, 168, 360
Mill, John Stuart, 293n100
Mind, 146, 147–148, 150, 185, 349. *See also* Depression; Imagination (fancies); Thoughts
"Minding Baby," xvii, 7, 28–29
   Sutherland and, 36
   Sutherland on, 34
Mistakes, 261
Moisture, 86–88, 174, 279, 280, 316–318. *See also* Water
   basics, 321–322
   bedding and, 174, 178, 362
Morality, 21, 311, 430
Morning treatment, 81, 313
Mortality, registration districts and, 104–105, 330
Mortality of the English Army (Nightingale), 40n1
Mothers, 33, 66, 428
   infant mortality and, 68
   ventilation and warming and, 79, 311

Mucus, 404
Music, 144

N

Narcotics, 228
Nature, 63, 149–150, 253, 303, 350
Nerves, 150, 151, 204, 351, 406.
    See also Irritability
New Sale of Food and Drugs Act
    of 1875, 419n2
Night air, 84–85, 314–315
Nightgowns, 174, 362
Nightingale, Florence
    basics, vii–viii
    biographies, 16, 43, 43nn37,
        287n20
    birth/death dates, 3
    Crimea, in the, 41n13, 93,
        287n36
    education, 24
    health of, 290n66
Nightingale Fund, 410
Nightingale School, 20
Nitrogen, 165
Noise
    babies and, 401, 405
    basics, 13, 125–144, 337–348
    carriages and, 285n12
    pets and, 209n
"Noise," 30
"Note as to the Number of
    Women Employed as
    Nurses in Great Britain,"
    7–8, 13
"A Note on Pauperism" (Nightin-
    gale), 295n123
*Notes of Matters Affecting the
    Health, Efficiency, and
    Hospital Administration
    of the British Army*
    (Nightingale), 288n41

Notes on Hospitals (Nightingale),
    12, 286n13, 290n62,
    413n1, 413n6
*Notes on Nursing for the Labour-
    ing Classes* (third ver-
    sion), 7–10, 21–29. See
    also Identification of edi-
    tions
*Notes on Nursing: What It Is, and
    What It Is Not* (first ver-
    sion), 5–6, 10–14, 13, 16,
    291n72. See also Identifi-
    cation of editions
*Notes on Nursing: What It Is,
    and What It Is Not*
    (Library Standard edi-
    tion) (second version),
    xvii, 14–21, 18–19,
    26–27. See also Identifi-
    cation of editions
"Note Upon Employment of
    Women," 7–8
"Note Upon Some Errors in
    Novels" (Nightingale), 20
Novello, Sabillo, 40n4
Novels, 20–21, 277–279. See also
    specific novels
Nurses. See also specific types of
    nurses
    ages of, 282n, 284t, 410
Nurses (*continued*)
    basics, 258–267, 290n69,
        395–401
    employment of, 282–283
    good, 253
Nursing, 63–66, 123–124,
    303–318. See also Profes-
    sionalism
Nutrition. See Cooking; Diges-
    tion; Eating (nutrition);
    Feeding; Food

O

Oat cake, 166, 359
Oats, 161, 357
Obedience, 263, 399
Objections to nursing, 250–257
Observation. See also Experience
    basics, 212–244, 258–267,
        382–393, 395, 408
    cultivating, 221–223,
        387–388
    doctors and, 167
    eating (nutrition) and, 355,
        358
    health and, 253
    hopes and, 376
    novels and, 278
    patients, by, 219–220, 386
    staring versus, 259
    ventilation, of, 309
    visitors and, 137, 202n, 344,
        377n
Odors
    basics, 322
    disinfectants and, 90, 318
    floors and, 188–189,
        192–193, 369, 371
    furniture and, 186, 192, 367
    God and, 316n
    surgery and, 245
    ventilation and, 274–275,
        310
The Odyssey (Homer), 287n29
"On Sudden Death in Infancy
    and Childhood" (West),
    13
Operas, 278
Opium, 268
Organization, 225
Ottley, Lucy J., 9–10
Overexertion, 137, 344

P

Paillasse, 413n6
Pain, 126, 337, 348
Paint, 113, 191, 333, 370
Paleness, 228, 234
Pathology, 253
Patience, 134–135, 194, 342–343,
    372
Payments to Nightingale, 10n
"People Overheard," 13
Peritonitis, 239, 266–267, 382
Perspiration
    babies and, 406
    basics, 372
    bathing and, 196, 198, 373,
        374
    bedding and, 362
    draughts and, 83, 314
    first edition (NN) and, 289n48
    observation and, 260, 397
    ventilation and, 364
Pets, 209n
Phlebitis, 99
Physicking, 250–251, 252,
    407–408
Physiognomy of disease,
    227–228, 291n77
Pickles, 162n, 357n
Pigsties, 322
Pillows, 180, 364
Plagues, 108
Pleurisy, 239, 264, 400
Plimsole (Plimsoll), Samuel, 426
Pneumonia, 264
Poetry, 26–27
Pollution, ix
Pound cake, 285n9
Poverty, 242, 295n123, 392, 411.
    See also Class issues
Precautionary principle, ix

Privies/chamber pots/water-closets, 87–89, 98, 316–318, 322, 421. See also Excreta
Professionalism, 18, 21, 49, 123–124, 283, 303. See also Calling, nurse's; Nursing
Progression of diseases, 231–233
Proofs, 12
Puerperal fever, 43n37
Puffing, 397
Pulmonary disease, 77–78, 102, 311–312
Pulses, 237–238, 239–240, 260, 266, 391, 392, 397
Punctuality, 153–154, 247, 266, 352
Punctuation, 17–18
Pyaemia, 97, 98, 240, 245

Q

Quain, R., 43n37
The Quarterly Review, 17
Questions, lazy, 220, 386, 400
Questions, misleading, 215–218, 221, 384–386
Quinine, 265, 400

R

Railway carriages, 91n
Rawlinson, Robert, 426n2
Readership, 11–12
Reading, 151, 271, 351, 394
Reading aloud, 141–143, 270, 346–347
Registration districts, 104–105, 330
Relapses, 232, 269, 277, 390
Religion, 244, 266–267, 268, 294n113, 382, 401. See also God

Reparative process, 64
Repletion, 153, 352
"Representative Women. The Free Nurse. Catherine Mompesson: Mary Pickard: Florence Nightingale" (Scott), 6
Reprints, 5, 6, 8
"Researches on Light—Sanatory—Scientific and Aesthetical" (Brewster), 289n55
Restoratives, 169, 285n4, 360
Revisions, 17
Rheumatic phthisicky, 294n119
Rheumatism, 309, 321
Rice, 357
Rickets, 95, 325
Robert-Houdin, J.E., 141, 287n30, 291n72, 346
Roberton, John, 286n15, 289n55
Rooms, 186–194, 367–372
Royal Hibernian School, 34, 38
Rubbing, 398
Rustling, 129–130, 339–340

S

Sago, 161, 357
Saint Thomas's Hospital, 4, 8, 14, 21, 31, 32, 410
Sancho Panza *(Don Quixote),* 270, 294n115
"Sanitary Condition of Hospitals and Hospital Construction" (Nightingale), 286n13
"Sanitary Construction of Hospitals" (Nightingale), 12
Sanitation. See Hygiene; specific remedies

Sarah Gamp *(Martin Chuzzlewit)* (Dickens), 19, 20, 21, 294n104
Sarcasm, 22
Scarlatina, 310n, 401, 421
Scarlet fever
    air and, 71, 79, 100, 306, 328
    children's epidemics and, 110, 310, 332
    construction and, 321
    drains/sewers and, 94, 324, 422, 425
    infection and, 108, 312, 331
    remedies, 421
    schools and, 38, 76
Schools
    basics, 277
    floors and, 369, 371
    health education and, 283
    management and, 336
    sewers and, 422, 425
    typhoid fever and, 420
    ventilation and warming and, ix, 76–77, 79, 310, 312
Schools of nursing, 20, 410–414
Science, 68–69
Scorbutic dysentery, 357n, 358
Scorbutic sores, 161, 163
Scott, Ingleby, 6
Scrofula, 95, 178, 289n52, 294n121, 325, 363
Scudder, J.M., 6
Scutari (district), 21, 93, 292n97, 324
Secretions, 260, 264, 400
Servants
    ages of, 284t, 411, 412
    babies and, 403
    basics, 95, 325
    bedrooms of, 100, 327–328

first edition (NN) and, xvi–xvii
    management and, 122–123
    noise and, 133
    Sutherland, J., and, 13
    training of, 98–99
Sewers. See also Drains
    basics, 323, 326, 420–426
    1875 manuscript and, xviii
    Sutherland and, 34, 36–38
    ventilation and, 70, 93, 191, 306, 321, 324, 370
    water and, 92–93
Sexism, 22, 40. See also Feminism; Women
Shakespeare, William, 268, 278, 290n65, 294n114
Shaking, 138, 344–345, 405
Shivers, 397
Shocks, 112, 333
Sinks, 93, 321, 324, 326, 423
Sitting, 181, 364
Skin
    baby, 404–405, 406
    basics, 195–198
    bathing and, 372–373, 374
    face, of, 234
    observation of, 227, 260, 261, 397
    rubbing and, 262, 397
Skretkowicz, Victor, vii
Sleep. See also Night air
    babies and, 401, 402, 403, 405
    basics, 125–126, 261–262, 337–338, 397, 399
    beds and, 179, 364
    children and, 247, 248, 275, 277
    coffee/tea and, 168, 359–360

convalescence and, 271
death versus, 263
eating (nutrition) and, 353n
education and, 429–430
information about, 216, 384
interruptions and, 136, 343
noise and, 125, 337
nurses', 124
observation of, 264
schools and, 76, 310
ventilation and, 308
ventilation/warming and,
    71, 75, 79, 102, 306, 308,
    312
Sloe-leaf (blackthorn) tea, 171,
    289n47, 360
Slop pails, 89–90, 317–318
Small-pox, 94, 107, 109, 324, 330,
    331
Smith, Beatrice Shore, 13
Smith, Robert Angus, 78, 91n,
    285n3
Smoke, 86, 310, 315
Smoking, 33, 427
Soap, 373, 374
Social determinants of health, ix
Social reform, 4
Soldiers, 102, 103, 169, 285n11,
    329. See also Military
    hospitals
Sores, 198, 374, 398
South, John Flint, 20
Speaking, 135, 342, 343. See also
    Communication; Whis-
    pering
Standing, 134, 135, 136, 213, 342,
    343, 383
Starch, 130, 340
Starvation, 154, 164, 219, 352,
    353, 358, 385

Statistics, 202n, 377n. See also
    Averages
Status of nurses, 18
Stewart, Dugald, 266, 294n110
Stimulants, 104, 260, 397
Strikes, 33
Style, writing, 11–12, 17–18, 22,
    23–24, 24–26, 28–29
Subsidiary Notes as to the Intro-
    duction of Female Nursing
    into Military Hospitals in
    Peace and in War
    (Nightingale), 286n13
Suet, 162n, 357n
Suffering, 64, 65, 303, 379
Sugar, 163, 357–358
Suggestions on a System of Nurs-
    ing for Hospitals in India
    (Nightingale), 31
Suicides, 116–117, 334–335
Superstitions, 226–227
"Supplementary Chapter" (NN),
    7, 18
Surgery, 117, 253, 269, 408
Surgical nurses, 245–246, 407
Surprises, 113–114, 135–136,
    333, 342, 405. See also
    Interruptions
Sutherland, John, Dr.
    basics, 41n13
    complaints to, 15
    doctors, on, 18
    first edition (NN) and, 11–13
    second edition (NN) and,
        30–31
    style, writing, and, 24, 27
    third edition (NNLC) and,
        33–38
Swallowing, 153, 352
Sweets, 163, 357–358

Swelling, 397
Sword and Gown (Lawrence), 21, 291n72, 292n97
Sympathy, 203
Symptoms, 64, 65, 303, 304

T

Table A, xvii, 105t
Tapioca, 161, 357
Tea
    basics, 167–172, 261, 359–360
    children and, 276, 418
    sloe-leaf (blackthorn), 171, 289n47, 360
    water for, 199
Teachers, 281, 283
Temperaments, patient, 225–226, 267
Thinking, 133, 342
Thirst, 168–169, 359–360
Thoughts, 185, 220, 349, 350–351, 386. See also Depression; Imagination (fancies); Mind
Throats, sore, 400, 404
Time, 266. See also Punctuality
Tobacco, 33, 427, 428–429
"Torino Fratelli Bocca, Librai di S.S.R.M." (Novello), 40n4
Trades' Unions, 33
Translations, 5, 15
Trust, 243–244
Truth, 30, 201, 214–215, 375–376, 383. See also Honesty
Typhoid fever, 34, 109, 238, 331, 392, 420, 422
Typhus, 109, 168, 331, 360

U

Unconscious patients, 261. See also Delirium

Unions, labor, 33
Union Schools, 411
Unkindness. See Kindness/unkindness
Unpublished additions (NN), xviii
Urination, 261, 264, 288n46, 397, 400

V

Vaccination, 94, 324
Variety, 145–151, 209, 230, 348–351, 371–372, 394–395
Vegetables, 161, 199, 408
Vehicles, 91n
Ventilation. See also Air; Wind; Windows
    basics, 107, 184, 306–318, 326, 330
    beds and, 177, 362–363
    construction and, 91–92
    eating (nutrition) and, 270
    furniture and, 371
    hospitals and, 286n15
    hygiene and, 94–95, 187, 192–193, 324, 367–368, 371
    management and, 112–113, 333
    sewers and, 324, 423–424
    walls and, 190–191
    warming and, 70–90, 320
Ventilators, 190, 251, 320
Views, 149, 350, 365
Virgil, 286n13
Visitors
    agitation and, 113–114, 333–334
    basics, 132, 136–137, 210–211

cheer and, 201, 207–208,
339, 375–382
convalescence and, 394
eating (nutrition) and, 156,
270, 354
food and, 394
noise and, 127–128, 339

W

Wages of nurses, 412
Walls, 190–192, 325, 326,
369–370. See also Paint
Warming
babies and, 401, 403–404
basics, 80–81, 126, 306–318,
338, 398
children and, 247, 274, 275
nursing and, 262
observation and, 261
surgery and, 245
ventilation and, 72–73, 74,
82, 248–249, 313–314
windows and, 75, 308
Washing. See Bathing
Water, 198–199, 320–321,
373–375, 374. See also
Drains; Moisture; Sewers;
Wells
Water-closets/chamber
pots/privies, 87–89, 98,
316–318, 322, 421. See
also Excreta
Wealthy. See Class issues
Web sites, xi
Wells, 92–93, 320–321
West, Charles, 13, 292n90
"What Food," 33
"What is a Nurse?", 7, 18, 22,
26–28
Whispering, 125, 127, 128, 292n,
337, 338, 339

Whitlows, 97–98, 326
Whitney blankets, 179, 289n54
Whooping cough, 110, 286n14,
332
Wills, 381
Wind, 285n2, 294n118
Windows. See also Ventilation;
Views; Wind
babies and, 403
basics, 71–76, 96, 306–312,
326, 399
beds and, 177, 183–184, 363,
366
doors and, 83–84, 314
fires and, 82, 306, 310, 314
noise and, 131–132, 341
pyaemia and, 98
scarlet fever and, 100, 328
stables and, 94–95,
324–325
variety and, 149, 348, 350
Wishing, 413n7
Women. See also Feminism; Sexism
digestion and, 162n
employment of, 7–8,
281–283
military hospitals and,
118–119
nursing and, 67, 250–257,
263–264, 305, 407
observation and, 224–225,
389
Workshops. See Factories
World Health Organization, x
World War I, 9
Wylie, James, 289n55

Y

Young ladies, 23, 69, 101–103,
305, 328–329, 377n